UNDERSTANDING
DECISION-MAKING
IN NURSING
PRACTICE

SAGE was founded in 1965 by Sara Miller McCune to support the dissemination of usable knowledge by publishing innovative and high-quality research and teaching content. Today, we publish over 900 journals, including those of more than 400 learned societies, more than 800 new books per year, and a growing range of library products including archives, data, case studies, reports, and video. SAGE remains majority-owned by our founder, and after Sara's lifetime will become owned by a charitable trust that secures our continued independence.

Los Angeles | London | New Delhi | Singapore | Washington DC | Melbourne

KAREN HOLLAND & DEBBIE ROBERTS

UNDERSTANDING DECISION-MAKING IN NURSING PRACTICE

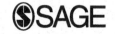

Los Angeles | London | New Delhi
Singapore | Washington DC | Melbourne

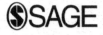

Los Angeles | London | New Delhi
Singapore | Washington DC | Melbourne

SAGE Publications Ltd
1 Oliver's Yard
55 City Road
London EC1Y 1SP

SAGE Publications Inc.
2455 Teller Road
Thousand Oaks, California 91320

SAGE Publications India Pvt Ltd
B 1/I 1 Mohan Cooperative Industrial Area
Mathura Road
New Delhi 110 044

SAGE Publications Asia-Pacific Pte Ltd
3 Church Street
#10-04 Samsung Hub
Singapore 049483

Editor: Alex Clabburn
Assistant editor: Ruth Lilly
Production editor: Vishwajeet Mehra
Copy editor: Michelle Clark
Proofreader: Thea Watson
Indexer: Judith Lavender
Marketing manager: Ruslana Khatagova
Cover design: Wendy Scott
Typeset by: KnowledgeWorks Global Ltd.
Printed in the UK

Library of Congress Control Number: 2022935605

British Library Cataloguing in Publication data

A catalogue record for this book is available from the British Library

ISBN 978-1-5264-2446-4
ISBN 978-1-5264-2447-1 (pbk)

At SAGE we take sustainability seriously. Most of our products are printed in the UK using responsibly sourced papers and boards. When we print overseas we ensure sustainable papers are used as measured by the PREPS grading system. We undertake an annual audit to monitor our sustainability.

Dedication

This book has been written for all those students learning to become nurses, supported by their mentors, supervisors and assessors in both university and practice settings.

The global COVID-19 pandemic has had a significant impact on all of them and evidence of this can be seen throughout the book, especially when decision-making on behalf of or with others has been challenging. The dedication to their roles and to those needing care has been made visible to a global audience.

In recognition of their valuable contribution throughout this unprecedented time, when making decisions of any kind has had an impact on both their personal and professional lives, we dedicate this book to all student and qualified nurses globally and thank them all for their dedication and commitment to the nursing profession.

Contents

List of Figures and Tables

Figures

Tables

About the Editors and Contributors

The Editors

Karen Holland is the Founding Editor of *Nurse Education in Practice* journal and a senior lecturer (Honorary) in the School of Health and Society, University of Salford. She has co-edited and authored seven books, two of which are in their 3rd Edition (both translated into Japanese). She has been a Series Editor of nursing books for two major publishers, focused on supporting student learning in practice. Her main interest and career experience is in the field of nursing education, and in particular curriculum development and evaluation, evidence-based teaching and learning as well as research-informed practice. Her most recent book, *Anthropology of Nursing*, reflects her long-standing interest and commitment to exploring how nursing itself can be viewed and understood through an anthropological lens. She has been the Subject Chair (Nursing and Health Professions) for the Elsevier Scopus Content Selection Advisory Board (CSAB) since 2010 and is a committed advocate for ethical publishing and authorship. Her 20 years as Editor/Editor in Chief of an international nurse education journal enabled her to support and promote scholarly publishing in the field of nursing education and practice. She is currently engaged in reviewing for a number of international nursing journals as well as writing and editing new books to enhance student nurse engagement in the practice of nursing.

Debbie Roberts has deep expertise in nursing, with more than thirty years' experience as a qualified nurse, and twenty years as a nurse academic for universities in Wales and England. Debbie's areas of teaching and research expertise include practice and immersive learning, as well as clinical simulation. She has a particular interest in linking research, teaching and innovation, ensuring that evidence-based teaching is used within nurse education and relevant research is embedded into the curriculum. Debbie supports PhD students and has examined several PhD candidates. Widely published in the field of nurse education, she has contributed to textbooks that are used as core texts in nurse education programmes in several countries. She has also published more than thirty peer-reviewed papers for international journals, with her work often cited by others, indicating the impact of her ideas on teaching and learning internationally. Debbie has established a wide range of national and international links through her work as an external examiner and, in 2019, she was nominated as one of the top 100 women in Wales in the inaugural Welsh Women's Awards, which celebrate those women who continue to thrive and excel at the forefront of their professions and make meaningful contributions to the country.

The Contributors

Angela Darvill was a Senior Lecturer in Children and Young People's nursing at the University of Huddersfield. Angela is a Senior Fellow of the Higher Education Academy, has over 20 years' experience in Higher Education and has been responsible for the education of nurses, mentors and lecturers. Angela's PhD was a study of newly registered children's nurses' transition into children's community nursing teams.

Angela Williams is a Senior Lecturer in Nursing (Adult), Wrexham Glyndŵr University – qualified as a nurse in 1985 and as a midwife in 1987, working in the London and Surrey area until she focused her career on health visiting. After working for several years in the London area she moved back to rural Wales to work as a community midwife and focused her experience on providing the highest quality of midwifery care. Angela moved into Higher Education in 2003 where she started her lecturing career as a senior lecturer in adult nursing in Wrexham Glyndŵr University. She has an interest in using e-learning to support the student experience, as well as using social media such as Twitter to enhance student engagement. Over the last couple of years using a blended approach to deliver nurse education has become a focus of her teaching style. In May 2016, Angela received the prestigious title of Queen's Nurse and in 2017 Angela received the Freedom of the City of London.

Dale Nixon is a Registered Learning Disability Nurse, qualifying in 2004. He started working with people with a learning disability in 1995, as a support worker before commencing his nurse training. Dale has had various roles in clinical practice including working as an acute liaison nurse for 10 years prior to moving into Higher Education in 2018. Since then, he has worked at the School of Nursing and Midwifery at Keele University as a Lecturer in Learning Disability Nursing. Dale is passionate in relation to the health inequalities of people with a learning disability as well as raising awareness and understanding of people with a learning disability across the programmes he teaches on, which include both undergraduate and post-graduate levels. He is a father, a Port Vale FC and real ale fan away from work.

Daniel Lucy has been a Registered Specialist Community Public Health Nurse since 2014. He has undertaken research with the Institute for Employment Studies to review the effectiveness of workplace interventions for common health problems.

Deborah Atkinson RN, MSc, BSc (Hons) is a senior nurse with more than 30 years' NHS experience practicing in urgent and emergency care. Previously, Deborah has held Executive and Consultant nurse roles, and has been qualified at advanced practice level since 2002. She has also completed a Professional Doctorate in Health and Social Care. Deborah currently works as a Clinical Development Lead with Health Innovation Manchester, supporting the delivery of safe patient care across the urgent and emergency care pathway. She has managed wide-scale system change across acute and primary care interfaces and works closely with commissioners and colleagues across the health and care economy to develop, deliver and evaluate innovative services to improve outcomes and experiences for patients.

Gareth Holland has been a qualified Mental Health nurse for 13 years, gaining experience in caring for people in a number of specialist mental health care fields. This has enabled him to develop his knowledge and expertise across a wide variety of scenarios in decision-making and management of care situations. Gareth is now a Senior Practitioner for Personality Disorder based in the community, having experienced the same role within an in-patient hospital environment. His main interest is improving access to appropriate care for people diagnosed with personality disorder whilst also enhancing his own professional knowledge and expertise in this specialist field of nursing practice.

Jane McGrath, after qualifying as a Staff Nurse almost 10 years ago, has predominantly worked in a Specialist Oncology Hospital which she holds very close to her heart. Her career as a newly qualified nurse began in an Acute Assessment Unit, and since then she has gone on to gain experience in many areas of nursing within an Oncology setting. More recently she became a member of the Covid Screening Team who were formed to respond to the Coronavirus Pandemic which she found very rewarding. Jane has now returned to her role as Endoscopy Nurse and caring for patients pre- and post-surgery. Her Grandfather's diagnosis when she was a teenager was the catalyst to her working in Oncology, and she would like to dedicate her contribution to this book to him.

Jenni Templeman is a senior lecturer and programme lead in the Faculty of Health and Social Care at the University of Chester. Jenni has written chapters for several books and is research active. Her PhD focused on 'an ethnographic study of critical care nurses' experiences following the decision to withdraw life-sustaining treatment from patients in a UK intensive care unit'.

Joanne Cleary-Holdforth is an Assistant Professor at the School of Nursing, Psychotherapy and Community Health, Dublin City University. A registered nurse and midwife with the Nursing and Midwifery Board of Ireland (NMBI), her clinical speciality was in nephrology, dialysis and transplantation. Following completion of her BSc and MSc in Nursing at the Royal College of Surgeons Ireland (RCSI), Joanne successfully undertook a post-graduate diploma in third level teaching and learning at the Dublin Institute of Technology and is a certified mentor in Evidence-based Practice from Arizona State University (USA). She has been passionate about EBP and nurse education throughout her career and has been teaching EBP at under- and post-grad levels for over 20 years. Joanne completed her PhD in 2020, with a thesis entitled 'A National Study Exploring Knowledge, Beliefs and Implementation of Evidence-Based Practice among Nurses, Midwives, Lecturers and Students in the Republic of Ireland'.

Louise Cogher MA(HE), PGDiP (HE), RNT, BA(Hons), DPSN, RNLD, FHEA is Professional Lead for Learning Disability Nursing, School of Nursing and Midwifery, Keele University. During her learning disability nursing career, she has held numerous positions, as well as managing services, both in England and overseas in Bermuda and Guernsey, the Channel Islands, across a range of settings. Her main areas of interest in clinical practice focused on health promotion and facilitation, person-centred planning facilitation, positive behaviour support, active support, and practice development. She moved to Higher Education in 2008 and has extensive experience in teaching learning disability nursing as well as public health in relation to the health inequalities of people with a learning disability and applied behaviour analysis at undergraduate and post-graduate levels. Louise is a post-graduate researcher undertaking Doctoral studies with a focus on women with learning disabilities' experiences of accessing midwifery services. Louise is a passionate advocate for Learning Disability Nursing and the people they have chosen to serve.

Marcia Kirwan is an Associate Professor in the School of Nursing, Psychotherapy and Community Health at Dublin City University. She qualified as a nurse from St. Bartholomew's Hospital and City University, London, and subsequently as a midwife from the University of Wales, Cardiff. She is an experienced educator, teaching across several undergraduate and post-graduate programmes, including nursing. Dr Kirwan has over 30 years nursing and healthcare experience including specialist nursing roles, and national leadership roles. Her research lies within three distinct but overlapping themes: patient safety, missed or rationed nursing care and nurse workforce planning, and her collaborations on this work extend across many European countries. The focus of this research is mainly on the impact of nurses and nursing on measurable patient outcomes.

Melissa Corbally is an Associate Professor in General Nursing at the University of Dublin, Trinity College. She has over 20 years of experience in educating nurses through creating and implementing simulated ward-based learning scenarios. She is passionate about fostering excellence in nursing practice and has also developed a framework for nursing assessment to assist student nurses in understanding this process more easily. In 2018, she was awarded a fellowship Ad Eundem of the Faculty of Nursing and Midwifery, Royal College of Surgeons Ireland for her contributions to nursing and nurse education. Her research interests are broad but include nursing assessment, prostate cancer nursing care, intimate partner violence, masculinities and marginalised genders. She has a particular interest in narrative methodology and the relationship between life stories and clinical decision-making.

Natalie Robinson is a Senior Lecturer in Children's Nursing with special interests in nurse decision-making and nurse autonomy. Natalie's interest in decision-making stems from her clinical background in Paediatric Critical Care. Natalie worked as a Matron in Paediatric Critical Care during the COVID 19 Pandemic and worked as part of a national group looking at reskilling workforces for redeployment in the pandemic. Natalie's research to date explores nurse confidence in 'making every contact count' by engaging in difficult conversations about lifestyle choices and health promotion. Natalie's leadership experience has led her to focus on supporting nurse engagement with quality improvement and explore how education and training can influence the quality and safety of patient care. Natalie's move into Higher Education is to focus on her development as an early career researcher and support the delivery of pre-registration nursing programmes and the advancement of the nursing profession. Natalie is a qualified Professional Nurse Advocate and is exploring the advancement of this role and how it supports nurse resilience and well-being.

Stephen Prydderch is a Registered Specialist Community Public Health Nurse with a background in Health Visiting. He has published in the area of preparing student nurses to be prescriber ready at the point of registration. At the time of writing, he was a Lecturer in Nursing at Bangor University, with a special interest in student experience.

Therese Leufer is an Assistant Professor at the School of Nursing, Psychotherapy and Community Health in Dublin City University. She has worked in nurse education for over 25 years both in the United Kingdom and Ireland. Her clinical speciality was in neurosurgical intensive care nursing. She completed a BSc (Hons) in Health Studies at London South Bank University followed by an MA in Higher Education at the University of Greenwich, London. Therese is a Fellow of the Higher Education Academy (FHEA) (UK) and a certified mentor in Evidence-based Practice from Arizona State University (USA). She has considerable experience in programme management coupled with a sustained commitment to teaching excellence. She has developed and delivered dedicated Evidence-based Practice (EBP) modules at master's level for over 20 years. She was awarded a Doctorate in Education (EdD) from the University of Bristol (UK) for a thesis entitled 'Tackling Evidence-based Practice in Nursing Education'.

Tony Warne has over 20 years of experience in mental health nursing and service management, gained through working in a variety of different specialist mental health service environments and contexts before being appointed Professor in Mental Health Care and Dean of School at the University of Salford in 2007. The focus of his research interest has been on inter-personal, intra-personal and extra-personal relationships, using a psychodynamic and managerialist analytical discourse. This research has centred on exploring the impact of such relationships on mental health nursing practice, policy, organisation and particularly nurse education and the preparation for practice. He has published extensively and is the Co-Editor and author of the books: *Using Patient Experience in Nurse Education* and *Creative Approaches to Health and Social Care Education.* He is currently Professor Emeritus at the University of Salford and was appointed Chair of Stockport NHS Foundation Trust in 2021.

Preface

Learning to be a nurse requires students to develop a set of skills and a knowledge base that will enable them to make the transition from being a learner to a qualified nurse. As with any transition, this can often seem a daunting prospect, and one where the student may ask, 'How am I ever going to learn all that I need to know to get through this course and become a qualified nurse?'

For student nurses, this experience entails learning in 'two worlds' – that of the university and that of the practice environment. Although there is a physical distinction between the two, it is important that the learning which takes place in one is integrated with the learning in the other.

These 'two worlds' require that students learn both separate and integrated sets of skills in order to qualify and be ready to take on further sets of skills in whatever nursing environment they are employed in. The skills that are discussed in the various chapters illustrate how, in many instances, they are built on pre-existing knowledge and experience, but many will also have to be adapted by student nurses when they are 'coping with the unknown'. This can occur in relation to facing a new environment each time they start a new placement, communicating with patients, their families and a large number of health and social care professionals. In addition, some have to deal with difficult and often complex situations, as well as distressing and stressful learning experiences.

At university, there are also situations that may be unknown, such as learning new study skills, working with others, searching and finding information, and managing 'academic' workloads.

It is every student's goal to complete their course with the required foundation knowledge and skills for the future, and it is an essential goal of this book to enable the student to gain these, for a successful learning and nursing experience in relation to decision-making. Decision-making is a critical element of day-to-day practice for any nurse working in a variety of health care environments. Decisions can be related to clinical care, ranging from helping a patient to decide what to eat (to ensure a balanced nutritional intake, essential for well-being) or deciding how best to feed the patient who has had a stroke, to more complex decisions, such as those required to resuscitate someone who has had a heart attack or support those with complex mental health needs. Central to all such decision-making is involving the patients or clients and, where appropriate, their family or carers.

It is important to note that in this book, reference to 'the patient' implies anyone who has a health care need and is from any age group. The term 'client' is also seen in relation to individuals, especially in literature referring to those within a mental health care environment.

Nursing decisions can also involve deciding how to prioritise workloads, what evidence to use for a care plan or deciding if you are competent to undertake a certain task. This may not directly involve the patient in the decision-making process but will fundamentally be affected either, by that evidence-base you have evaluated and determined underpins best practice, to the way it then supports the delivery of the planned care.

To engage in effective decision-making, the student requires a set of skills underpinned by the most appropriate knowledge and best evidence, which they need to acquire during the course of their learning. In its new standards, *Future Nurse: Standards of proficiency for registered nurses*, the Nursing and Midwifery Council (NMC, 2018a) recognises the importance of decision-making skills when registering as a nurse.

This can be seen throughout all the seven platforms, where to achieve outcomes such as, for example, being an accountable professional (platform 1) it explicitly states that registered nurses: 'act professionally at all times and use their knowledge and experience to make evidence-based decisions about care' (2018a: 7).

Our aim in this book is to facilitate the learning experience of the student by providing them with an insight into real-world examples of decision-making in action. These are supported by a foundation of knowledge that they will be required to use along with their own experience, and which is fundamental to achieving the key competencies and proficiencies of the NMC Standards (2010 and 2018a).

It is anticipated that the book will support student learning throughout their programme of learning and will meet students' needs with regards to the foundation skills and knowledge required for effective decision-making in all fields of practice.

The book does not, however, provide answers to specific clinical or health-related problems, such as the clinical outcome of giving the correct medication to a patient or how to recognise when a patients' blood pressure is too high. Rather, it seeks to support students in becoming more confident and comfortable with the process and skills of decision-making, including:

- when to make effective clinical judgements.
- how to use frameworks and pathways to follow specific decision-making possibilities.
- how and when to use a wide range of evidence (including patients' views) to underpin a decision-making pathway.
- making it clear what the difference is between decision-making 'for' and 'in' nursing practice; this is essential, as not all decisions have a 'clinical' component (that is, in the direct nursing care sense or involving a nursing intervention).

In the book we look broadly at the process of making decisions, including the following aspects:

- The seven platforms of the NMC standards of proficiency (2018a) are addressed in specific chapters, but also important topics for practice, such as leadership and management, communication, professional values and nursing practice will be addressed throughout the book as appropriate.
- General issues underlying clinical decision-making are discussed in the chapters on each of the four fields of nursing practice, such as working in partnership with service users in mental health. However, for specific clinical information, readers should consult a clinical skills and clinical nursing textbook that will form essential reading for their modules or their programme.
- The use of evidence of all kinds is an essential theme throughout the book, from consideration of physical evidence to that based on reflective practice and intuition.
- Given the major importance of the global pandemic caused by the COVID–19 virus, for both qualified nurses and nursing students, we have made appropriate additions to the text in relation to its impact on learning and teaching as well as patient care. In addition, we have been able to include an extra chapter that focuses on the impact of the COVID–19 virus, as a global pandemic, on nurse education.

This book will establish a clear relationship for the student between theoretical concepts underpinning the principles of decision-making and the realities that they will face in both an academic and practice context. To facilitate this, the book has been written in three parts, each building on the basic principles of decision-making relevant for that section.

Overview

Part 1 Decision-Making: Theory and Practice

The focus in this part is on the theoretical and evidence-base underpinning decision-making for nursing. Students are encouraged to interact with the chapter content, through engaging with a number of activities and case studies.

Chapter 1 Principles of Decision-Making for Practice
Chapter 2 Making Decisions as a Student: Decision-making Opportunities
Chapter 3 Using Evidence for Decision-making
Chapter 4 Reflection and Learning from Decision-Making
Chapter 5 Ethical Issues and Decision-Making in Practice
Chapter 6 Communication Skills and Decision-Making in Practice

Part 2 Decision-Making in Practice

Part 2 will focus on the four fields of practice where student nurses will be undertaking their practice, learning and engaging in the decision-making required to register as a qualified nurse in that field. These could include reference to leadership and management in relation to care situations.

In addition, the chapters bring together the wider aspects of decision-making for professional practice, especially linked to specific NMC Standards. Case studies or scenarios are included as a means of exploring various options that a nurse can make with regards to patient and service users' care.

Chapter 7 Decision-Making in Mental Health Nursing
Chapter 8 Decision-Making in Children's and Young People's Nursing Practice
Chapter 9 Decision-Making in Learning Disability Nursing
Chapter 10 Decision-Making in the Field of Adult Nursing

Part 3 Decision-Making for Health Care

This part focuses on specific areas of health care where nurses have an increasing responsibility for ensuring patient safety and managing risk, as well as promoting health. These have been noted in the NMC Standards (2018a) in particular as key areas for ensuring that future qualified nurses have the knowledge and skills as well as competence in decision-making to lead and manage the delivery of effective practice and evidence-based outcomes. There is also a specific focus, when appropriate, on the potential impact of a pandemic situation on decision-making in practice. This includes both hospital and community environments. Although some decisions, of course, are very specific to the context of the current COVID-19 pandemic, aspects of them would be implicit in any future situations where similar decisions were required.

Infection control on the level that nurses have experienced, in 2020–22 for example, has come to envelop both hospital and community in a more integral way, along with a heavy reliance on the involvement of the population at large. This particular period of time became a global health care situation regarding student and qualified nurses, as well as the multidisciplinary health and social care teams they work in.

Chapter 11 Decision-Making for Risk Assessment and Patient Safety in Practice
Chapter 12 Decision-Making in Complex Situations in Practice
Chapter 13 Decision-Making for Promoting Health and Preventing Ill Health in Practice
Chapter 14 Decision-Making and Nursing Education in a Global Pandemic

It is appreciated that the book focuses primarily on the UK education context, given that the professional body (NMC) changes would have a major impact on the future of nursing in this country (NMC, 2018a). However whenever possible, reference is made to situations which actually traverse all international contexts where student nurses learn to become qualified nurses.

Scenarios may refer to different professional body requirements, but it is recognised that many of these will be familiar to nurses in other countries due to the inherent understanding of what nursing care and practice means. Holland (2020) refers to this as a nursing culture and although there will be specific social and cultural contexts in which nursing exists, as well as the different level of professional decision-making nurses have in certain countries, the basis of nursing work and therefore their practice in caring for patients will resonate with an international reader.

Due to the nature of the COVID-19 virus and the ability of people to travel the world via many different routes, the world began to be impacted by what has turned out to be not only a new species of virus but also one of the most infectious and deadly to human beings.

The impact on the need for nursing staff to care for people in hospitals and community settings made it necessary to have as many qualified nurses, supported by other health care workers, to be able to care for them. The pace of infections as well as the critical nature of the illness caused by the virus, outpaced the number of nurses available.

Decision-making situations multiplied and as a result the NMC, working with the Department of Health (DOH) and the university education sector, made a decision (seen as a short-term solution) to enable changes to be made to the regulations governing the mandatory requirements of a nursing programme / curriculum, leading to the registration of student nurses in the UK. (See Chapter 14 for further details.)

The learning experiences of some student nurses across the UK now required the development of a set of skills and knowledge which were integral to professional care that had never before been seen or experienced by the majority of the health care workforce.

Making decisions in this context therefore came to be of critical importance, both clinically and ethically, but also had to be encompassed by the continuation of a high level of professional care. To enable additional understanding of the impact of the pandemic on learning and practice, we have added several articles specifically related to this impact. (See Further reading sections and Web resources in all chapters, and especially Chapter 14.)

We wish to note here that the original text had been prepared and was ready to take forward to final review and subsequent publication in March 2020. However, as we all now know, the COVID-19 virus arrived and had a huge impact on the personal and professional lives of nurses and student nurses worldwide. The focus of this book is still on the principles of decision-making outlined in the individual chapters. We could not, however, not include reference to one of the biggest challenges to our society in the UK – and, indeed, globally – that there has ever been. We hope that you will appreciate that although there is research still being conducted internationally on the impact of COVID-19 on both student learning and qualified nurses in practice, it will take some years for a new body of evidence on this subject to emerge and underpin future practice and have an impact on curricula and practice learning. What we offer in this book is a starting point, as we have begun to pull together evidence that is available to help us, and you, raise an awareness of the outcomes of this global event and to understand what has been happening during the pandemic in nurses' education and learning in clinical practice.

The addition of Chapter 14 is part of this starting point especially to enable those whose pathway to becoming a qualified nurse was interrupted by the pandemic, which challenged the health and social care services and universities to engage in major national decision-making that was focused not only on managing and making decisions on the risk to patients and ensure their safety but also to the whole of the workforce which was now tasked with their overall care delivery and management.

As a result of these challenges the student nurse learning journey, and indeed other health care students, such as from medicine, physiotherapy, midwifery or radiography, has been severely impacted but it will be some time before the full picture emerges.

As noted at the beginning of this Preface, learning to become a nurse can be seen as a daunting prospect, to the 'beginner or novice' student nurse, regardless of how and where that learning is taking place. We hope, however, that by exploring many of the decision-making challenges that you, as a student nurse, may face on your journey to becoming a qualified nurse, that the chapters in this book offer you support and guidance as to safe practice options and develop your confidence in making decisions in the future.

Karen Holland and Debbie Roberts

Note

You will note that the terms 'patient' and 'client' appear in certain chapters and literature discussed. The use of one term rather than the other reflects the preferred option for the people being cared for as well as the context of the decision-making situation being described and discussed. However, we wish to convey that these terms in no way detract from the importance of considering everyone as an individual.

We would also like to acknowledge that throughout the book we have aimed to use the gender neutral (they/them/their) instead of he or she, but occasionally have used the pronouns 'he' or 'she', with the intention that they are used in a general sense and not to describe a specific client group. We fully recognise the importance of referring to people individually as they wish to be known. This is an important aspect of communicating effectively with a person during their overall care delivery and assessment of their individual needs.

Students may also note that the referencing style used in this book may not appear in the same citation style as the one being used by their university for their assignments and projects. The system in use here is the APA 7th Edition. Please ensure that if you cite or use this book as a reference source to support your academic assignments that you use the system in use in your university and accurately reflect the message being conveyed by the chapter authors.

References

Holland, K. (2020). *Anthropology of Nursing: Exploring cultural concepts in practice.* Abingdon: Routledge.

Nursing and Midwifery Council (NMC) (2018a). *Future Nurse: Standards of proficiency for registered nurses.* London: NMC.

Acknowledgement

This book has been written at an unprecedented time in the history of global health, with the COVID-19 pandemic in turn impacting on our initial deadlines for completion and publication. To get to this stage would not have been possible without the commitment of both of us as co-editors, to ensure that students had a book that was as up to date as we could make it, and also ensure that the content reflected what had also been happening in their learning environments and their journey to becoming a registered nurse. We believe we have managed this with the help of the SAGE team as a whole with their support and encouragement to maintain momentum during a period of instability and the unknown and subsequently to getting the book to production with all that entails. Special thanks go to Alex Clabburn, Senior Commissioning Editor who has been on the journey with us from the beginning and to Ozlem Merakli, Editorial Assistant, and Laura Walmsley, Senior Commissioning Editor, for their support at various times on the same journey. We also wish to thank the production team overall and, in particular, for his never-ending patience and support, Vishwajeet Mehra, Production Editor, who has managed to get us to this final step of publishing the book.

Special thanks also go to all our chapter authors who have undertaken this same journey with us and pulled out all the stops to pick up their chapters again when still affected by what Schon would call the 'swampy lowlands' of their practice. We thank them for their commitment. Thanks also go to those colleagues who began an earlier 'book' journey with us focused on the importance of decision-making skills for student nurses and we continue to be grateful for their contribution to the ongoing evidence-based narrative.

Given the unprecedented time that student nurses have had to manage their lives, as well as everyone involved in their learning journey, we also wish to acknowledge the major contribution that the Nursing and Midwifery Council has made to ensuring their safety and well-being, and through doing so, ensured that those they worked with and learnt from as well as those they cared for were assured of the same.

PART 1

DECISION-MAKING: THEORY AND PRACTICE

This part of the book will focus on the theoretical and evidence-base underpinning decision-making for nursing. It is important that you are able to understand the rationale for making different kinds of decisions, as well as ensure that, whenever possible, your decisions are underpinned by an evidence base. Being able to understand the evidence for your decisions is not enough however to change or develop further your decision-making skills, which is why there is a focus on reflection and reflective practice in the book. Reflecting on your experiences in a structured way can help you to identify a different way of making similar decisions or alternatively, it can help you to use that experience and to apply the learning to a range of other decisions.

1

PRINCIPLES OF DECISION-MAKING FOR PRACTICE

Karen Holland and Debbie Roberts

Chapter objectives

The aims of this chapter are to:

- outline the principles of decision-making in an 'enabling learning' culture;
- consider why learning to make decisions is an important part of learning to become a nurse;
- consider the skills and knowledge necessary for effective decision-making in both practice and university learning settings;
- consider what is known about decision-making as a student nurse.

Introduction

The focus of this book is on acquiring decision-making skills to apply in nursing practice. As such, it will become apparent that not only is it essential for student nurses to learn what those skills are, but it is also equally important that they learn to become competent and proficient in making decisions. These are essential parts of becoming a qualified nurse.

As individuals, we make decisions of one form or another on a daily basis. We have to make basic decisions, such as what time to get up in the morning, what to wear, who is going to take the children to school or what to eat for breakfast. On the surface, such decisions do not appear to require major consideration but, for some people, even these seemingly basic decision-making situations can cause immense stress. This can result from the very act of making a decision or from having to take into account the context or impact of a decision on others. Your ability to become a confident decision maker in your nursing practice, however, will be dependent on the decisions that you make as a student at university and in your daily life. Some of the situations in which making decisions may have an impact on all aspects of your learning to become a nurse will be discussed in Chapter 2.

This chapter is concerned initially with the underlying principles of decision-making as a student nurse. It explores why it is important and necessary to learn about decision-making and how to make decisions. It will also focus on what has been shown in the literature about decision-making, as both a student and a qualified nurse and, most importantly, what you need to achieve to meet the Nursing and Midwifery Council's (NMC) (2018a) *Future Nurse: Standards of proficiency for registered nurses* and, in some contexts, the competencies in the NMC's (2010) *Standards for Pre-registration Nursing Education*. Later chapters will focus on the application of some of this learning to specific practice contexts and situations. In particular, Chapter 14 shows how the COVID-19 global pandemic had an impact on the learning experience of student nurses, especially the introduction of the initial NMC's *Recovery Standards* in July 2020 and, later, the *Recovery and Emergency Programme Standards* in February 2021 (since updated as NMC, 2022).

Student nurses learning to become qualified nurses are assessed at various points during their course of study by experienced practitioners who have also completed a course to become practice assessors (NMC, 2018b).

So where to begin? For students studying in the United Kingdom (UK), we begin with the NMC's *Standards of proficiency for registered nurses* (NMC, 2018a) and the Standards for education and training (NMC, 2018b). Those of you studying in other countries can use the outcomes outlined in this book as a guide and consider your own country specific professional body requirements on decision-making skills alongside those that apply in the UK. Because nursing is a global profession, however, and regardless of the country in which you are learning to become a nurse, the content of the chapters may also be of use to you to access the relevant requirements and expectations of a qualified nurse with regards to decision-making. Also given the way in which qualified nurses' cross international borders to work, this will give you an added insight into what may be expected of you should you choose to work in another country on qualifying.

We will initially consider what the requirements are of the NMC in the UK with regards to ensuring that future nurses are able to practice safely as a registered nurse.

The Requirements of the Nursing and Midwifery Council Standards (2010 and 2018a)

In view of the importance of decision-making to both your learning as a student in university and practice settings, and your need to achieve a successful outcome of becoming a graduate registered nurse, it may be a good place to begin with the difference between the two most recent sets of educational standards: competencies to be achieved following the 2010 curriculum and proficiencies to be achieved following implementation of the 2018 Standards from September 2020 in all nursing curricula in UK universities. The NMC are still publishing them both at the present time along with many different resources of value for students and their mentors and supervisors (see Web resources). Given the crossing over between the two sets of expected outcomes in practice and related graduate awards, decisions regarding students and their ongoing studies and practice assessments were determined to be the province of the individual university in consultation with the students.

Since March 2020, however, the COVID-19 pandemic has had a major impact on student and qualified nurses, in particular regarding assessment of learning at universities and in practice settings (see Chapter 14 for a more detailed explanation). We decided, therefore, to include explanations of both sets of standards to be achieved by a qualified nurse, especially given that many new clinical supervisors in practice may have only just qualified and achieved the NMC's 2010 competencies.

A brief overview only is given here as you may encounter references in your ongoing learning experiences to both competencies and proficiencies.

The NMC (2010) Standards comprise of four main 'domains': each of which require the student nurse to be able to learn how to make decisions that are underpinned by an evidence base and a clear decision-making pathway. These domains cover the following areas:

- professional values
- communication and interpersonal skills
- nursing practice and decision-making
- leadership, management and team working.

The domains, as well as having a generic standard of competence that applies to all student nurses regardless of their intended field of practice (Adult nursing, Learning Disability nursing, Children's nursing or Mental Health nursing – see Chapters 7–10), also have field-specific competencies that have to be achieved by the end of students' programmes of learning in both practice placement and university assessments (NMC (2010) *Standards for Pre-registration Nursing Education* – see the Web resources section at the end of this chapter for the link). You will see aspects of all these domains and their outcomes in the revised 2018 Standards, as they were considered essential prerequisites for registration as a future qualified nurse.

The NMC (2018a) Standards comprise seven platforms:

1. Being an accountable professional;
2. Promoting health and preventing ill health;
3. Assessing needs and planning care;
4. Providing and evaluating care;
5. Leading and managing nursing care and working in teams;
6. Improving safety and quality of care;
7. Coordinating care.

These platforms encompass outcome statements of proficiencies that have been developed to apply across all fields of practice and care settings. (Full details of these platforms and proficiency outcomes can be found in the NMC Standards (2018a) – see the Web resources section at the end of this chapter.)

Discussing the difference between competence and proficiency is outside the word limits of this chapter but a reference to the work of Patricia Benner (1984) in From *Novice to Expert* can be found in the reference list and recommended reading in the context of expectations of a qualified nurse. Some pre-registration curricula may have used this model as a framework for student learning experiences and many of you will already be familiar with her work from your studies.

To be able to make decisions applicable to these NMC outcomes you will need to understand the various principles underpinning the decisions that you will be required to make as a student nurse learning to become a qualified nurse, as well as to know why they are appropriate for certain decisions and not for others. Part 1 of this book, including this chapter, is intended to give you this theoretical foundation while also ensuring that we discuss their relationship with the actual reality of practice contexts.

The Principles of Decision-Making and their Relevance to Learning to Become a Qualified Nurse

If you are expected to achieve the NMC's competencies, many of which require decision-making of one sort or another, then it is important to consider the different types of decisions that you can make, as well as the theoretical principles underpinning them. You will note references to these throughout this book. In addition, you will find many articles and books that refer to 'clinical decision-making' – that is, decision-making in situations that require a decision to be made based on either a set of clinical data related to a patient, which can be analysed to make a 'clinical' decision (such as administering pain relief following assessment of a patient's needs and cues from the patient, indicating pain) or, alternatively, on the basis of the best evidence from research, which can lead to changes in what decisions are made in clinical practice (such as what type of pain relief can be given to a patient in pain). All of these are 'clinical', in the sense that they are decisions made with regard to the direct care of patients. (Please note that there will be times when one of the terms 'patient' or 'client' or 'service user' is the preferred option, in particular when a clinical decision about direct care is to be discussed.)

One could argue that any decision made in a clinical environment that has a direct or indirect impact on patient care could be considered an example of clinical decision-making. Regardless of the type of decision-making, there will always be a possible positive or negative outcome, which will depend on the information available on which to base the decision.

In Chapter 2, we look at a broad range of decision-making opportunities and options with which you will be faced as a student nurse studying for a degree in nursing, combined with registration as a qualified nurse. In Chapter 3, we will look at how you can use evidence of different kinds to help in the decision-making process; in Chapter 4, we focus on how you can learn from decision-making through reflection – which appears to be a central core of most students' curriculum. Chapter 5 focuses on the fundamental ethical issues in the decision-making process, an understanding of which is an essential prerequisite to becoming an accountable registered nurse. Chapter 6 explores the importance and relevance of effective communication skills in decision-making. These six chapters establish the essential foundation of a future nurse's practice and where there has to be a strong relationship between knowledge and skills to ensure successful attainment of proficiencies (competencies) for qualifying as a nurse.

So how do you learn to make decisions and what underpins the decision-making process that you undertake?

Theories about Decision-Making: the Basics

Here, we introduce you to the basics of decision-making, so that you can consider how decisions are made in practice. It is important to remember, however, to undertake further reading to add depth to your learning (see the Further reading section at the end of this chapter for some suggestions).

The three main theories about decision-making, according to Aston et al. (2010: 7), are the:

- information-processing model
- intuition model
- cognitive continuum theory.

Although other authors, such as Thompson and Dowding (2009) and Standing (2010), expand on these three models, the basic principles of them all are the same. They are mainly used in the context of clinical decision-making rather than as the principles of decision-making generally. You may, however, come across terms such as 'hypo-thetico-deductive reasoning' (Thompson and Dowding, 2009: 63), which follows several 'different stages of reasoning when making judgements and decisions'. In essence, it consists of four basic stages:

1. 'cue acquisition' – collecting clinical information;
2. 'hypothesis generation' – at which point, possible options may be considered based on the data gathered;
3. 'cue interpretation' – when the data is examined more closely and, together with the 'whole picture', used to consider a revised decision or possibility;
4. 'cue evaluation' – the stage when you may decide that, despite having an idea as to what you need to do or what the problem could be, a rethink is needed and perhaps some more data is required or even that you need to repeat your data collection, to check its accuracy.

After going through these stages, you will be able to make a more definite decision, based on the best possible clinical data available.

Jones (1996) outlines an important relationship between other skills that are required in relation to the decision-making process, such as 'critical thinking' and 'critical analysis' (Tappen, 1989). These, she defines as follows:

> *Critical thinking* is a skill developed in looking for alternative solutions to prob-lems and adopting a questioning approach. *Critical analysis* is a tool used in critical thinking and may involve asking the following questions:
>
> *   What is the central issue?
> *   What are the underlying assumptions?
> *   Is there valid evidence?
> *   Are the conclusions acceptable?

These questions help analyse the steps in the decision-making process. (Jones, 1996: 3)

Both critical thinking and critical analysis are key concepts throughout the book, and examples of situations in which these are used by students and their mentors/ practice supervisors in practice will be explored, as well as examples of their use in aca-demic learning in the university. Both are skills that can be taught and learnt and are considered essential for the graduate qualified nurse of the future; along with decision-making skills, they underpin the clinical and managerial leadership roles that will be expected of that nurse.

Two additional terms associated with decision-making in practice are 'clinical rea-soning' and 'clinical judgement'. We will define them briefly here, to help to identify the links between them and the decision-making process but will return to them later in this chapter.

- Clinical reasoning is defined by Levett-Jones et al. as: 'a logical process by which nurses (and other clinicians) collect cues, process the information, come to an understanding of a patient problem or situation, plan and implement interventions, evaluate outcomes and reflect in and learn from the process (Hoffman, 2007). It is not a linear process but can be conceptualised as a cycle of linked clinical encounters' (2010: 516).
- Clinical judgement, according to Benner et al., refers to: 'the ways in which nurses come to understand the problems, issues or concerns of clients/patients, to attend to salient information, and to respond in concerned and involved ways' (1996: 2).

Tanner (2006) subsequently developed a clinical judgement model that consists of four phases – noticing, interpreting, responding and reflecting – that Lasater describes as 'the major components of clinical judgement in complex patient care situations that involve changes in status and uncertainty about the appropriate course of action' (2007: 497). Tanner concluded from her research that 'reflection on practice is often triggered by a breakdown in clinical judgement and is critical for the development of clinical knowledge and improvement in clinical reasoning' (2006: 204). This concept of 'reflection' in the decision-making process, and its use and experience, is discussed in more detail in Chapter 4.

In addition to these decision-making processes and problem-solving tools, there are other frameworks that we can use to determine when certain types of decision-making are more appropriate than others. The three main frameworks discussed in the literature are the:

- information-processing model
- intuition model
- cognitive continuum theory model.

We will now explore these briefly as they relate to decision-making situations in which student nurses will be involved and will offer additional reading for more in-depth analysis of the use of each framework in nursing practice. We will explore these theories of decision-making mainly in the context of clinical decision-making rather than decision-making generally, which is explored in Chapter 2.

Types of Decisions Made using the Information-processing Model

The information-processing theory of how we make decisions is based on how we manage information, obtained both in the short and long term. You will start your nursing course with a store of information gathered from several sources and experiences. You will then be given new information that, initially, you will store in your short-term memory. Eventually, as you begin to learn additional information, that initial material will be stored in your long-term memory (Aston et al., 2010).

An example that Aston et al. (2010: 7) offer is one from practice: 'When a nurse assesses a patient for the first-time information is gained and immediately placed in short-term memory. This then "triggers" certain cues that cause information retrieval from the long-term memory.' As you progress in your course of study, and as you acquire new knowledge and skills and, at the same time, gain experience in a variety of clinical placements, you will accumulate a great deal of information that will be retained in your long-term memory. Meeting a new situation for the first-time, such as a new patient with a new life health history, may well 'trigger' this information that has, effectively, been kept 'in storage' until such time as it becomes apparent that it might be valuable in helping you to care for this new patient or in understanding his or her health problem – even though, on a personal level, he or she is new to you.

Of course, in nursing, as in any life experience, this one theory of how we use information is not the only way to explain how we make decisions and, often, we use a number of different theories to explain how we arrive at taking a particular action in nursing practice.

Types of Decisions Made using the Intuition Model

As with the information-processing theory of decision-making, our use of intuition in nursing is also based on information of previous similar experiences that is triggered by the present situation. Benner et al. (1996: 142) talk about the 'expert practitioner', who makes decisions based on 'intuitive' links between what he or she is observing and what his or her subsequent response is.

Imagine, for example, that, as a student nurse during your first placement, you observed a situation in which a patient returning from theatre collapsed and had to be resuscitated. His symptoms and the physiological observations, which you had been involved in observing with your mentor or practice supervisor, clearly indicated that he had suffered a heart attack following surgery, but he had no previous history that would indicate this as a possible outcome.

In your third year, you are again on placement in a surgical ward and bringing a patient, who has had chest surgery, back from the operating theatre with a theatre nurse. You are observing the patient as you are returning with him from the recovery room, and you note a change of face colour; he also begins to be agitated and complains of some chest pain.

You take his pulse immediately and note that it is irregular. Your 'intuition', based on your past experience in a surgical ward, as well as other experiences of the unexpected during other placements, tells you that something is 'not right' with this patient. His clinical condition, as well as the fact that he is telling you about his chest pain, is con-firming your 'intuitive' concern about this patient. A decision is required immediately: you are aware from that first experience of how quickly the patient could deteriorate. You decide (along with the qualified theatre nurse, who you have had to persuade, because she assumed from her knowledge of his chest surgery that his current prob-lem resulted from that surgery) that he needs immediate care and both agree to take him back immediately to the recovery area of the operating department, where he can obtain immediate medical care and intensive monitoring of his observations. It is then diagnosed that he has, in fact, had a heart attack or myocardial infarction of some kind.

As you become more experienced after qualifying as a nurse, you will develop what could be called 'holistic knowing' – that is, the ability to see the 'bigger picture' (Ben-ner et al., 1996) making connections between what you see then and there (that is, immediately) and your previous experience, to conclude that 'something is not right'. You might also say that you are using information stored in your memory, as well as previous experience and intuitive knowing, but these are very different types of decision-making. Aston et al. state that these two forms of decision-making 'may be regarded as two ends of a spectrum as a means of decision-making', but 'in reality, most nurses utilise a mixture of the two elements in their decision-making' (2010: 7).

Benner's (1984) research, examining the clinical performance of beginning and expert nurses, sought to determine and understand any differences between them. The outcome of her study is one that has had a major impact on our understanding of not only what happens after a nurse has qualified, but also assists us in determining what skills and knowledge a student nurse must gain along the journey from novice to qualified nurse stage. Of particular importance is how they learn to make decisions.

Blum offers a case study of a student nurse's clinical practice experience, demon-strating what she calls the 'Benner intuitive–humanistic decision-making model in action' (2010: 303). In this example, the student was experiencing some practice and academic learning, as well as personal difficulties and the faculty member managed to work through a difficult situation through a shared decision-making process over a period of time. Complete Activity 1.1 to reflect on this student's experience.

Activity 1.1

1. Access C. Blum (2010), Using the Benner intuitive–humanistic decision-making model in action: A case study, *Nurse Education in Practice*, 10(5), 303–307.
2. Read the paper and consider the experience of the student, Jade.
3. Consider how important it is to look at the impact of your own personal and learning experiences on how you make decisions in relation to others.
4. Discuss with one of your supervisors how they can offer you opportunities to learn decision-making skills as part of your practice learning goals to becoming proficient in caring for patients.

Learning how to manage shared decisions is an essential outcome of the NMC's (2018a) platform 3 (3.4) and platform 4 (4.2) proficiencies.

The stages that Benner identified which could enable us to understand the difference between being competent and being proficient (as a qualified nurse) can be seen in her explanation of these as found in her research. Both can be seen as describing and achieving safe practice as an outcome for a qualified nurse, with increasing confidence and expertise being gained from lengthier periods of experience.

Stage 3: Competent

Competence is demonstrated by a nurse who has been working in the same job and in the same or similar situations for about two or three years and has begun to have confidence that their actions are now based on experience of same or similar situations. For Benner, the:

> competent nurse lacks the speed and flexibility of the proficient nurse but does have a feeling of mastery and the ability to cope with and manage the many contingencies of clinical nursing. The conscious, deliberate planning that is characteristic of this skill level helps achieve efficiency and organisation. (1984: 27)

Stage 4: Proficient

'Proficiency', for Benner, is when qualified nurses have progressed beyond competence, to look at situations as wholes rather than focusing on different smaller parts of a situation, that is, not seeing the whole. Having such a perspective, they can make a decision when a less experienced or novice nurse may think, 'how did they get to decide on the decision they made as I could not see how they did it so quickly – what did they have to know to be able to make that decision?' The proficient nurse because of their 'experienced-based ability to recognise whole situations', has learnt from experience 'what typical events to expect in a given situation and how plans need to be modified in response to these events' (Benner, 1984: 28). They use some inherent rules learnt in order to make decisions. Benner calls these 'maxims', which guide them when making decisions.

Benner's final stage of Expert is where a nurse can be observed making a decision where there is an immediate grasp of a situation they encounter and with it an immediate 'knowing' that something is wrong and at the same time knowing what they need to do in terms of decision-making. The expert no longer relies on the guiding rules, as it were, to connect things up to make the appropriate decision but appears to 'intuitively' know how to manage the making of many decisions in their total context.

We can also draw on Benner's explanations of these stages in a nurse's practice by observing how good mentors or practice supervisors help student nurses learn to make decisions while caring for patients. They unpack the 'whole' of a situation and explain all the parts so that students are then able to see what they have to learn. We liken this to the fact that qualified nurses practice in 'wholes' and student nurses learn in parts, as they do not yet have the experience alongside the appropriate knowledge and skills to be able to deliver that totally holistic care.

Types of Decisions Made using the Cognitive Continuum Theory

Alongside the two other decision-making theories described above is what Thompson and Dowding call the 'cognitive continuum model of decision-making' (2002: 12). This theory is that there is a spectrum, with intuitive decisions at one end, and information-processing and analysis at the other (Aston et al., 2010). The types of decisions made using this theory arise only when evidence-based protocols are being used. Holland and Roxburgh state that these are, 'in basic terms, steps laid down which are to be followed when making a decision for a range of situations' (2012: 53). They cite the examples of 'clinical procedure steps for infection control practice or a directive for a major disaster' and a study by Rycroft-Malone et al., which 'showed that qualified nurses used other kinds of information to help them make decisions even where protocol-based care was in place and showed a range of decisions rather than following a standardised approach' (2009: 55).

Nursing practice is, it might be argued, an unpredictable environment, given that each patient and each nurse–patient encounter is unique and, therefore, an unknown in terms of specific decision-making situations. However, even as a student nurse on your very first placement, you are able to draw on certain life experiences, on new information of various patient health problems, knowledge of physiology, and knowledge of how people live and of different cultural needs, as well as numerous other kinds of experiences and knowledge.

An excellent example of how this can be used is when communicating with both patients and your peers, who started their nursing course with you. Communicating with people is an essential requirement of being a nurse and the NMC requires all students to fulfil a range of communication competencies (NMC, 2010) and, in 2018, it added a specific skills set regarding communication and relationship management 'that a newly registered nurse must be able to demonstrate in order to meet the proficiency outcomes' (NMC, 2018a: Annexe A).

See Activity 1.2 to explore some decision-making models a little further.

Activity 1.2

Consider how you would use intuition and information-processing models involving communicating in the following situations.

1. A service user, who regularly comes to the school of nursing, and you meet during a teaching session in the classroom, has come to talk to you about her experience of health care. She has become very upset about her past experience in a certain local hospital while talking to you.
2. A student in your tutor group is very quiet during one of the teaching sessions about bereavement and dying. He is sitting next to you, and you notice that he has begun to cry.

In the first situation, you may have considered intuitively that the lady must have had a 'poor' experience of health care to make her that upset and you may realise that you will need to make and communicate a decision regarding whether she needs to stop telling her story. You may also begin to recall that this local hospital she is talking about had been in the newspapers the previous year because of standards of care. Recalling this information will enable you to put the two issues together and to reassure the service user, as well as to ask another student to request the teacher to return to the classroom as this would be a pre-arranged and shared decision in such a situation.

In the second situation, you may use intuition that 'something is not right' with the other student, as he started to cry during the teaching session, but also because you recall something he said to you earlier about a parent's illness.

Recalling this information, as well as the information that you have about the grieving process, will help you to make a decision to suggest quietly to the student that he might like to leave the class and offer to accompany him. (Also, at the beginning of the session, the teacher had said that, not knowing students' 'situations', she would understand if the session were to trigger some memories that may upset them and so would fully understand if they were to leave the classroom. She offered that either she or a friend of the student might accompany them.)

Decision-Making as a Student Nurse: the Essential Knowledge and Skills

Given that nurses make decisions every day about the care of their patients and clients, as well as decisions that affect their own personal and professional practice, it is important to consider how student nurses learn to make decisions during their experience of learning to become a qualified nurse. The NMC (2010) makes it very clear that student nurses are expected to demonstrate their competence in decision-making in relation to nursing practice, so are to be taught and learn these skills during their programme of study toward becoming a qualified nurse. This is to involve learning in clinical placements, as well as in clinical simulation teaching sessions, and be underpinned by an evidence-based understanding of decision-making theories. We all make decisions every day, from a simple one, such as when to get up in the morning, to more complex ones, such as what to do if you find a patient collapsed at home.

Box 1.1 gives an extract from the NMC (2010) about competencies in decision-making in all fields of practice in relation to 'Domain 3: Nursing practice and decision-making'. There are also examples in Box 1.2 from the NMC (2018a) proficiencies, as they relate specifically to the outcomes of decision-making.

Box 1.1

NMC (2010) *Standards for Pre-registration Nursing Education*, Domain 3: Nursing practice and decision-making

Generic standard for competence

All nurses must practise autonomously, compassionately, skilfully and safely, and must maintain dignity and promote health and wellbeing. They must assess and meet the full range of essential physical and mental health needs of people of all ages who come into their care. Where necessary they must be able to provide safe and effective immediate care to all people prior to accessing or referring to specialist services irrespective of their field of practice. All nurses must also meet more complex and coexisting needs for people in their own nursing field of practice, in any setting including hospital, community and at home. All practice should be informed by the best available evidence and comply with local and national guidelines. Decision-making must be shared with service users, carers and families and informed by critical analysis of a full range of possible interventions, including the use of up-to-date technology. All nurses must also understand how behaviour, culture, socioeconomic and other factors, in the care environment and its location, can affect health, illness, health outcomes and public health priorities and take this into account in planning and delivering care. (NMC, 2010: 17)

Field standard for competence (Adult)

Adult nurses must be able to carry out accurate assessment of people of all ages using appropriate diagnostic and decision-making skills. They must be able to provide effective care for service users and others in all settings. They must have in-depth understanding of and competence in medical and surgical nursing to respond to adults' full range of health and dependency needs. They must be able to deliver care to meet essential and complex physical and mental health needs. (NMC, 2010: 17)

Field standard for competence (Children)

Children's nurses must be able to care safely and effectively for children and young people in all settings and recognise their responsibility for safeguarding them. They must be able to deliver care to meet essential and complex physical and mental health needs informed by deep understanding of biological, psychological and social factors throughout infancy, childhood and adolescence. (NMC, 2010: 44)

Field standard for competence (Learning disability)

Learning disabilities nurses must have an enhanced knowledge of the health and developmental needs of all people with learning disabilities, and the factors that might influence them. They must aim to improve and maintain their health and independence through skilled direct and indirect nursing care. They must also be able to provide direct care to meet the essential and complex physical and mental health needs of people with learning disabilities. (NMC, 2010: 35)

Field standard for competence (Mental health)

Mental health nurses must work with people of all ages using values-based mental health frameworks. They must use different methods of engaging people, and work in a way that promotes positive relationships focused on social inclusion, human rights and recovery, that is, a person's ability to live a self-directed life, with or without symptoms, that they believe is meaningful and satisfying. (NMC, 2010: 22)

Complete Activity 1.3 to familiarise yourself further with the competencies relating to decision-making in the standards.

Activity 1.3

In order to explore the types of decision-making situations that qualified nurses need to demonstrate read the generic standard for all fields of practice and the specific one(s) for the fields of practice (see Box 1.1) and then the same for Standards for proficiency (see Box 1.2).

1. Consider, in particular, the knowledge and skils required to meet these identified parts of the 'Generic standard for competence':
    a. Decision-making must be shared with service users, carers and families and informed by critical analysis of a full range of possible interventions, including the use of up-to-date technology. (NMC, 2010: 17)
    b. All nurses must also meet more complex and coexisting needs for people in their own nursing field of practice, in any setting including hospital, community and at home. All practice should be informed by the best available evidence and comply with local and national guidelines. (NMC, 2010: 17)
    c. They must assess and meet the full range of essential physical and mental health needs of people of all ages who come into their care. (NMC, 2010: 17)

In relation to the first point (a.), we can see that the action of decision-making is to be shared with others and that the student is expected to critically analyse a range of possible interventions, including those involving technology. In essence, this competence involves evaluating the evidence base for decision-making in relation to nursing interventions.

The critical analysis of evidence is normally a requirement of an academic essay, which may focus on demonstrating that students have reviewed the evidence on a topic or intervention, judged the positives and negatives involved, and supported their views with 'relevant literature and current research' (Duffy et al., 2009). Critical analysis is not about criticising evidence; there must be an element of balance between the positives/benefits and the negatives/drawbacks, and you must use evidence to support your views. In the reality of clinical practice and making a decision such as whether one kind of nursing practice is more beneficial to the patient than another, nurses rely heavily on the fact that their decision will be based on an accurate and informed critical analysis and evaluation of the evidence that has been available to them.

In relation to the second point (b.), we see here again the link between decision-making and evidence-based practice (see Chapter 3 for more detail). The NMC makes it clear that this has to be the best available evidence – ensuring again that this has been well evaluated by those providing it, whether it is a journal article, a book, or a policy document.

In the third point (c.), we can see the importance of assessing the needs of people, any decisions relating to their care depending very much on the nurse's ability to assess their needs in the first instance and then to follow that with the ability to meet the person's 'essential physical and mental health needs'. This requires decision-making skills informed by knowledge of numerous health problems and underlying physical or mental causes, and, most importantly, how they are often interlinked in some way.

Once you have critically analysed the evidence available, you will then need to demonstrate how you decide on which information and evidence to use to inform your decision. (See Chapter 3 for EBP and decision-making.)

This is where critical thinking skills come into play. You may have the best evidence available, but now have to decide how best to use this to help the patient or client for whom you are caring. Applying best evidence cannot be undertaken in isolation from a range of other factors, such as the care environment, your own skill set, any cultural factors that may have an impact on patients' needs or the possible actions and decisions that may be required of other health care professionals. Nurses need to 'sift' through all these factors in order to be able to base their decisions on 'best' evidence. This sifting, or selecting, and making a judgement is critical thinking.

As a student nurse, you will more than likely question, when observing qualified nurses in practice, how and why they decide that a particular action is the best choice at one time, for example when undertaking oral hygiene of a patient, but then, in a similar situation the next day, the nurse makes a completely different decision. In this situation, you are likely to find that the scenario and the evidence may remain the same – that is, how to undertake oral hygiene and what to use to clean the mouth – but that the patient is different (the first patient may have been elderly, while the second is young) and that multiple other factors are consequently different, leading to a different decision.

Critical analysis and critical thinking, therefore, are closely linked in terms of skills that you need to acquire to become a competent practitioner. During your course of study in both university and practice placements, you will develop and integrate knowledge and experience, and you will achieve these skills by the end of your graduate programme. These two skills are also said to be indicative of a graduate education and Girot (2000), basing her views on a range of evidence, uses the terms 'problem-solve, reason logically, analyse information and form conclusions' as a way of defining critical thinking.

Now read the Standards for proficiency outcomes in Box 1.2 and complete the Activity indicated.

Box 1.2

Examples of outcomes to be achieved from three platforms (NMC, 2018a)

Platform 1: Being an accountable professional

1.8 demonstrate the knowledge and skills, ability to think critically when applying evidence and drawing on experience to make evidence informed decisions in all situations. (2018a: 8)

1.9 understand the need to base all decisions regarding care and interventions on people's needs and preferences, recognising and addressing any personal and external factors that may unduly influence your decisions. (2018a: 8)

Platform 3: Assessing needs and planning care

3.4 understand and apply a person-centred approach to nursing care, demonstrating shared assessment, planning, decision-making and goal setting when working with people, their families, communities and populations of all ages. (2018a: 14)

Platform 4: Promoting and evaluating care

4.2 work in partnership with people to encourage shared decision-making, in order to support individuals, their families and carers to manage their own care when appropriate. (2018a: 17)

Complete Activity 1.4 to set learning goals that will enable you to achieve the proficiencies required.

Activity 1.4

1. Read the examples of outcomes (NMC, 2018a) given in Box 1.2. These are some of the proficiencies that a newly qualified nurse has to have attained.
2. Consider how you could achieve these in your next placement with the guidance of your practice supervisors.
3. Consider the care given to a person in your last placement. What key skills and knowledge did you need to be able to make decisions to ensure the best evidence-based care was going to be given to that person?
4. Discuss with your practice supervisors how they can support you in terms of learning opportunities to enable you to achieve your learning goals with regard to decision-making for the care of *one* person at your next placement.
5. You may also wish to consider here the implications and impact COVID-19 has had on your knowledge and skills that are necessary to care for patients within your learning placement. (See Chapter 14 for further information.)

You will already have a practice assessment schedule that you will have discussed with your personal tutor prior to going to your next placement. Each university and practice partnership will have developed their own unique or shared practice assessment documentation to support learning and assessment in practice environments where students are undertaking placements. Decision-making in relation to patient care is not an isolated event: working in a team to determine ongoing care is very much at the centre of shared person-centred care. For an example of a practice assessment schedule that can be accessed online, see the Web resources section at the end of this chapter.

Clinical Reasoning, Clinical Judgement and Decision-Making

We have noted that two other phrases used in conjunction with 'critical analysis' and 'critical thinking' are 'clinical reasoning' and 'clinical judgement'. Levett-Jones et al. state that, 'in the literature the terms clinical reasoning, clinical judgement, problem-solving, decision-making and critical thinking are often used interchangeably' (2010: 516). However, they also cite Elstein and Bordage (1991), who view clinical reasoning as 'the way clinicians think about the problems they deal with in clinical practice. It involves clinical judgements (deciding what is wrong with the patient) and clinical decision-making (deciding what to do)' (Levett-Jones et al., 2010: 516).

We can begin to see a possible way of differentiating between all these terms when it comes to learning to make decisions in clinical practice and, of course, in your other academic work. Clinical decision-making can be seen as the end point, when you are seen to take an action of some kind based on a range of other skills deriving from critical thinking, critical analysis, clinical reasoning and clinical judgement.

Levett-Jones et al. offer a framework for clinical reasoning called the 'five rights of clinical reasoning', based on a PhD study by Hoffman (2007) (one of the authors) who explored how students and qualified nurses made decisions 'when caring for patients in an intensive care unit' (Levett-Jones et al., 2010: 516). The initial thinking strategies that Hoffman found were as follows:

- describe the patient situation;
- collect new patient information;
- review information;
- relate information;
- recall knowledge;
- interpret information;
- make inferences;
- discriminate between relevant and irrelevant information;
- match and predict information;
- synthesise information to diagnose or identify a problem;
- establish goals;
- choose a course of action;
- evaluate (Levett-Jones et al., 2010: 516).

The 'five rights' of clinical reasoning in relation to student nurses and how new or novice nurses can apply them are 'the ability to collect the right cues and take the right action for the right patient at the right time for the right reason' (Levett-Jones et al., 2010: 517). See Levett-Jones et al. (2010) for a diagrammatic view of the clinical reasoning process and Chapter 2 in this book.

Tanner undertook a major review of the evidence on clinical judgement in nursing, on which she based 'an alternative model of clinical judgement' (2006: 204). She concluded that there were five key themes arising from this evidence:

1. clinical judgements are more influenced by what nurses bring to the situation than the objective data about the situation at hand
2. sound clinical judgement rests to some degree on knowing the patient and his or her typical pattern of responses, as well as engagement with the patient and his or her concerns
3. clinical judgements are influenced by the context in which the situation occurs
4. nurses use a variety of reasoning patterns alone or in combination and the culture of the nursing care unit
5. reflection on practice is often triggered by a breakdown in clinical judgement and is critical for the development of clinical knowledge and improvement of clinical reasoning (Tanner, 2006: 204).

Conclusion

We can see, from an exploration of the evidence available to us with regards to definitions and explanations of what decision-making entails as a qualified nurse, what a student nurse has to learn and what skills he or she has to gain to become an effective caring decision maker in practice. These skills have to be underpinned by an evidence base, not only in terms of the knowledge underpinning the rationales for decision-making at any level, but also the increased importance of developing critical analysis and critical thinking skills in both theory and practice. These skills are essential, along with an in-depth knowledge of patient care situations and experiences, to developing clinical reasoning and clinical judgement skills, all of which underpin the effectiveness of decision-making in nursing practice. Integrating what is learnt in theory and clinical simulation environments with what is then experienced in the context of clinical practice will ensure the successful development of decision-making skills, allowing you to become the competent practitioner that you must be to become a registered graduate nurse. We will be exploring many of these definitions and examples from practice throughout the book.

References

Aston, L., Wakefield, J. and McGown, R. (eds) (2010). *The Student Nurse Guide to Decision Making in Practice*. Maidenhead: Open University Press.

Benner, P. (1984). *From Novice to Expert: Excellence and power in clinical nursing practice*. Menlo Park, CA: Addison-Wesley.

Benner, P., Tanner, C., and Chesla, C. A. (1996). *Expertise in Nursing Practice: Caring, clinical judgement and ethics*. New York: Springer.

Blum, C. A. (2010). Using the Benner intuitive-humanistic decision-making model in action: A case study. *Nurse Education in Practice*, 10(5): 303–307.

Duffy, K., Hastie, E., McCallum, J., Ness, V., and Price, L. (2009). Academic writing: Using literature to demonstrate critical analysis. *Nursing Standard*, 23(47): 35–40.

Girot, E. A. (2000). Graduate nurses: Critical thinkers or better decision makers? *Journal of Advanced Nursing*, 31(2): 288–297.

Hoffman, K. (2007). A comparison of decision-making by 'expert' and 'novice' nurses in the clinical setting: Monitoring patient haemodynamic status post abdominal aortic aneurysm surgery. Unpublished PhD thesis, Sydney University of Technology, Sydney (available online at: https://opus.lib.uts.edu.au/handle/10453/21800, accessed 3 August 2022).

Holland, K. and Roxburgh, M. (2012). *Placement Learning in Surgical Nursing: A guide for students in practice*. Edinburgh: Baillière Tindall Elsevier.

Jones, R. A. P. (1996). Processes and models. In R. A. P. Jones and S. Beck (eds), *Decision Making in Nursing*. Albany, NY: Delmar. pp. 3–24.

Lasater, K. (2007). Clinical judgement development: Using simulation to create an assessment rubric. *Journal of Nursing Education*, 46(11): 496–503.

Levett-Jones, T., Hoffman, K., Dempsey, J., Jeong, S. Y.-S., Noble, D., Norton, C. A., Roche, J. and Hickey, N. (2010). The 'five rights' of clinical reasoning: An educational model to enhance nursing students' ability to identify and manage clinically 'at risk' patients. *Nurse Education Today*, 30(6): 515–520.

Nursing and Midwifery Council (NMC) (2010) *Standards for Pre-registration Nursing Education*. London: NMC.

Nursing and Midwifery Council (NMC) (2018a). *Future Nurse: Standards of proficiency for registered nurses*. London: NMC.

Nursing and Midwifery Council (NMC) (2018b). *Realising Professionalism: Standards for education and training Part 1: Standards framework for nursing and midwifery education*. London: NMC.

Nursing and Midwifery Council (NMC) (2022). *Current Recovery Programme Standards*. London: NMC.

Rycroft-Malone, J., Fontenla, M., Seers, K. and Bick, D. (2009). Protocol-based care: The standardisation of decision making. *Journal of Clinical Nursing*, 18(10): 1490–1500.

Standing, M. (ed.) (2010). *Clinical Judgement and Decision Making in Nursing and Inter-professional Health Care*. Maidenhead: Open University Press.

Tanner, C. A. (2006). Thinking like a nurse: A research-based model of clinical judgement in nursing. *Journal of Nursing Education*, 45(6): 204–211.

Tappen, R. (1989). *Nursing Leadership and Management: Concepts and Practice*, 2nd edn. Philadelphia, PA: S. A. Davis Co.

Thompson, C. and Dowding, D. (eds) (2002). *Clinical Decision Making and Judgement in Nursing*. Edinburgh: Churchill Livingstone.

Thompson, C. and Dowding, D. (eds) (2009). *Essential Decision Making and Clinical Judgement for Nurses*. Edinburgh: Churchill Livingstone/Elsevier.

Further Reading

Abdulmohdi, N. (2019). Investigating nursing students' clinical reasoning and decision making using high fidelity simulation of a deteriorating patient scenario. Unpublished PhD thesis, Anglia Ruskin University, UK (available online at: https://arro.anglia.ac.uk/id/eprint/704906, accessed 3 August 2021).

Anton, N., Hornbeck, T., Modlin, S., Haque, M. M., Crites, M. and Yu, D. (2021). Identifying factors that nurses consider in the decision-making process related to patient care during the COVID-19 pandemic. PloS ONE, 16(7): e0254077.

Cameron, M. E., Schaffer, M. and Park, H. (2001). Nursing students' experience of ethical problems and use of ethical decision-making models. *Nursing Ethics*, 8(5): 432–447.

Gummesson, C., Sunden, A. and Fex, A. (2018). Clinical reasoning as a conceptual framework for interprofessional learning: A literature review and a case study. *Physical Therapy Reviews*, 23(1): 29–34.

Manetti, W. (2019). Sound clinical judgement in nursing: A concept analysis. *Nurse Forum*, 54: 102–110.

Von Colln-Appling, C. and Giuliano, D. (2017). A concept analysis of critical thinking: A guide for nurse educators. *Nurse Education Today*, 49: 106–109.

Web Resources

All Wales *Practice Assessment Document and Ongoing Record of Achievement* – includes descriptions of updated roles related to student learning in practice: https://nurse-mentors.bangor.ac.uk/documents/ALL%20WALES%20PRACTICE%20 ASSESSMENT%20DOCUMENT.pdf (accessed 20 June 2022).

Hoffman et al.'s clinical reasoning cycle – clinical reasoning scenario using this model: www.youtube.com/watch?v=OxKILfnHM1k (accessed 20 June 2022).

NHS Scotland effective practitioner resources: www.effectivepractitioner.nes.scot.nhs.uk/clinical-practice.aspx (accessed 20 June 2022). There is also one focused on decision-making in practice: www.effectivepractitioner.nes.scot.nhs.uk/clinical-practice/clinical-decision-making.aspx (accessed 20 June 2022).

Nursing and Midwifery Council (NMC) (2010) *Standards for Pre-registration Nursing Education*: www.nmc.org.uk/globalassets/sitedocuments/standards/nmc-standards-for-pre-registration-nursing-education.pdf (accessed 20 April 2022).

Nursing and Midwifery Council (2018a) *Future Nurse: Standards of proficiency for registered nurses*: www.nmc.org.uk/globalassets/sitedocuments/standards-of-proficiency/ nurses/future-nurse-proficiencies.pdf (accessed 20 April 2022).

Nursing and Midwifery Council (2018b) *Realising Professionalism: Standards for education and training Part 1: Standards framework for nursing and midwifery education*: www. nmc.org.uk/globalassets/sitedocuments/standards-of-proficiency/standards-framework-for-nursing-and-midwifery-education/education-framework.pdf (accessed 20 April 2022).

Nursing and Midwifery Council (2022) *Current Recovery Programme Standards* (updated January 2022) – these (and the *Emergency Standards,* removed on 30 September 2021) relate to student learning in practice and at university for pre-registration nurses and are applied to all nursing programmes: www.nmc.org.uk/globalassets/sitedocuments/ education-standards/current-recovery-programme-standards.pdf (accessed 20 June 2022).

2

MAKING DECISIONS AS A STUDENT: DECISION-MAKING OPPORTUNITIES

Debbie Roberts

Chapter objectives

The aims of this chapter are to:

- consider the principles of decision-making in the context of undertaking a course of study;

- consider the various general decision-making situations that will have an impact on your learning to become a nurse;
- consider the types of decisions that you will be required to make in relation to clinical placements and your role as a student nurse;
- consider the different ways in which academic and practice staff can help you to achieve your goal of becoming a qualified nurse.

Introduction

This chapter introduces the underlying principles of decision-making. You will be encouraged to consider decision-making in two contexts: as a student in university, together with decision-making as a student nurse in practice (see Chapter 1). Nurses make decisions all the time with one study suggesting that nurses can make decisions every 30 seconds (Bucknall, 2000).

Decision-making is widely regarded to be a combination of interpersonal, technical and cognitive skills. It is important to stress that decision-making skills do not develop by chance and, as a student, you will have to develop your decision-making skills in readiness for taking decisions as a qualified nurse. Like all other skills, decision-making should be practised regularly so that you improve over time.

Following a major consultation with registrants and key stakeholders, the Nursing and Midwifery Council (NMC) published a new set of educational standards in 2018. The standards consist of four key documents:

- *Future Nurse: Standards of proficiency for registered nurses* This document provides the NMC's vision for the role of the nurse in the twenty-first century and describes the contribution of nurses to health and health care. According to the NMC, nurses of the future will require 'The confidence and ability to think critically, apply knowledge and skills, and provide expert, evidence-based, direct nursing care' (2018a: 3). The role of the nurse and the associated proficiencies are grouped under seven platforms:

  1. Being an accountable professional;
  2. Promoting health and preventing ill health;
  3. Assessing needs and planning care;
  4. Providing and evaluating care;
  5. Leading and managing nursing care and working in teams;
  6. Improving safety and quality of care;
  7. Coordinating care.

  Throughout the pre-registration nurse education programme, students will be working towards becoming the future nurse described within this document.

Decision-making is associated with all the seven platforms and, as a student, you will be expected to demonstrate that you are making progress towards the proficiencies described there and be able to develop and refine your decision-making ability. (See the Web resources section at the end of this chapter for the link to this, the first of the five documents.)

- *Realising Professionalism: Standards for education and training Part 1: Standards framework for nursing and midwifery education* (2018b) (See the Web resources section at the end of this chapter for the link to this first part of the new educational standards.)
- *Realising Professionalism: Standards for education and training Part 2: Standards for student supervision and assessment* (2018c) This part of the standards sets out the expectations for the learning, support, supervision and assessment (of theory and practice) of students in the practice environment. The standards describe how students should be supported to learn in practice settings and introduces two new roles – namely, those of practice supervisors and practice assessors. (See the Web resources section at the end of this chapter for the link to this second part of the new educational standards.)
- *Realising Professionalism: Standards for education and training Part 3: Standards for pre-registration nursing programmes* (2018d) This part of the standards outlines what are known as programme standards, which are specific to each pre-registration or post-registration programme. The legal requirements for all pre-registration nursing education programmes are described in this document. (See the Web resources section at the end of this chapter for the link to this final part of the new educational standards.)

As seen in Chapter 1, the above standards include both direct and indirect reference to decision-making skills and knowledge, which it is expected that students will acquire during their clinical placement learning and by engaging with the underpinning theoretical and evidence-based background during their university studies. The focus to this book is on these two aspects of decision-making.

What Is Nursing Decision-Making?

There are several terms in the literature that are often used interchangeably. You will see terms such as 'decision-making', 'problem solving', 'clinical reasoning' or 'clinical judgement', as well as others that are used when writers are discussing how and why nurses respond to clinical situations in particular ways (see Chapter 1 for more details).

Koharchik, Caputi, Robb and Culleiton (2015), writing from a North American perspective, suggest that effective, patient-centred decision-making hinges on adept clinical reasoning and, more importantly, that such reasoning is essential if professional standards are to be maintained. Koharchik and colleagues state that:

Clinical reasoning involves applying ideas to experience in order to arrive at a valid conclusion and is the term most widely used to describe the way a health care professional analyses and understands a patient's situation and forms conclusions. (2015: 58)

As we saw in Chapter 1, it is generally recognised that problem solving skills and decision-making skills are not the same. Problem solving is a broader phase of the decision-making process if it is used in decision-making at all. The first stage might involve framing the issue as a problem – in other words, acknowledging that a 'problem' exists. A problem must then be analysed (the problem solving part) before a range of possible actions to be taken is identified and a suitable solution selected from those identified (the decision-making part).

Problem solving is a process through which you develop an understanding of the situation in order to make changes. Problem solving will involve intrapersonal factors (your own motivations – to be a good person, for example), interpersonal factors (those that apply to others, such as a patient in pain) and extra-personal factors (perhaps in relation to your profession or institution), because all will have an impact on the outcome. People balance these factors in different ways and that is why we solve problems in different ways. It is also why we make different decisions.

Decision-making is widely regarded to be a combination of interpersonal, technical and cognitive skills. For that reason, this book focuses on broad principles of decision-making, as it is not possible to provide exemplars or rules for all situations in all circumstances.

In order to start this process of developing decision-making skills generally, we can begin by looking at how we already use these in non-clinical situations.

Decision-Making During a Course of Study

Life is full of decisions that must be made. However, for the most part, we do not really stop and think about them in our daily lives. In other words, these decisions could be said to be unconscious or 'tacit' (see the Further reading section at the end of this chapter).

The journey to becoming a student of nursing begins much earlier than your first day at university. In the first instance, what made you decide to become a nurse? Was it a family tradition, with members of your family having been nurses or in related health professions, or was it something else? This decision would be influential in your journey to becoming a nurse. Once you decided that you wished to join the nursing profession it would influence both your school and college pathways. The next step is to decide to apply when the time is right to do so.

Having applied and been accepted on to a pre-registration nursing programme at university, you will gradually be equipped with the knowledge, skills and professional attitudes to become a qualified nurse in whichever field of practice you have elected to pursue. But how did you decide which university you wanted to attend? Perhaps you made some pragmatic decisions, choosing whichever university was closest to where you live or that had placements near to where you live? Alternatively, you may have made a conscious decision to study away from your home town. You may also have investigated whether or not individuals graduating from your university have found gainful employment. Perhaps you looked carefully at the facilities on offer at different universities and considered which would provide you with the best academic or pastoral support. You may have looked at what previous students have said about particular universities as part of the annual National Student Survey.

You will then have weighed up a number of different factors and they will have influenced your decision as to where to study and also gain relevant practical experience. Complete Activity 2.1 to reflect on your decision process.

Activity 2.1

1. Think back to your reasons for choosing the university at which you are studying. Consider all the information that you gathered, as well as any personal issues that you took into account when making your decision.
2. What major changes did you have to make in your life before starting the course?
3. How did these impact on others in your social and family groups?
4. What was the most important decision you had to make to achieve your ambition to learn to become a nurse?
5. What did you think was going to be the biggest challenge for you?

While on your university course, you will experience a range of approaches to learning and teaching, as well as different environments. It is likely that you will be expected to undertake some form of group work (either formally or informally). Indeed, as a graduate, many employers will expect that you will be able to work collaboratively and effectively with other people from a wide range of backgrounds and countries around the world. You may be expected to undertake small projects or assessments in groups; giving presentations, devising reports and written work; these activities may be classroom based or via an online or virtual environment.

Activity 2.2

1. During a directed study session at university, you are asked by your lecturer to work in a group of five with your peers to deliver a presentation on preparing for your first practice placement.

2. Think about what is required for the group to produce the final presentation.
3. Consider all the roles that people might undertake in this activity: agreeing a plan, finding information, delegation of jobs to do, bringing information back to the others and deciding which information you will keep and which you will reject and so on.
4. Think about your strengths and how you will establish your role in the group.

Group work can be an excellent way to learn together, but sometimes this kind of activity can be difficult. An example could be that there is someone in the group who likes to lead and take control, which can stifle creativity or supress some individuals' ideas. There might also be times when some individuals do not deliver what they had agreed to at the beginning of a planned task and, potentially, create feelings of resentfulness among other members of the group.

What is clear from these examples is that one of the first tasks in the decision-making that a small group has to undertake when allocated a specific task is to identify the roles for people and the expectations of each person.

Being a Student Nurse in Clinical Practice: Ensuring Self-care and Safe Practice

Student nurses in the UK divide their time equally between university (class-based activity) and learning as a student in (clinical) practice. Practice based learning opportunities can take place in a wide variety of health and social care settings: hospitals, community hospitals, community settings, specialist services and many more. You will work and learn alongside other students (your peers), registered nurses and possibly nursing associates, as well as health care support workers in caring for patients or clients. As part of the new NMC educational standards, student nurses are expected to learn how to support the learning of others, which includes when they have to make decisions. The new standards apply to all care settings and all areas of practice (that is, all four fields of practice in the UK), and had to apply to all curricula for students commencing their programme from September 2020. In relation to supporting others, one of the outcome statements (platform 1, 1.5), which all nurses are required to have achieved at the point of registration, is to:

> understand the demands of professional practice and demonstrate how to recognise signs of vulnerability in themselves or their colleagues and the action required to minimise risks to health. (NMC, 2018a: 8)

Clinical practice can be a fast-paced, emotionally charged, stressful environment, which can place great demands on you physically and emotionally. You will see people when they are anxious, in pain, depressed, unable to communicate, when they have received bad news or who are approaching the end of their life. In any of these circumstances, as a student, you are expected to learn and practice ethical principles and be compassionate in the care that you provide. Given the nature of practice as described, you will also be vulnerable, and expected to recognise the impact of being at risk yourself, which could have a negative impact on your ability to be effective as a decision maker.

How, then, do students learn to develop the ability to offer compassionate care, which will encompass supporting patients to make decisions, but at the same time be aware of colleagues who may have difficulties engaging in such sharing. Complete Activity 2.3 to learn more about how to do this.

Activity 2.3

1. Access and read the paper by K. Curtis (2014), Learning the requirements for compassionate practice: Student vulnerability and courage, *Nursing Ethics*, 21(2): 210–223.
2. Consider your own learning journey, as it relates to compassionate practice, and what kinds of decisions you had to make.
3. Consider each of the key themes revealed in the study by Curtis and relate these themes to how you are feeling about being able to provide compassionate care.

The paper in Activity 2.3 outlines the nature of the progression in learning how to provide compassionate care. This is important, because, like many nursing skills, compassion may have to be learned. It should not be assumed that everyone is able to practice with compassion at a high level at the point of starting their journey as a student nurse. The study by Curtis (2014) shows that some students had concerns about their ability to engage in and maintain compassionate practice. In particular, think about the point raised by Curtis, that students should learn 'how to learn from their experiences rather than blame themselves when ideals are difficult to uphold' (2014: 218).

At the time of writing, the world has been experiencing a pandemic, which has had a major impact on the work and lives of nurses globally. It is evident from the various social media sites linked to nursing, as well as the developing evidence base of the effects of the COVID-19 virus on the work of nurses, that learning to become a nurse has increased in terms of the vulnerability and risk to self and others. (see Chapter 14).

McGeehin Heilferty, Phillips and Mathios (2021) describe the mental fatigue and impact of the pandemic on the journey to becoming a nurse. Their study, which analysed 56 letters written by student nurses at the height of the pandemic in 2020, describes some of the challenges to both the university and practice learning aspects of being a student nurse during that time. The students used a range of strategies to help them to cope, including drawing on family and friends to promote their resilience, which is an essential prerequisite to underpinning effective decision-making.

Resilience during the pandemic was of the utmost importance, given the changing nature of the clinical environment where students undertook their placements. Amsrud, Lyberg and Severisson (2019) explored how nurse educators could support the students' development of resilience based on a synthesis of qualitative research. They stated that the first step towards this was to ensure that students had access to a culture characterised by trustworthiness (Amsrud et al., 2019). See Activity 2.4 to think about these aspects of your experiences. Make some notes that you can return to later to determine if anything has changed.

Activity 2.4

1. Think about the informal support mechanisms that are available to you, such as family and friends, as well as the formal university-based ones.
2. Think about what triggers might lead you to seek support.
3. Have you developed resilience to be able to make decisions in both your daily and professional life?
4. What has had the most impact on you?

During the pandemic, student nurses (as well as many health and social care colleagues) have experienced increased exposure to death and dying (McCallum. et al., 2021). Poignantly, McCallum et al. noted:

> Nurses are ringing relatives to update them or talking on video calls to try and support relatives who are not able to visit and are having to hear the worst news through a remote platform. Understandably people are angry, and some are taking this anger out on nurses who are advocating for the patient while also acting as the messenger. Throughout all this, nurses are coping with their own feelings of grief and yet are continuing to come into work, continuing to provide professional nursing care. (2021: 2)

The sheer number of people who have died during the pandemic has had an impact on registrants and student nurses alike. Galvin, Richards and Smith (2020) undertook a longitudinal cohort study investigating inadequate preparation regarding death and dying in nursing students and considered their findings in relation to the possible implications post COVID-19 pandemic. Their conclusions were that:

> it is not the increase in death and dying per se that causes mental health difficulties but that it is instead the experience of high levels of death and dying in combination with inadequate preparation. (2020: 1)

Complete Activity 2.5 to consider what support you have or may need.

Activity 2.5

1. Access and read the review by L. J. Thomas and S. H. Revell (2016), Resilience in nursing students: An integrative review, *Nurse Education Today*, 36: 457-462.
2. Start to identify all the potential sources of support (formal and informal) that you might be able to draw on if you felt stressed during a clinical placement.
3. How might you start the process of seeing a difficult day as a challenge and an opportunity to overcome barriers? Who or what from your list above might be the most able or available to provide support?
4. What strategies can you start to develop to minimise stress?
5. Start to think about what actions you will take to obtain the range of support that you may need as a student nurse.

You might find it useful to make some notes for this activity that can be shared with your personal tutor or academic supervisor when setting new learning goals.

The Impact of the Learning Environment on Student Self-care

Nursing care is delivered around the clock in a variety of placement settings. Thus, student nurses are expected to engage in learning through clinical practice experiences throughout the twenty-four hours of each day and throughout the entire week.

Adjusting to the expectations of shift work can be difficult, as eating and sleeping patterns can often be disrupted. Gifkins, Johnson and Loudoun (2018) used a case study approach to capture differences and similarities in food choices and eating patterns between twelve experienced and nine inexperienced nurses while working shifts. The Australian study revealed that nurses from both groups experienced increases in snacking and craving food while at work generally, but predominantly during night shifts. Nurses from both groups also consumed more caffeine (mostly through tea and coffee) while on night shifts. However, an increase in caffeine consumption can interfere with sleep.

James, Butterfield and Tuell, in their study of student nurses' sleep patterns and the impact of shift work on safe practice, concluded that 'sleepiness can impair nursing students' confidence in their ability to practice safely' (2019: 547). This had implications not only for their self-care needs but also on their making decisions confidently, in terms of giving care to patients. These implications were categorised as having an impact in relation to preventing adverse events to patients (such as giving injections) and preventing injuries to themselves (occupational health, such as ensuring safe lifting practices were employed).

Imagine that you are allocated for two-weeks of 'work' duty, with four-night shifts over a two-week period (which is a pattern of four-night shifts on and three off each week). If you have already undertaken this type of shift pattern, consider the questions in the past tense - that is, 'What did you do?'

1. What can you do to prepare for the two weeks in terms of your dietary choices during that time?
2. Is there anything you can do to maximise the likelihood of sleeping well during the two weeks, to your environment or your diet? For example, will you decide to maintain your usual pattern of eating your main meal of the day at 18.00 even when on night shift?
3. Will you decide to exercise more or less during the two weeks when you will be doing night shifts?

You may want to think about the environment where you sleep. If you usually like complete silence in order to get to sleep, will the room be quiet enough during the day or will you need some earplugs? Light can also be an issue, as many people like complete darkness to sleep. Maybe some blackout blinds or a sleep mask would help?

In the study by Gifkins, Johnson and Loudoun (2018), the nurses from both the less experienced and the most experienced group would snack more and skip meals due to fatigue, although they believed that this was detrimental to their health and well-being. In addition, the nurses all indicated that they could not drink enough fluids while on night duty (shifts) so most kept bottled water with them at all times, even while on shift.

In terms of your well-being, it is important to think about how you can maximise self-care and avoid the pitfalls of missing meals, dehydration and fatigue. The study by Gifkins, Johnson and Loudoun emphasises the need for individuals to establish 'what works for me' (2018: 817). To do that, find a regime of eating, drinking, sleeping and exercise that works for you while maximising your health.

Decision-Making in Nursing Practice: The Student Experience

As seen earlier, making decisions in relation to how you can ensure that your practice is safe, and you can access as much support as possible when undertaking a practice learning placement is dependent not only on your own self but that of many others. In particular, those that are tasked with your learning pathway, including teaching you knew skills and knowledge. These are discussed in various chapters in the book as relevant, but to begin your thought processes in preparation for placement learning, consider Activity 2.7 and what role everyone plays in your journey to becoming a qualified nurse.

Activity 2.7

1. Write down the type of placement you will be going to next and the kinds of patient care experiences you are likely to experience there. Summarise the information, as if you were explaining it to another student.
2. Imagine the first hour at the placement. Write down what you think will happen after you arrive.
3. Write down the first three decisions that you might have to consider during this time.

You may have noted the following decisions:

- what you might discuss and decide on with your practice assessor and practice supervisor when you meet them for the first time;
- whether to ask any questions about the patients/clients you will be caring for that day;
- whether to ask for your shift hours as soon as the morning report has been given (about the patients you will be caring for that day);
- who you will be working with that day and what your role will be in the team?

Now think about your answers to Activity 2.7 in relation to the following types of decisions described in Chapter 1. What do you have to consider before making the decision to act on any of your four choices? Your answers will very much depend on whether you have considered the 'cues', either in the context of care and what is actually happening around you; what evidence you are 'picking up' about whether or not it is a good time to be asking any questions; how busy your mentor is; what is happening with the patients in your care; whether your shift hours might simply be read from the 'off duty' rota on the noticeboard in the staff area of the ward or community office.

The frequency of decision-making in nursing practice is dependent on five inter-related factors, which are the:

- clinical environment;
- patients who can be found within that environment;
- nurses' perceptions of their clinical role;

- operational autonomy;
- degree to which they see themselves as active and influential decision makers (Thompson et al., 2004).

The study by Thompson et al. (2004) demonstrates three levels of what they term 'decisional complexity', meaning that nurses often have to respond to clinical situations by making quick decisions and often the decisions they need to make are complex. The study showed that student nurses take more time to collect information on which to base their decisions than experts, who spend less time than student nurses seeking information to reduce uncertainty in their decision-making. So, remember that decision-making as a student nurse may not be as fluid and speedy as the decision-making that will emerge as you develop your expertise and remember the time you take to collect information on which to base your decisions is important and should not be underestimated.

As part of your pre-registration nurse education programme, you may be introduced to examples of computerised decision support systems (CDSS), which are used in clinical practice and or in clinical skills laboratories, though there they may be known as interactive computerised decision support frameworks (ICDSF) (Hoffman et al., 2011). CDSS or ICDSF have been developed to help nurses and other health care workers, as a guide to bedside decision-making. It is thought that such computerised systems are helpful when large volumes of complex information have to be considered and a rapid decision is required. Computerised systems can help students to model the way that more experienced nurses think, approach a clinical problem and find potential solutions. Hoffman et al. (2011: 589) present a model of clinical reasoning, which is represented as a cycle, reflecting the cyclical nature of nursing care.

Hoffman et al. point out that the parts of the 'clinical reasoning cycle are not clear cut and in reality, the steps merge and the boundaries between them are often blurred with nurses moving back and forth between some steps and merging others' (2011: 588). Nonetheless, this visual representation of the way in which some clinical decisions are arrived at may be useful in helping you to plan your learning in placement by using the same process to identify those decisions you identified earlier. For example, underpinning knowing what illnesses patients might have would be this cyclical process, starting at the top of the cycle – 'Consider the patient situation' – then moving to the next – 'Collect cues/information' – then onwards, working your way through the next three, to making a decision either with or for the person – the 'Take action' step.

This model can also be of value in supporting students' ability in identifying and managing clinical situations with patients, identified by Levett-Jones et al. (2010) as 'the five rights of clinical reasoning'. You will note that in Activity 2.8, there is an example related to the cause of the pandemic, which has had such an impact on the delivery of nursing care and health care generally. Given the pattern of the virus and its continued persistence in society generally at the time of writing, it is important

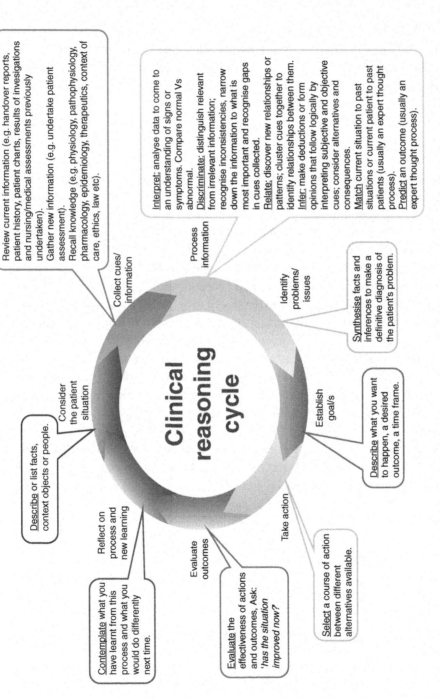

Figure 2.1 Model of clinical reasoning (Hoffman et al., 2011, reproduced with permission of the authors).

From Hoffman, K., Dempsey, J., Levett-Jones, T., Noble, D., Hickey, N., Jeong, S., Hunter, S. and Norton, C. (2011). The design and implementation of an Interactive Computerised Decision Support Framework (ICDSF) as a strategy to improve nursing students' clinical reasoning skills. *Nurse Education Today*, 31(6): 587–594.

that we include possible scenarios that students will already have been exposed to. Those who have not can still engage in discussion with their peers in general terms and regarding what is known about the nature of infection control during a pandemic. We have also included an additional chapter (Chapter 14), that begins to focus on student learning and decision-making related to disasters, such as a pandemic.

Activity 2.8

1. Access and read the paper by T. Levett-Jones et al. (2010), The 'five rights' of clinical reasoning: An educational model to enhance nursing students' ability to identify and manage clinically 'at risk' patients, *Nurse Education Today*, 30(6), 515–520.
2. Watch the video on clinical reasoning (see the Web resources section at the end of this chapter for the link).
3. Consider the required information and actions needed in using the cycle (as described and seen in the paper) in an environment where:
   a) the patients all had symptoms of COVID-19 but were not critically ill
   b) another environment where the patients were in an intensive care environment
   c) an elderly care environment where patients with memory difficulties were diagnosed as having symptoms of COVID-19. All were tested and clinically diagnosed as having COVID-19.
4. Undertake a review of literature focusing on student learning during the COVID-19 pandemic and share your findings with your peers. Identify the major decision-making challenges at the following levels:
   (a) global
   (b) national
   (c) personal and professional.

Conclusion

This chapter has focused on examples of learning opportunities related to decision-making as a student nurse. It is an introduction to this subject and, along with the other chapters in Part 1 of this book, will establish a foundation of knowledge that can be used to underpin your practice. Your ability to make the right decisions will develop over the course of your learning journey towards becoming a qualified nurse. It is important that you make decisions based on the best evidence available at the time and, of course, that your decisions do no harm to yourself, to your colleagues or, most importantly, to those patients and clients you will be learning to care for and with whom you will be working.

References

Amsrud, K. E., Lyeberg, A. and Severinsson, E. (2019). Development of resilience in nursing students: A systematic qualitative review and thematic synthesis. *Nurse Education in Practice*, 41: 102621.

Bucknall, T. (2000). Critical care nurses' decision-making activities in the natural clinical setting. *Journal of Clinical Nursing*, 9(1): 25–35.

Curtis. K. (2014). Learning the requirements for compassionate practice: Student vulnerability and courage. *Nursing Ethics*, 21(2): 210–223.

Galvin, J., Richards, G. and Smith, A. P. (2020). A longitudinal cohort study investigating inadequate preparation and death and dying in nursing students: Implications for the aftermath of the COVID-19 pandemic. *Frontiers in Psychology*, 11: 2206.

Gifkins, J., Johnston. A. and Loudoun. R. (2018). The impact of shift work on eating patterns and self-care strategies utilised by experienced and inexperienced nurses. *Chronobiology International*, 35(6): 811–820.

Ha, L. and Pepin, J. (2018). Clinical nursing leadership educational intervention for first-year nursing students: A qualitative evaluation. *Nurse Education in Practice*, 37–43.

Hoffman, K., Dempsey, J., Levett-Jones, T., Noble, D., Hickey, N., Jeong, S., Hunter, S. and Norton, C. (2011). The design and implementation of an interactive computerised decision support framework (ICDSF) as a strategy to improve nursing students' clinical reasoning skills. *Nurse Education Today*, 31(6): 587–594.

James, L., Butterfield, P., and Tuell, E. (2010). Nursing students' sleep patterns and perceptions of safe practice during their entrée to shift work. *Workplace Health and Safety*. Volume: 67 issue: 11, page(s): 547-553. Accessed 24.5.22 via: https://journals.sagepub.com/doi/pdf/10.1177/2165079919867714

Koharchik, L., Caputi, L., Robb, M. and Culleiton, A. L. (2015). Fostering clinical reasoning in nursing students: How can instructors in practice settings impart this essential skill? *The American Journal of Nursing*, 115(1): 58–61.

Levett-Jones, T., Hoffman, K., Dempsey, J., Jeong, S. Y.-S., Noble, D., Norton, C. A., Roche, J. and Hickey, N. (2010). The 'five rights' of clinical reasoning: An educational model to enhance nursing students' ability to identify and manage clinically 'at risk' patients, *Nurse Education Today*, 30(6), 515–520.

McCallum, K. J., Walthall, H., Aveyard, H. and Jackson, D. (2021). Grief and nursing: Life and death in the pandemic. *Journal of Advanced Nursing*, 77(5): 2115–2116.

McGeehin Heilferty, C., Phillips, L. J. and Mathios, R. (2021). Letters from the pandemic: Nursing student narratives of change, challenges and thriving at the outset of COVID-19. *Journal of Advanced Nursing*, 77(8): 3436–3445.

Nursing and Midwifery Council (NMC) (2018a). *Future Nurse: Standards of proficiency for registered nurses*. London: NMC.

Nursing and Midwifery Council (NMC) (2018b). *Realising Professionalism: Standards for education and training Part 1: Standards framework for nursing and midwifery education*. London: NMC.

Nursing and Midwifery Council (NMC) (2018c). *Realising Professionalism: Standards for education and training Part 2: Standards for student supervision and assessment.* London: NMC.

Nursing and Midwifery Council (NMC) (2018d). *Realising Professionalism: Standards for education and training Part 3: Standards for pre-registration nursing programmes.* London: NMC.

Royal College of Nursing (2012). Quality with compassion: The future of nurse education. *Report of the Willis Commission on Nursing Education.* London: Royal College of Nursing.

Thomas, L. J. and Revell, S. H. (2016). Resilience in nursing students: An integrative review. *Nurse Education Today*, 36: 457–462.

Thompson, C., Cullum, N., McCaughan, C., Sheldon, T. and Raynor, P. (2004). Nurses, information use, and clinical decision making – the real world potential for evidence-based decisions in nursing. *Evidence Based Nursing.* 68–72. https://ebn.bmj.com/content/ebnurs/7/3/68.full.pdf (accessed 24 May 2022).

Further Reading

Attenborough, J., Reynolds, L. and Nolan, P. (2019). Reflecting on our history: The nurses that roared: nurses from history who found their voices and challenged the status quo. *Creative Nursing*, 25(1): 67–73.

Forsberg, E., Ziegert, K., Hult, H. and Fors, U. (2016). Assessing progression of clinical reasoning through virtual patients: An exploratory study. *Nurse Education in Practice*, 16(1): 97–103.

Nibbelink, C. W. and Brewer, B. B. (2018). Decision-making in nursing practice: An integrative literature review. *Journal of Clinical Nursing*, 27: 917–918.

Sandford, S., Schwartz, B. and Khan, Y. (2020). The role of tacit knowledge in communication and decision-making during emerging public health incidents. *International Journal of Disaster Risk Reduction*, 50(2): 101681.

Swift, A., Banks, L., Baleswaran, A. et al. (2020). COVID–19 and student nurses: A view from England, *Journal of Clinical Nursing*, 29(17–18): 3111–3114.

Thompson, C., Aitken, L., Doran, D. and Dowding, D. (2013). An agenda for clinical decision making and judgement in nursing research and education. *International Journal of Nursing Studies*, 50(12): 1720–1726.

West, M., Bailey, E. and Williams, E. (2020). *The Courage of Compassion: Supporting nurses and midwives.* Report commissioned by the RCN Foundation, published by the King's Fund, London.

Web Resources

Hoffman et al.'s clinical reasoning cycle – clinical reasoning scenario using this model: https://www.youtube.com/watch?v=OxKILfnHM1k (accessed 2 June 2022).

International Council of Nurses (2021) *Nurses: A voice to lead: A vision for future healthcare, International Nurses Day 2021 resources and evidence*: www.icn.ch/system/files/documents/2021-05/ICN%20Toolkit_2021_ENG_Final.pdf (accessed 2 June 2022).

NHS Health England (2020), Student support guidance during COVID-19 outbreak: www.hee.nhs.uk/sites/default/files/documents/Student%20support%20guide%20master%20.pdf (accessed 2 June 2022).

NHS Health England (2020) Nursing and Midwifery COVID-19 Catalogue of Change: Supporting newly qualified nurses, midwives and new team members. *Case study: Learning identified by the CNO National Shared Professional Decision-Making Council*: www.england.nhs.uk/nursingmidwifery/shared-governance-and-collective-leadership/nursing-covid-19-catalogue-of-change/supporting-newly-qualified-nurses-midwives-and-new-team-members (accessed 2 June 2022).

Nursing and Midwifery Council (NMC): (2018a) *Future nurse: Standards of proficiency for registered nurses*: www.nmc.org.uk/globalassets/sitedocuments/education-standards/future-nurse-proficiencies.pdf (accessed 24 January 2022).

Nursing and Midwifery Council (NMC): (2018b) *Realising Professionalism: Standards for education and training Part 1: Standards framework for nursing and midwifery education*: www.nmc.org.uk/globalassets/sitedocuments/education-standards/education-framework.pdf (accessed 24 January 2022).

Nursing and Midwifery Council (NMC): (2018c) *Realising Professionalism: Standards for education and training Part 2: Standards for student supervision and assessment*: www.nmc.org.uk/globalassets/sitedocuments/education-standards/student-supervision-assessment.pdf (accessed 24 January 2022).

Nursing and Midwifery Council (NMC): (2018d) *Realising Professionalism: Standards for education and training Part 3: Standards for pre-registration nursing programmes*: www.nmc.org.uk/globalassets/sitedocuments/education-standards/programme-standards-nursing.pdf (accessed 24 January 2022).

Nursing and Midwifery Council (NMC): (2021) *NMC statement: Enabling student education and supporting the workforce*: www.nmc.org.uk/news/news-and-updates/statement-enabling-student-education-and-supporting-the-workforce (accessed 24 January 2022).

3

USING EVIDENCE FOR DECISION-MAKING

Joanne Cleary-Holdforth and Therese Leufer

Chapter objectives

The aims of this chapter are to:

- consider the value and importance of evidence-based practice (EBP) in decision-making;
- examine all aspects required to determine what is the best available evidence;
- further develop your searching and critical appraisal skills.

Introduction

This chapter focuses on the value and importance of evidence-based practice (EBP) in any decision-making involving patient and client care. It examines all aspects of what is required to determine that the evidence on which the decision-making will be based is the best available, including developing your searching and critical appraisal skills. The chapter also describes how you can improve these skills to achieve the necessary standards relevant to your stage of learning and, eventually, those essential for becoming a registered nurse. The ability to make clinical judgements and decisions that enhance and support effective patient care outcomes, as well as deliver that care in a holistic way, will depend on the underpinning knowledge and practice evidence that you, as a future qualified nurse, will use.

From reading Chapters 1 and 2 you will have gained much information about the principles of decision-making, as well as why they are so important for your nursing practice. As you progress in your nursing career, it will be invaluable to know when to:

- make decisions;
- take decisive action;
- call a doctor or refer a patient to another health professional;
- withhold a particular medication;
- recommend an alternative nursing intervention.

It is equally imperative that you understand why you are making these decisions and where you might go to find the information that you need to underpin them.

The Nursing and Midwifery Council (NMC), in *Realising Professionalism: Standards for education and training Part 3: Standards for pre-registration nursing programmes*, specifies clearly that student nurses must be afforded learning opportunities to enable them to 'develop and meet the *Standards of proficiency for registered nurses* to deliver safe and effective care to a diverse range of people' (2018d: 10). In its *Future Nurse: Standards of proficiency for registered nurses* (2018a), the NMC sets out seven key areas, or 'platforms', that cover specific outcomes student nurses must achieve at the point of registration. This chapter will focus on platform 4: Providing and evaluating care, as it is directly related to your future role as a registered nurse in leading evidence-based decision-making and compassionate and safe practice. The statement concerning what is required for platform 4 is presented in Box 3.1 that follows.

The seven platforms are supplemented by two 'annexes A and B' that reflect what is expected of a newly registered nurse in terms of knowledge and capability to deliver safe, proficient care at the start of their career. Annexe B focuses specifically

---

Box 3.1

Platform 4: Providing and evaluating care (NMC, 2018a)

Registered nurses take the lead in providing evidence-based, compassionate and safe nursing interventions. They ensure that care they provide, and delegate is person-centred and of a consistently high standard. They support people of all ages in a range of care settings. They work in partnership with people, families and carers to evaluate whether care is effective, and the goals of care have been met in line with their wishes, preferences and desired outcomes. (2018a: 16)

---

on nursing procedures that nurses must demonstrate they can perform safely on registration. This is the annexe that is relevant to platform 4 in particular, outlining the procedures for the planning, provision and management of person-centred nursing care. An example is listed in Box 3.2 and a link to the full Annexe documents can be found in the Web resources.

Box 3.2

Annexe B, Part 2: Procedures for the planning, provision and management of person-centred nursing care (NMC, 2018a)

3. Use evidence-based, best practice approaches for meeting needs for care and support with rest, sleep, comfort and the maintenance of dignity, accurately assessing the person's capacity for independence and self-care and initiating appropriate interventions,
   3.1 observe and assess comfort and pain levels and rest and sleep patterns
   3.3 use appropriate positioning and pressure-relieving techniques. (2018a: 33)

In order to deliver best practice effectively in the planning, provision and management of person-centred nursing care, nurses need to be equipped with specific knowledge and skills for evidence-based practice at the earliest possible opportunity (Leufer and Cleary-Holdforth, 2009; Leufer, 2020). In this chapter we will discuss the use of evidence-based practice to support the clinical decisions in your delivery of nursing care. We will provide you with a practical framework and approach to evidence-based clinical decision-making that will enable you to access all the relevant information from the appropriate sources, which you can rely on to ensure the best possible care for your patients.

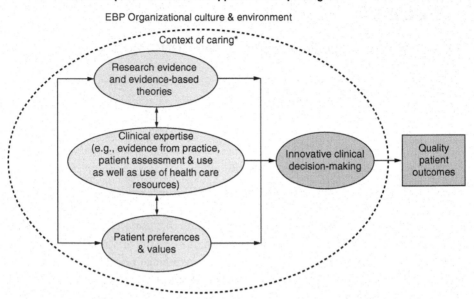

The conceptual framework to support the EBP paradigm

EBP Organizational culture & environment

* The context of caring allows for individualisation of the patient provider relationship

Figure 3.1   The conceptual framework to support the EBP paradigm (Melnyk and Fineout-Overholt, 2019, reproduced with permission of the authors).

Reproduced with permission from Melnyk and Fineout-Overholt (2019). *Evidence-Based Practice in Nursing and Healthcare: A Guide to Best Practice*, 4th edn. Philadelphia, PA: Wolters Kluwer Health/Lippincott, Williams & Wilkins.

Evidence-Based Practice: What Is it?

What, then, is evidence-based practice (EBP) and why are we reading and hearing about it more and more?

EBP has gained global momentum among various health care professional groups since its original inception in the early 1970s. Cleary-Holdforth (2020) considers it to be both a concept and a process, indicating its dynamic and evolving nature. This is similarly reflected by Melnyk and Fineout-Overholt (2019) who urge caution regarding how quickly health care practices can become outdated in the absence of current best evidence. Evidence-based practice is 'an holistic approach to care delivery that places the individual patient at its core' (Cleary-Holdforth and Leufer, 2009: 286).

Frequently mistaken to mean 'research utilisation' alone, EBP encompasses three core elements, of which research or evidence utilisation is only one. The remaining two core components are clinical expertise and patients' preferences and values. EBP is therefore a partnership between clinicians of various professions, patients and the best available evidence to inform decision-making in care settings and optimise patient outcomes. To put it simply, EBP is an approach that takes into account key influential factors to help make decisions regarding patients' care. These factors include:

- patients' preferences or opinions;
- the nurses'/clinicians' experience and expertise;
- relevant evidence from research, expert reports or significant organisations.

All these factors contribute to a patient care decision that will provide the best results for patients. It has been argued by authors such as Walsh and Ford (1994) that, in their view (See Fig.3.1), nursing care was based on 'ritual' and/or the personal preferences of medical consultants/ward sisters. Others, however, urge caution regarding such statements and argue that clear evidence of ritual in its widest context needs to be considered (see Holland, 2020).

An individual nurse's expertise and/or experience were not always influential in the decision-making around patient care. In our view, there were practices that were not always grounded in 'sound evidence' and decisions about clinical care were not often queried in terms of why practice was changed, or indeed why it was not. It must be noted, however, that consideration has to be given to the context in which care practices were developed over time, and that these took place because of the evidence available at the time.

Nurses in the 1940s, 1950s, 1960s and, indeed, later, for example, did not knowingly choose care and treatments that may cause the patient any 'harm'. Examples include the routine rubbing of alcohol on patients' buttocks, in the belief that such rigorous friction, coupled with a drying substance, would somehow prevent the development of pressure sores; the topical application of egg white and oxygen therapy to established pressure sores, in the belief that this would heal them; and the use of 'Edinburgh university solution of lime' (Eusol) for wound desloughing, which has courted immense controversy over the years (Tingle, 1990). These are just a few of the practices that we, and some of your tutors, would have witnessed in our respective student nurse training.

To support the ongoing development of research in nursing care, the Royal College of Nursing launched 'The Study of Nursing Care' series of reports in 1966, after being invited to undertake research by the then Ministry of Health (UK). This research provided pieces of evidence that are still important today and they are often referred to in research papers. For example, 'The unpopular patient' by Felicity Stockwell, 'Nurse – I want my mummy!' by Pamela Hawthorn or 'Nil by mouth?', a descriptive study of nursing care in relation to pre-operative fasting by Stephanie Smith (see the Web resources section at the end of this chapter for the link to PDFs of these studies, which can be downloaded from the RCN's website, from its library catalogue, special collections). To explore some of these historical research issues further, work through Activity 3.1.

Activity 3.1

1. Visit a relevant database (examples can be found later in this chapter) and undertake a search for current evidence in relation to the following practices:
   - the routine rubbing of alcohol into patients' buttocks to prevent the development of pressure sores;
   - the use of Eusol for wound desloughing.
2. Reflect on the nature of the evidence that may have been used to underpin these practices in the past. Consider the alternatives that were also options at the time, in the 1960s and 1970s.
3. Access and read the review by S. Church and P. Lyne (1994), Research-based practice: Some problems illustrated by the discussion of evidence concerning the use of a pressure-relieving device in nursing and midwifery, *Journal of Advanced Nursing*, 19: 513-551.
4. Consider the evidence provided in the review and why the authors concluded that there was insufficient evidence on which to base best practice decisions in the use of pressure-relieving cushions in pressure ulcer prevention. In particular, they considered that decisions were made on clinical judgement and not research findings.

Questioning such practices at that time was not encouraged, and the culture and historical background of nursing largely compelled nurses to 'follow orders.' EBP, however, actively encourages questioning and values the ongoing accessing and critical appraisal of evidence to scrutinise practice and the pursuit of improved patient outcomes. Jolley (2020) suggests that EBP enables the 'weeding out' of ineffective practices, and the identification and implementation of improved ones. This highlights the importance of ensuring balance in our thinking when considering the rationales for patient care. While the evidence supporting a particular practice may not be highly visible or, indeed, readily accessed, this does not always mean that a particular practice is not based on evidence or, indeed, that it does not have value for patient care.

EBP is also concerned with the standard of care delivery and how evidence is used to inform clinical decisions (Aveyard and Sharp, 2017). According to Melnyk and Fineout-Overholt (2019), it is a process comprised of seven easy-to-follow steps (See Table 3.1) that guides nurses from their initial question about an aspect of patient care through to making the most appropriate decision for the individual patient, plus its implementation, evaluation and dissemination.

So far, we have considered evidence in the context of how it is used to underpin practice/care decisions that demonstrate that there are clear steps and outcomes, which can be traced to a scientific basis. However, it is important before going further that we have a foundation of understanding as to what we actually mean by 'evidence' and how that then becomes an essential core component of evidence-based practice. It is important that students and qualified nurses understand that their decision-making in practice has to be based on a clear evidence-base, in order to ensure that they deliver safe and ethical care. We will now explain some of the key terms associated with EBP.

Table 3.1 The steps taken in the evidence-based practice (EBP) process (Melnyk and Fineout-Overholt, 2019).

0	Cultivate a spirit of enquiry within an evidence-based practice (EBP) culture and environment.
1	Ask the burning clinical question in PICOT format.
2	Search for and collect the most relevant and best evidence.
3	Critically appraise the evidence (that is, rapid critical appraisal, evaluation and synthesis).
4	Integrate the best evidence with one's clinical expertise and the patient's/family's preference and values in making a practice decision or change.
5	Evaluate outcomes of the practice decision or change based on evidence.
6	Disseminate the outcomes of the EBP decision or change.

Evidence

The meaning of the word 'evidence' in its broader application is 'something which provides ground for belief or disbelief' (*Collins Concise Dictionary and Thesaurus*, 1995: 318). However, the evidence to which we refer is that which should be used to underpin practice in the nursing context. In the context of nursing, then, what is evidence?

Melnyk and Fineout-Overholt, long-time active proponents of EBP, define evidence as 'a collection of facts that are believed to be true' (2019: 9). They further classify this into 'internal' and 'external' evidence, which, respectively, are evidence generated from practice and that generated from research. Examples of evidence from practice (internal evidence) and how it can be generated include outcomes from quality improvement projects involving patients, clinical audits on various aspects of patient care delivery and the results of outcomes measurements on patient interventions (Black and Jenkinson, 2009; McDonnell et al., 2007; Melnyk and Fineout-Overholt, 2019; Thompson, 2003).

External evidence, however, is generated by conducting formal research studies or clinical trials to investigate or explain a particular phenomenon relating to an aspect of patient care. Examples might be a research study to explore the experience of 'phantom pain' in patients who have undergone a below-knee amputation (Desmond et al., 2008) or a study to test the relationship or link between cigarette smoking and lung cancer (Centre for Disease Control and Prevention, 2011). These are just two examples of how evidence from research used to answer clinical questions can contribute to decisions about patient care.

From this it is clear that there is more than one source of evidence on which we can draw on to underpin practice. In fact, Turner et al. (2017) suggests that there are numerous sources of evidence, including diverse forms of information, such as research findings; professional opinion; patient experience; clinical guidance and local data or context. In certain circumstances, such as the COVID-19 global pandemic, the best or only evidence available to health care professionals may be that which is generated internally or guidance from appropriate authorities, such as the World Health Organisation, or early or preliminary research (Borges do Nascimento et al., 2020; Cotton et al., 2020; Kim, 2020; Giles et al., 2021).

To consider wider sources of evidence, complete Activity 3.2.

Activity 3.2

1. Access and read the article by W. Xu, A. D. Towers, P. Li and J. Collett (2006), Traditional Chinese medicine in cancer care: Perspectives and experiences of patients and professionals in China, *European Journal of Cancer Care*, 15(4): 397-403.
2. Consider how traditional Chinese Medicine (TCM), as shared by participants in this study, provided evidence that supported its benefits in the management of their cancer. In particular, consider the way in which long-standing cultural beliefs supported their decisions to use TCM practices in their own care.

With the spotlight placing emphasis on different sources and types of evidence used to underpin decision-making, the role of the patient/stakeholder in shared decision-making is brought into clear focus (Turner et al., 2017). Patients, as the recipients of the care being decided on and delivered, must, wherever possible, be central to the decision-making process. Individual patient preferences and idiosyncrasies will influence care planning and decisions. It is imperative, therefore, that individual patients' voices are heard and influence the care that they receive if the true meaning of 'individualised patient care' is to be realised.

Individualised care is a two-way process, and it is imperative that the patient is involved in decisions affecting his or her health and well-being (Rycroft-Malone and Bucknall, 2010; Turner et al., 2017). It is not only about the nurse perceiving the patient as an individual human being. While adopting that approach is important, it is also about the nurse hearing and respecting the very valuable and pertinent perspective and input offered by the patient. Patients (and their carers) are a very significant, but perhaps underutilised, resource. They are, however, a resource input that EBP recognises and values as a core component in its approach to underpinning decision-making in the delivery of patient care. Such decision-making cannot happen in a vacuum or in isolation from the real-life situations that are the contexts of care. Crucial factors in this regard – such as the particular setting, patient profile, ward philosophy and culture, and the organisation of care delivery in the particular facility, among others can potentially have a huge influence on how decisions are reached about patient care delivery. To explore this further, complete Activity 3.3.

Activity 3.3

1. Consider how the context of care has had a major impact on patient and carer involvement in decision-making during the COVID 19 pandemic. Include both hospital and community settings.
2. What new evidence have you had to learn about and use during your placements to be able to practice safely as a nurse while also delivering the best possible care?
3. Visit Health Education England's website and, over time, access the range of resources provided specifically for nurses, midwives and allied health professionals to support them via e-learning during the pandemic situation (see the Web resources section at the end of this chapter for the link).
4. Access and read the article by N. Anton, T. Hornbeck, S. Modlin, M. M. Haque, M. Crites and D. Yu (2021), Identifying factors that nurses consider in the decision-making process related to patient care during the COVID-19 pandemic, *PLoS ONE*, 16(7): e0254077. Think about the points that focus on decision-making related to patient care during the COVID-19 pandemic.

The Evidence-Based Practice Process

As outlined in Table 3.1, the EBP process is comprised of seven clear steps (Melnyk and Fineout-Overholt, 2019: 17). On close consideration of the steps taken in the EBP process, you may, like us, feel that there appear to be similarities between these and the steps of the nursing process (Holland and Rees, 2010) – that is, assessment, planning, implementation and evaluation. Indeed, this is clearly reflected by the NMC in its *Future Nurse*: *Standards of proficiency* (2018a), platforms 3 and 4, which are 'Assessing needs and planning care' and 'Providing and evaluating care'. As you may appreciate from the nursing process, before you embark on delivering any patient care, you must first take a step back, assess the patient and the situation, and ask yourself, 'What does my patient need?' and 'What is the best course of action in this context?' This, in essence, is the first step on the road to clinical judgement and decision-making.

Many theories exist in relation to clinical judgement and decision-making, as you discovered in Chapter 1. However, for practice to be influenced by such theories, thereby, arguably, narrowing the theory–practice gap, they need to be 'accessible, understandable, relevant and applicable' (Standing, 2017: 11). In other words, they need to make sense to nurses in the context of their practice. With this in mind, we will offer Standing's explanations of both 'clinical judgement' and 'clinical decision-making', to ensure that we have a shared understanding of these terms as they are used in the rest of this chapter.

Clinical Judgement and Decision-Making

'Clinical judgement', as defined by Standing, is 'informed opinion (using intuition, reflection and critical thinking) that relates observation and assessment of patients to identifying and evaluating alternative nursing options' (2017: 7). It can be argued that intuition, reflection and critical thinking are largely subjective and invisible in nature. Intuition, in particular, has attracted much debate and controversy over the years with regard to its legitimacy as a basis for decision-making and, indeed, to come to a general consensus on what exactly it is (Benner and Tanner, 1987; Cioffi, 1997; Pellegrino, 1979; Thompson and Dowding, 2009). However, it is clear from Standing's definition that decision-making is underpinned by a combination of these subjective components *and* the more tangible, explicit or 'scientific' components, such as physiological observations and assessments of patients.

Standing goes on to emphasise how clinical judgement is applied in the clinical decision-making process 'to select the best possible evidence-based option to control risks and address patients' needs in high-quality care for which you are accountable' (2017: 8). This process of clinical judgement and decision-making clearly draws on a number of key components, such as intuition, reflection and critical thinking, to underpin your decision regarding which is the best course of action for patients. The steps in the EBP process, outlined in Table 3.1, facilitate this by helping you to ask the relevant patient care questions and guiding you to and through the available evidence, thereby enabling you to select the best available evidence to underpin your patient care decisions with confidence.

As is clear from Table 3.1, there is a logical order to the steps of the EBP process. Similar to the nursing process, it will always begin with a question. To get the information you need on which to base your clinical judgement and decision, you need to ask the right questions. Ideally, the information that you are seeking should be the best-quality evidence available, to ensure that you will deliver the best possible care. To this end, there are levels of evidence that are ranked in order of their quality and potential usefulness to practitioners. These levels are well documented and are frequently referred to as a 'hierarchy of evidence'.

Once you have gathered the best-quality, most relevant evidence that you can, you must determine its usefulness by assessing its quality. Depending on the conclusions you reach as to its quality, which involves critical review (Rees, 2010), you will be in a position to decide what to do next. There are two possible outcomes at this point. First, you may find that the evidence you have reviewed indicates that the standard of care you are currently delivering is consistent with best practice, in which case you will simply continue with this practice. Alternatively, this evidence might point towards the need to change or amend existing practice in some way – to ensure that it is the most up-to-date care and is consistent with international standards, for example. When a change in practice is implemented, it is imperative that the results are closely monitored and measured to ascertain whether or not the desired results are achieved. This is akin to the 'evaluation' step in the nursing process and provides the opportunity to take stock. If the desired outcomes are not achieved, then it is essential that you return to the first step of the EBP process, reflect carefully on the desired outcome(s) and revisit the components that underpinned your clinical judgement (perhaps your intuition or critical thinking around aspects of the situation) in coming to that decision(s). It may at this point be necessary to rearticulate your clinical question, either with a different focus or level of specificity. Indeed, it may even be the case that a new question is warranted. In this way, the EBP process, similar again to the nursing process, can become cyclical in nature and application.

Consider this EBP process and your own practice by completing Activity 3.4.

Activity 3.4

1. Access and read the article by E. Stewart (2006), Nursing guidelines: Development of catheter care guidelines for Guy's and St Thomas, *British Journal of Nursing*, 15(8): 420-425, which considers one example of how the process of EBP has been operationalised or implemented in practice - in this instance, to underpin the development of new catheter care guidelines for an NHS trust.
2. The importance of having the best available evidence related to catheter care for nurses can then be considered in relation to the Royal College of Nursing's (2021) Guidelines in its booklet *Catheter Care: RCN guidance for nurses* (see the Web resources section at the end of this chapter for the link). There, a body of evidence has been developed to support decision-making in relation to catheter care.
3. Finally, consider how you have used this evidence in the RCN's guidance in your own practice involving catheter care.

The Steps of Evidence-Based Practice for Decision-Making

Decision-making plays an integral role in nursing practice, and, during the course of your career, you will find yourself in situations where you need to make different types of decisions, that could be classed as 'routine', 'responsive' and 'emergency'. It has been suggested that different types of decisions are informed by different types of judgements (Standing, 2017; Thompson and Dowding, 2009).

- In a *routine* situation, you can take a considered approach to decision-making, because you have the luxury of time and access to resources, including senior colleagues, policies, protocols and, if necessary, published materials that you can consult to help you reach decisions and plan or deliver care.

- There will also be situations that you did not anticipate and, therefore, have no plan in place – that is, a *responsive* situation. This type of situation requires more of a 'thinking on your feet' approach and draws on a variety of sources of judgement types, such as personal experience, peers, the patient(s) and the context.
- A third type of situation that you may encounter in practice is an *emergency*, which demands prompt and confident decision-making to maximise the outcome for the patient, as far as possible. This situation can take you very much by surprise, because not only is it unplanned but it is also usually spontaneous and urgent in nature, requiring immediate action. For example, as a qualified nurse you may be undertaking a drug round where you are required to administer prescribed medications to your patient. However, your patient (who normally accepts his medications without hesitation) refuses to take them on this occasion for some reason. You will need to respond to this situation by thinking quickly and deciding the best course of action to address this unanticipated scenario. In this type of situation, decisions are often underpinned by intuition and reflection in action (Schön, 1983), and with the benefit of peers as a resource, together with the patient and the local context, or any combination of these (reflection is discussed in more detail in Chapter 4). This type of decision needs to be made very quickly and almost without thinking. Thompson and Dowding (2009) describe such decisions as 'fast and frugal'.

Examples of these three types of decisions are outlined in Table 3.2. In some cases, like these, you will not have much time to make your decision; in others, such as the routine example, you will be in a position to give it much more thought. EBP plays a vital role in all types of clinical decision-making. Therefore, it is imperative to develop the skills required to engage in this process, to foster good judgement and decision-making practices as you progress in your nursing career.

We will now explore each of the seven steps in the EBP process, reaffirming the importance and relevance of evidence for making decisions and the types of evidence that are the most suitable for this, but first complete Activity 3.5 in preparation.

Activity 3.5

1.   Before reading the seven steps involved in EBP, consider the types of decisions outlined in Table 3.2. In relation to each one, reflect on your experiences in clinical practice and provide examples of each type of decision that you have encountered. Consider also how those decisions were made and what 'evidence' informed or facilitated them.
2.   In particular, note what type of knowledge - for example, physiological, ethical or patient knowledge - was necessary to understand your decision-making and that of others in the examples.
3.   Consider how the context or environment in which they took place had an impact on how you could make a decision related to the patient's situation.

Table 3.2 Examples of types of decisions nurses need to make in practice.

Routine decision making	You are a student nurse at a practice placement and are concerned that the taking and recording of patients' physiological observations scheduled for 10 a.m. are often not undertaken at that time, as a result of other activities on the ward, including meeting patients' hygiene needs, doctors' rounds, medication rounds, patients leaving the ward for investigations/procedures and so on. You consider the possibility of suggesting a trial change to this policy, bringing the 'observations round' forward to 8 a.m. from 10 a.m. You have seen this change applied on another ward and it seems to allow for more timely and efficient monitoring and recording of observations. This reflective, perhaps intuitive, clinical judgement may need to be supported by consulting other sources of advice, including peers, patients and the relevant literature on this subject, making a decision on this issue.
Responsive decision making	As a qualified nurse, you are undertaking a 'drug round', during which you are required to administer prescribed medications to your patient. Your patient, who normally accepts his medications without hesitation, today refuses to take them. You will need to respond to this situation by thinking quickly and deciding the best course of action to address this unanticipated scenario.
Emergency decision making	Examples could include a patient collapsing, the outbreak of a fire requiring evacuation, a cardiac arrest or a confused, aggressive patient, to mention only a few. You will need to respond immediately and appropriately to such situations.

Steps in the Evidence-Based Practice Process

Step 0: Cultivate a Spirit of Enquiry

While this step may seem to be more of an organisational strategy than an individual one, it is important to acknowledge that we all have our part to play in this regard. A culture and environment in which practitioners are happy and comfortable enough to raise questions about the current standard of care or practice promotes such a spirit of enquiry among individuals within an organisation.

When management and senior staff are seen to welcome questions about current practice and suggestions for how patient care could perhaps be enhanced, there is an 'openness' to enquiry and to embracing EBP. It is important also that an organisation's management team is seen to support its practitioners in the development of the skills necessary to advance this spirit and culture of enquiry and, indeed, to operationalise EBP in the form of practice development initiatives.

From an individual practitioner's perspective, it is prudent that they embrace this culture and avail themselves of every opportunity offered to develop the necessary knowledge and skills to enable them to contribute actively to it and to enhancing patient care. Carter et al. (2018) offer an insight into interventions to achieve EBP and a culture of enquiry among nurses.

As a student nurse, you will be working and learning alongside your practice supervisors or mentors and other practitioners, who should be actively encouraging this spirit and culture of enquiry. As part of this learning experience, complete Activity 3.6.

Activity 3.6

1. Based on your knowledge and understanding of EBP, as well as what you believe a spirit or culture of enquiry to be, reflect on your clinical placements to date and ask yourself if you have seen or experienced it in any of these environments.
2. What do you believe characterises a spirit of enquiry in a clinical setting?
3. How is a spirit of enquiry demonstrated in your current placement? If you believe that this is not promoted there, list the reasons why you think this might be? What contribution do you think you could make to cultivating a spirit of enquiry if you had responsibility for supporting students?
4. Discuss with your mentor or supervisor how you can gain an opportunity to develop your EBP skills in practice to meet the NMC's competencies or proficiencies that will be part of your final placement assessment. (This will be determined as well by your own university's practice assessment requirements and whether or not you are being assessed at the main progression points.)

Step 1: Ask the Important Clinical Question

As we noted earlier in this chapter, the starting point in this process is the articulation of an important clinical question. Where do these questions emerge from? Many of them arise from day-to-day practice when nurses find themselves asking questions such as:

*   'Is there not a better way of doing this?'
*   'There must be a better dressing for this wound that will speed up healing and reduce the frequency of dressing changes?'
*   'I wonder if music therapy might reduce my patient's anxiety levels or episodes of challenging behaviour?'

All of these require nurses to make decisions of some kind. Nurses are prompted to ask these kinds of questions because they are engaging actively in patient care every day and motivated to do their best for their patients. Other questions will be triggered by specific conditions, particular patient needs, or experiences encountered, or indeed where new or alternative interventions are being considered.

To develop these ideas or questions that emerge from practice to a point at which they can be articulated, or 'asked aloud', so that the process of answering them might begin, it is important that you begin by writing something down – on paper or electronically – giving due consideration to the specifics of what you are asking.

This is the start of a very essential step in EBP, in which you work on developing a clear question relating to the aspect of practice about which you wish to enquire. This important clinical question needs to be one that will readily allow you to search for information or evidence on databases, for example, and one to which you can realistically find an answer. In other words, this question needs to be 'searchable' and 'answerable', so that it will yield, or allow you to get to, the information that you need. There are established frameworks in existence that will help you to construct questions in this way, including the PICOT question format (see page 56). First, complete Activity 3.7, as you will need to refer to your answers later in this chapter.

Activity 3.7

1. Consider a question about an aspect of your practice that relates to patient care. Such questions are the starting blocks for clinical judgement and decision-making in practice and are crucial if clinical practice is to evolve and improve over time. Your question may be one that you are asking in the process of completing an assignment, a dissertation or systematic literature review.
2. In your own words, construct and write down the question* that you wish to ask.
3. Enter the keywords, or key search terms, from your question into a database of your choosing (for example, the Cumulative Index to Nursing and Allied Health Literature (CINAHL) and see how many 'hits', or results, you obtain from your search.
4. Determine how many of these hits appear irrelevant or unrelated to the question that you asked.

* Note that you will need to refer to this question later in the chapter, after looking at the PICOT format for framing clinical questions.

A clinical question needs to be well considered, focused and reasonably specific. If you have taken sufficient time to make notes or to prepare in the manner indicated, you will be well on your way to framing your question.

For newcomers to the EBP process, this step can, at first, seem arduous and time-consuming. However, developing a well-articulated clinical question is time well spent and pays significant dividends in the end. If this step is rushed, it is likely that the search will not be specific enough, yielding an abundance of literature in the results, making the task of reviewing it all unmanageable, so leading to an unsuccessful outcome. This can be disheartening and frustrating, leading to nurses running the risk of wanting to abandon the search for an answer to their question.

As a student, it is important to understand how clinical questions are asked. That way, when evaluating evidence to underpin practice (engaging in a critical review), you can at least have an understanding of how the questions asked by researchers were determined and, ultimately, how the findings of their investigations answered it.

To help you with the process of writing a searchable answerable question, there are many evidence-based question-framing tools that you can use (Cormack, Gerrish and Lathlean, 2015; Craig and Smyth, 2012; Melnyk and Fineout-Overholt, 2019). These will help you to break down your question, identify its important elements and guide you as to where to place due emphasis in it. Melnyk and Fineout-Overholt (2019) recommend using a tool known as the 'PICOT format' to do this.

Asking your question using the PICOT format

The 'PICOT format' is comprised of five individual components or elements, all of which need to be carefully considered when constructing the question. Each element must be clearly identified to enable the drafting or construction of a searchable, answerable question.

Each of the five letters of the mnemonic denotes a component of the question that should be considered when writing it. The components, as described by Melnyk and Fineout-Overholt (2019: 40), are as follows:

- P for population, or disease, of interest (details such as age, gender, ethnicity or comorbidity, intellectual disability or mental health considerations).
- I for intervention, or range of interventions, of interest (therapy, exposure to disease, risk behaviour, such as smoking).
- C for comparison intervention or issue of interest (alternative therapy, placebo or current practice, absence of disease or absence of risk behaviour, such as being a non-smoker). On occasions, a 'comparison' is not applicable, but the 'context' may be more relevant (for example, a particular clinical setting, such as a hospice or community setting).
- O – for outcome of interest (expected outcome from a therapy, such as improved or faster healing or reduced episodes of challenging behaviour, improved self-belief or esteem levels).
- T for time involved to demonstrate an outcome (such as the time expected for a smoking cessation intervention to work, with the smoker having stopped smoking).

Within the PICOT format, several question templates are provided to help you to construct your specific clinical question. These include templates for intervention-type questions, prognosis-type questions, diagnosis-type questions, aetiology-type questions and meaning-type questions, such as those supplied by Melnyk and Fineout-Overholt (2019). It must be stressed at this point that no one question template is appropriate in every context. For example, if the clinical question were to relate to a

relatively unexplored area of nursing practice – such as the experience of women living with multiple sclerosis – there would be no 'intervention' as such, nor would you
be comparing it to anything; the focus would be purely on the 'issue' that is the lived
experience of this one group of women. In this instance, the meaning template (Melnyk and Fineout-Overholt, 2019: 44) would be more appropriate and useful, because
the 'I' component relates to an issue of interest rather than an intervention and the 'C'
component (comparison or context) is neither important nor relevant.

PICOT offers a clear framework for developing a clinical/practice question, which
in turn facilitates the best way in which to search and find the evidence, through
ensuring that the right 'key words' are formulated and then used in the database
searches. To demonstrate how a framework such as PICOT can help you to articulate
your clinical question in a useable way (which will be searchable and answerable), we
will use an example of a clinical question that might be raised.

Constructed or written before applying the PICOT format, the question might be
phrased as follows:

> How often should patients who are confined to bed rest be moved from their
> previous position?

If we look at this question more closely, it will become apparent that it lacks
the detail and specifics needed to guide and execute a strategic and fruitful search.
In its current state, if you were to go to the computer to search relevant databases, you would be highly likely to yield thousands of hits on the general area of
'patients confined to bed'. The majority of this information would be irrelevant,
lack quality and not provide an answer to your question. Remember, a computer is
only as useful or helpful as the 'instructions' that you give it.

The importance of taking the time necessary at this stage to get your question
right cannot be overemphasised. In the example question that we have provided, the
crucial elements that are seen as absent using the PICOT format are the intervention,
comparison, outcome and time.

The only element that is visible to some degree is the **population**. However, even
this lacks focus and the specific details necessary to guide a meaningful search. The
information that is provided here in relation to the population is 'patients who are
confined to bed', which is very vague. There is no indication of the age profile, setting
or presenting and/or underlying diseases that help to refine the question and, therefore, the subsequent search.

Here is an example of how our question could be phrased in a more focused and
refined manner:

> For patients who have had a stroke and are confined to bed (P) what is the
> effect of two-hourly turns (I) on skin integrity (O) compared to four-hourly
> turns (C) over the course of one month (T)?

As you can see, the question now contains all the elements of the PICOT format. In this particular scenario, these elements produce a clearly defined question in preparation for step 2 of the EBP process. In the case of some clinical questions or those in relation to particular settings, it may not always be essential or warranted to include the comparison (C) element, such as the following:

> How do mothers (P) who have been diagnosed with postnatal depression (I) perceive the impact of this condition on their ability to bond with their babies (O) in the first year post delivery (T)?

Similarly, it may not always be appropriate to include a time (T) dimension, as the following example question illustrates:

> Are users of mental health services (P) who have a history of (deliberate) self-harm (I) at increased risk of completed suicide (O) compared to individuals without a history of (deliberate) self-harm (C)?

Irrespective of the clinical question that you are asking or the clinical background from which you are coming, it is important to invest time and effort in formulating a good question that has a clear structure and contains the necessary elements of the PICOT format. As previously indicated, the comparison and time elements of this format do not always need to be included. However, the **population, intervention** and **outcome elements** must always be included and clearly defined. Formulating your questions strategically using a framework like PICOT renders the next step of the EBP process infinitely easier, as you will now see from working through Activity 3.8.

Activity 3.8

1. Consider the question that you wrote down about an aspect of your field-specific practice for Activity 3.7.
2. Using the PICOT format outlined above, rethink your question and the keywords that you might now use.
3. Enter these (perhaps revised) keywords into a database of your choosing (for example, CINAHL) and see how many hits your search yields this time.
4. Ascertain, at a glance, how many of these hits appear irrelevant or unrelated to the question that you asked.
5. Have you found any difference in the quantity and/or quality of the results that you have obtained this second time round – that is, for the question formulated using the PICOT format?

Completing Activity 3.8 will help to develop your evidence-searching skills, which are essential to most types of academic assignment, which are required to be underpinned by an evidence-base.

Step 2: Search for and Collect the Most Relevant and Best Evidence

The type of evidence that you need will be determined by the clinical decision that is to be made. For example, whether it is how to manage the anxiety of patients undergoing general anaesthetic pre-operatively or how to manage the pain control needs of patients post-operatively.

There are a number of questions that you may wish to ask yourself in advance of conducting your search. These are essential questions that will point you in the right direction to obtain the evidence necessary to underpin the clinical decision. A sample of such questions is presented in Table 3.3.

Good planning and developing of that initial evidence-searching question is essential for *effective* decision-making when searching the relevant databases or other possible web-based resources. It is important to have a well-articulated, searchable, answerable question prior to consulting these databases. Some of you reading this chapter may already have been asking the question: what is classed as a 'database'? Examples of databases commonly used include the following:

- Cumulative Index of Nursing and Allied Health Literature (CINAHL)
- Excerpta Medica Database (Embase)
- American Psychological Association's PsycINFO
- Medline
- Scopus
- Database of Abstracts of Reviews of Effects (DARE)
- Cochrane Library
- Dissertation Abstracts Online (DAO)
- Google Scholar.

Table 3.3 Factors to consider when undertaking a search for evidence.

What is the nature of the decision to be made?	Is it a clinical problem/an issue with a real patient focus? Is it an assignment requirement, such as a hypothetical scenario or the outcome of a review of the literature?
Is there a time constraint/urgency involved in this decision?	
What kind of evidence do I need?	For example, do I need to consult research or evidence-based practice guidelines or local policy? Do I need quantitative or qualitative evidence? What contribution can peers offer to this decision? What patient-related factors need to be considered?

It may be worth noting at this point that an invaluable source of help in this area is the subject librarian at your affiliated library, who can help to guide you on how to search the relevant databases in the most efficient way possible. Find your nearest library or the one best for you to access in Activity 3.9.

Activity 3.9

While at your clinical placement, find out whether there is a library in the area. This could be a library in the training and education centre at a hospital or community health centre or the main library in your town or city. Make a point of visiting the library early on in your placement (discuss doing so with your mentor first) and find out what resources are available and what access to resources is available to you as a student nurse.

In addition to the databases listed, there are several other excellent web-based resources to guide you through the process of undertaking the search for the most relevant and best available evidence. In order to do this, you will need to input keywords, or key search terms, into the database to commence your search. The benefit of having structured your clinical question using a format such as PICOT is that you immediately have to hand within your question the words that can serve as these key search terms to steer your database search. Similar to step 1 in the EBP process, planning and conducting your database search may initially seem challenging or perhaps unexciting. However, it too offers significant outcomes, particularly when you become more proficient and start to find that your searches yield highly relevant, good quality evidence, with the number of articles or pieces of evidence yielded being in single digits rather than the hundreds or thousands that can result from poorly steered searches.

Now that you have collected your evidence, the next step is to decide on its quality and usefulness in terms of answering your question. In other words, will the information that you now have to hand provide answers that will help you in your decision-making regarding the care of your patient? To answer this question may, at this stage, seem quite a daunting task. Perhaps a good place to start is to understand what is meant by the terms 'evidence' and 'quality evidence' in the context of this searching and reviewing activity.

A common perception is that if evidence is to be deemed of 'good quality', it must be derived from robust scientific research in hospitals or laboratories, such as clinical trials involving experimental approaches – perhaps a clinical trial of a new drug to ascertain its effects and/or side-effects. However, quality evidence exists in many different guises and includes studies that are not experimental in nature, such as an exploration of the experience of parenting a child who has a profound intellectual disability.

You will notice a clear difference in the focus and type of results that you might expect to emerge from these last two examples. This is largely a result, or a reflection of the different approaches used to answer different types of questions and can be grouped loosely into two research approaches: quantitative and qualitative research.

The nature of the question being asked will often dictate which is the most appropriate research approach for obtaining the information (data) needed to answer it and, ultimately, to make a decision in practice. In the case of the drug trial, for example, clear, decisive, unbiased data and results collected from large numbers of subjects are needed. This data must be objective, not influenced by individual or group opinions, interests or experiences. This quantitative approach may appear somewhat impersonal because of its precision, but that is where its strengths lie as a means of answering such questions. There are minimal margins for error because drugs, potentially, can cause significant harm to patients or else have little or no therapeutic effect.

The data required to answer the question concerning the experience of parenting a child with a profound intellectual disability are of a very different kind. Such qualitative data, for example, focus on the life experiences of particular individuals from their personal perspectives. Therefore, this data must be personal in nature and usually collected in person directly from smaller numbers (normally) of participants who have direct experience of the phenomenon of interest – in this case, they would be parents of children with a profound intellectual disability. It is the personal, but in-depth and very detailed, viewpoints of the participants that yield the answer to the question. It is the personal account that gives a qualitative approach to research its strength and uniqueness.

To practice working out which kind of data you need to answer your research questions, complete Activity 3.10.

Activity 3.10

Consider the following questions.

1. Does education about contraception reduce unwanted pregnancies in young people who live in socially deprived areas?
2. Why do young people who live in socially deprived areas have a higher incidence of unwanted pregnancies?
3. What are the perceptions of young people living in socially deprived areas of unprotected sex and contraceptive use?

Now answer the questions below for each of the questions above.

1. What is the nature of the question being asked?
2. Do I need quantitative (such as numerical data) or qualitative (more narrative-type data) evidence?
3. Do I need to consult expert authorities, research, EBP guidelines or local policy?
4. What contribution can professional peers make to this decision?
5. What patient-related factors need to be considered?

Whether the evidence you have collected is qualitative or quantitative, you will still need to ascertain its quality and usefulness. To help you with this there are tools known as 'hierarchies of evidence' (see section Clinical judgement and decision-making, pg. 50), which present different types of evidence in ranked order according to their quality and those that a number of EBP proponents recommend (Cleary-Holdforth and Leufer, 2008; Gerrish and Lacey, 2006; Guyatt and Rennie, 2002; Melnyk and Fineout-Overholt, 2019). Many of the hierarchies available combine quantitative and qualitative evidence together in a single hierarchy. Rees (2010), for example, advocates the use of a hierarchy that combines both qualitative and quantitative evidence to help when making a judgement about the quality and usefulness of the evidence that you have collected.

Combined hierarchies can often present all qualitative evidence in one single category, which tends to be ranked low down on the hierarchy. This does not acknowledge or give credence to the many different research approaches within the qualitative domain and, arguably, does not reflect the strength and potential contribution of the evidence generated by this approach. Such a combined hierarchy places greater value and emphasis on the scientific form of evidence, potentially to the detriment of qualitative evidence.

As you may appreciate, there are significant differences between quantitative and qualitative research approaches and to reflect these differences, separate hierarchies of evidence should be used. For examples of a single quantitative and a single qualitative hierarchy of evidence, respectively, see the resources given in Table 3.4.

Such single hierarchies of evidence provide separate ranking systems for judging quantitative and qualitative evidence respectively in terms of their quality and usefulness. Each hierarchy contains a list of various research designs within each of the research approaches, which you may or may not be familiar with. In the event that you are not familiar with some or all of these terms, the best resource to use to inform yourself is a good research textbook. You will be able to access some of these at your university library directly and through online access to the library e-books.

With these hierarchies to hand, you can map your respective pieces of evidence against the appropriate hierarchy and determine at what level each piece can be rated. In the first instance, however, you will need to decipher what type of evidence best answers the kind of question you are asking. For example, if your question concerns

Table 3.4 Examples of single hierarchies of evidence.

A hierarchy of qualitative evidence	Fineout-Overholt, E., Melnyk, B. M. and Schultz, A. (2005). Transforming health care from the inside out: Advancing evidence-based practice in the 21st century. *Journal of Professional Nursing*, 21(6): 335–344.
A hierarchy of quantitative evidence	Joanna Briggs Institute's Levels of Evidence (available online at: https://jbi.global/sites/default/files/2019-05/JBI-Levels-of-evidence_2014_0.pdf, accessed 25 January 2022).

Table 3.5 Levels of evidence to answer different clinical questions (adapted from Fineout-Overholt, 2019).

Types of clinical questions: Examples	Levels of evidence
Intervention questions In intellectual disability clients who have challenging behaviour (P), what is the effect of music therapy (I) on reducing challenging behaviour (O) compared to alternative behavioural interventions (C)?	• Systematic reviews and meta-analyses of all existing evidence, including all RCTs. • Single RCTs. • Controlled trials without randomisation. • Case-control and cohort studies. • Systematic review/meta-synthesis of qualitative or descriptive studies. • Single qualitative or descriptive studies. • Expert opinions by authorities and/or expert committees.
Prognosis questions For HIV-positive women (P), does the use of bottle feeding (I) compared to breastfeeding (C) their newborns in the first six months postnatally (T) predict the risk of developing mother-to-child transmission of HIV (O)?	• Meta-analysis of cohort or case-control studies. • Single cohort or case-control studies. • Single case studies.
Meaning questions What are the perceptions (O) of patients with a new diagnosis of cancer (P) of the manner in which their diagnosis was communicated to them (I)?	• Meta-synthesis of qualitative studies. • Single qualitative or descriptive studies. • Expert opinion by authorities and/or expert committees.

the effectiveness of a treatment or intervention, you will usually look for a systematic review of randomised controlled trials (RCTs) or one such trial, if these levels of evidence are available. To illustrate this further, see Table 3.5. This needs to be done in advance of critically appraising your evidence to determine the usefulness and potential contribution of each piece to answering your question and whether there may be some that you can simply discard at this point.

Practise using single hierarchies for decision-making by completing Activity 3.11.

Activity 3.11

The NMC's (2018a: 16) platform 4: Providing and evaluating care', outcome 4.6 states that registered nurses need to be able to 'demonstrate the knowledge, skills and ability to act as a role model for others in providing evidence-based nursing care to meet people's needs.'

1. Review the single hierarchies referenced in Table 3.4. Consider how they can help you to achieve the above outcome.
2. During your next placement, identify an area of practice that you can use to help demonstrate how you are able to achieve this NMC outcome when being assessed by your mentor or practice assessor.
3. Determine how you will be able to demonstrate that you have gathered the evidence, what the evidence is and how it relates to the area of practice chosen. (Include the evidence in your portfolio of practice learning experience.)

Step 3: Critically Appraise the Evidence

By now, you will have successfully formulated a relevant clinical question to your area of practice and found what you believe is the best available evidence with which to answer this question. You may also be in a position to discard any evidence of a lesser quality or that is inappropriate for the focus of your clinical question. The next step – that is, critically appraising the evidence that does have merit for answering your question – may at first appear to be a daunting prospect. However, if you have used a clear strategy for searching and finding, then choosing, the best evidence, it does not have to be as challenging as it may first appear.

There are many ways in which you can approach this task but using an appropriate critical appraisal tool will provide you with a list of pertinent questions that you need to answer in relation to your evidence. An example of one of these for either a qualitative or quantitative study can be found in Rees (2010: 178–180).

Practice using a critical appraisal tool of your choice to work through Activity 3.12.

Activity 3.12

1. Access these tools and review the different sections to be considered for critical review of the evidence that you have found and which you consider appropriate for answering the question that you have written. (It is not the purpose of this chapter to focus on this in detail, because we are considering how the evidence-base itself is important for decision-making.)
2. As you use the tools, give particular consideration to how the review questions help you to determine:

   - whether the results of the study are valid (*validity*);
   - what the results are (*reliability*);
   - whether the results will help you in caring for your patients (*applicability*).

It is evident from the considerations listed in Activity 3.12 that a reasonable level of research knowledge, including the principles and processes of both qualitative and quantitative research approaches, is needed to understand what is being asked and to be able to answer them. It will therefore be prudent to consult a good research textbook and have one with you when engaging in a general critical appraisal. Cleary-Holdforth and Leufer state that 'answering these questions enables nurses to ascertain the value of a given study in their day-to-day practice, thereby enabling them to *make informed decisions* about patient care in the clinical setting' (2008: 45). You will find it helpful to complete Activity 3.13 to engage with this process.

Activity 3.13

1. Consider an aspect of nursing care from the field of practice in which you are particularly interested - oral hygiene, for example.
2. Search for two articles about your chosen area - one qualitative, one quantitative. Using the critical appraisal tools in Holland and Rees (2010: Chapter 7) or similar recommended ones, try to undertake your own preliminary critical appraisal of these articles.
3. When you have completed this exercise, reflect on how the critical appraisal tools helped you in making sense of your chosen articles.
4. What was your final decision on the value of these papers for helping you to understand some of the evidence available on the chosen topic?

* Note that this is a good activity to undertake for those of you who will be completing an assignment involving a similar exercise or a possible dissertation in your final year of study.

Step 4: Integrate the Best Evidence with your Own Clinical Expertise and the Patients' Preferences and Values in Making a Practice Decision or Change

At this stage, having critically appraised your evidence, you will now be in a position to decide on one of two options. Either the evidence will indicate that the current practice in your clinical setting is consistent with other national or international standards, in which case you will continue with this practice and no change to it will warranted; or the evidence may indicate that your practice is not entirely in keeping with national or international standards, in which case some change in practice may be needed. (It is important to highlight here that, as a student nurse, you will not yet have ultimate decision-making authority and will need to liaise closely with your assigned mentor or supervisor who would need to be a qualified nurse.)

Where a change in practice has a direct impact on an individual patient, it is paramount that the evidence and the subsequent professional recommendations arising from it are discussed with the patient so that they can articulate their preferences and values, which must be considered and integrated into the decision-making process. Indeed, it is the ethical duty of all health care professionals to keep patients fully informed and involved in the decision-making process around their care (Cleary-Holdforth, 2017; Melnyk and Fineout-Overholt, 2019).

What do you do if the evidence appears to indicate that a change in practice is warranted? Consider the following scenario and possible learning experience that you may encounter in a clinical placement and consider the options to support decision-making in Activity 3.14.

Activity 3.14

Brief scenario: A recently completed audit of the care setting in which you are working has demonstrated a stark increase in reported medication errors during the previous calendar year. This is a cause for serious concern among the multidisciplinary team (MDT) members working in the area. A working group comprised of members of this team has been set up to discuss the findings and to consider how best to tackle the problem. You are invited to attend because your mentor is a member of the working group.

Reflecting on the definition of EBP and its core elements, consider the types of evidence that may be helpful in addressing this problem and informing the eventual decision-making and outcome for patient care. Here is one definition of EBP to consider:

> Evidence-based practice is an holistic approach to care delivery that places the individual patient at its core. It is far more than research utilisation alone and is a partnership between interprofessional clinicians, patients and the best available evidence to optimise patient outcomes. (Cleary-Holdforth and Leufer, 2009: 286)

When an appropriate course of action has been agreed and decided on, it is imperative that a collaborative approach is employed, and key steps are taken to ensure a smooth transition when adopting the change in practice. Consideration must also be given at this stage to how the outcomes of the implemented change will be measured and what these outcomes will be compared to, so as to ascertain whether patient care has benefited, or standards have improved as a result. Complete Activity 3.15 to consider how you could go about making a change in nursing practice.

Activity 3.15

Consider your role as a student nurse who has just undertaken and completed an assignment for which you searched, obtained and critically appraised evidence on an aspect of nursing practice.

On a subsequent clinical placement, you find that qualified nurses in that area are engaging in practice that is contrary to what you found (through your assignment) to be the best available evidence.

1. On reflection, how might you, as a student, address this difference in practice?
2. Discuss possible options with your mentor or practice supervisor.

Step 5: Evaluate Outcomes of the Practice Decision or Change Based on Evidence

Having implemented the change in practice that was deemed necessary based on the evidence obtained and reviewed, it is essential, subsequently, to measure the outcomes or results of this change. Outcome(s) measurement can take many forms and consider many aspects. Some examples of outcomes measurement can include patient satisfaction surveys, decreased cost of care or length of stay, physiological measures (such as blood pressure, aerobic fitness, reduced infection rates or improved wound healing rates), psychological measures (such as levels of anxiety, quality of life, levels of depression), functional improvement (such as improved gait or ambulation, return to independence) or outcomes such as nursing retention, improved staff morale or job satisfaction.

The purpose of doing this is three-fold. First, you want to determine if the outcomes of the decision to change practice in your workplace mirror the outcomes of that change in the evidence. Second, evaluating the outcome will allow you to inform future decision-making around nursing practice and patient care regarding that aspect of care. If the outcomes are positive or if the desired outcomes have been achieved, then clearly the decision will be taken to continue with this new practice for as long as it continues to work or until new evidence recommends further change. Third, if the outcomes are not as expected and the desired results of the change have not materialised, it is essential to investigate why this is the case. This may involve re-examination of the initial questions and further evidence to ensure successful decision-making outcomes.

It is worth noting here that, in advance of undertaking an assignment or dissertation that requires you to ask or answer a clinical question, it is important to consider what the nature of the question is and the desired end result. This will help you to articulate your question and to plan and direct your assignment.

Step 6: Disseminate the Outcomes of the Evidence-Based Practice Decision or Change

In order to maximise the learning that has been achieved through the EBP process that has led to and informed the implementation of a change in practice, it is imperative that this learning experience and its outcome are shared with as many interested parties as possible. To this end, nurses, including student nurses, can and should make efforts to disseminate their results so that other practitioners can learn from them, and, in turn, many more patients can benefit from this work. Examples of how and where nurses can disseminate their work are in-house study days, journal clubs, conference presentations (both poster and oral presentations) and professional publications. Although a daunting prospect, many students are now engaging in these, either on their own, or with their mentors or tutors. Complete Activity 3.16 to see how you might go about participating in such activities.

──Activity 3.16──

1. Access and read K. Holland and C. Rees (2010: 248-285) to see how students can disseminate their learning, including how to present the findings of their work. Alternatively, your own university may have its own guidance and related learning resources which you can access.
2. Consider how you would present your work to the other students in your seminar group.
3. It may be possible to undertake a similar exercise at your placement, where evidence can be presented on one aspect of patient care that you have explored, and think would add to student learning but also enable you to achieve competence in presentation skills and communication.

Conclusion

This chapter has focused on the value and importance of EBP in any decision-making involving patient and client care. It has examined all aspects of what is required to determine what evidence is the best available, including developing your searching and critical appraisal skills, as well as how these can help you to achieve the necessary NMC standards of proficiency relevant to your stage of learning and, eventually, those essential for becoming a registered nurse (2018a).

Making clinical judgements and decisions that enhance and support effective patient care outcomes, as well as delivering that care in a holistic way, will depend on the underpinning knowledge and practice evidence that you, as this future qualified nurse, will use.

References

Anton, N., Hornbeck, T., Modlin, S., Haque, M. M., Crites, M. and Yu, D. (2021). Identifying factors that nurses consider in the decision-making process related to patient care during the COVID-19 pandemic, PLoS ONE 16(7): e0254077.

Aveyard, H. and Sharp, P. (2017). *A Beginner's Guide to Evidence Based Practice in Health and Social Care*, 3rd edn. Buckingham: Open University Press.

Benner, P. and Tanner, C. (1987). How expert nurses use intuition. *American Journal of Nursing*, 87(1): 23–31.

Black, N. and Jenkinson, C. (2009). Measuring patients' experiences and outcomes. *British Medical Journal*, 330: 2495.

Borges do Nascimento, I. J. et al. (2020). Novel coronavirus infection (COVID-19) in humans: A scoping review and meta-analysis. *Journal of Clinical Medicine*, 9(4): 941.

Carter, E. J., Rivera, R. R., Gallagher, K. A. and Cato, K. D. (2018). Targeted interventions to advance a culture of enquiry at a large, multi-campus hospital among nurses. *The Journal of Nursing Administration*, 48(1): 18–24.

Center for Disease Control and Prevention (2011). State-specific trends in lung cancer incidence and smoking: United States, 1999–2008. *Morbidity and Mortality Weekly Report*, 16(60): 1243–1247.

Church, S. and Lyne, P. (1994). Research-based practice: Some problems illustrated by the discussion of evidence concerning the use of a pressure-relieving device in nursing and midwifery, *Journal of Advanced Nursing*, 19: 513–551.

Cioffi, J. (1997). Heuristics, servants to intuition, in clinical decision making. *Journal of Advanced Nursing*, 26(1): 203–208.

Clark, M. (2002). Pressure-redistributing cushions: The Cinderella of support surfaces? *Nursing Times*, 98(8): 59.

Cleary-Holdforth, J. (2017). Evidence-based practice: An ethical perspective. *Worldviews on Evidence-based Nursing*, 14(6), 429–431.

Cleary-Holdforth, J. (2020). 'A national study exploring knowledge, beliefs and implementation of evidence-based practice among nurses, midwives, lecturers and students in the Republic of Ireland'. PhD thesis, Dublin City University, School of Nursing, Psychotherapy and Community Health (available online at: http://doras. dcu.ie/24919, accessed 24 January 2022).

Cleary-Holdforth, J. and Leufer, T. (2008). Essential elements in developing evidence-based practice. *Nursing Standard*, 23(2): 42–46.

Cleary-Holdforth, J. and Leufer, T. (2009). Evidence-based practice: Sowing the seeds for success. *Nurse Education in Practice* (guest editorial), 9(5): 285–287.

Collins Concise Dictionary and Thesaurus (1995). London: HarperCollins.

Cormack, D., Gerrish, K. and Lathlean, J. (eds) (2015). *The Research Process in Nursing*, 7th edn. Oxford: Wiley-Blackwell.

Cotton, S. et al. (2020). Proning during COVID-19: Challenges and solutions. *Heart and Lung*, 49(6): 686–687.

Craig, J. V. and Smyth, R. L. (eds) (2012). *The Evidence-based Practice Manual for Nurses*, 3rd edn. Edinburgh: Churchill Livingstone Elsevier.

Desmond, D., Gallagher, P., Henderson Slater, D. and Chatfield, R. (2008). Pain and psychosocial adjustment to lower limb amputation amongst prosthesis users. *Prosthetics and Orthotics International*, 32(2): 244–252.

Fineout-Overholt, E., Melnyk, B. M. and Schultz, A. (2005). Transforming health care from the inside out: Advancing evidence-based practice in the 21st century. *Journal of Professional Nursing*, 21(6): 335–344.

Gerrish, K. and Lacey, A. (eds) (2006). The research process in nursing, 5th edn. Oxford: Blackwell Publishing.

Giles, M.L., Gunatilaka, A., Palmer, K., Sharma, K. and Roach, V. (2021) Alignment of national COVID-19 vaccine recommendations for pregnant and lactating women: Alineación de las recomendaciones nacionales de la vacuna de la COVID-19 para las mujeres embarazadas y lactantes. *Bulletin of the World Health Organisation*, 99(10): 730–746. DOI: https://doi.org/10.2471/BLT.21.286644

Guyatt, G. and Rennie, D. (2002). *Users' Guides to the Medical Literature*. Chicago, IL: American Medical Association Press.

Holland, K. (2020). *Anthropology for Nursing*. Abingdon: Routledge.

Holland, K. and Rees, C. (2010). *Nursing: Evidence-based Practice Skills*. Oxford: Oxford University Press.

Jolley, J. (2020). *Introducing Research and Evidence-based Practice for Nurses*, 3rd edn. Abingdon: Routledge.

Kim, Mi-Na (2020). What type of face mask is appropriate for everyone-mask-wearing policy amidst COVID-19 pandemic? *Journal of Korean Medical Science*, 35(20), e186. DOI: https://doi.org/10.3346/jkms.2020.35.e186

Leufer, T. (2020). Teaching core EBP skills to postgraduate nursing students. *Worldviews on Evidence-Based Nursing*, 17: 404–405. https://doi.org/10.1111/wvn.12431

Leufer, T. and Cleary-Holdforth, J. (2009). Evidence-based practice: Improving patient outcomes. *Nursing Standard*, 23(32): 35–39.

McDonnell, N., Kwei, P. and Paech, M. (2007). A disposable device for patient-controlled intravenous analgesia: Evaluation by patients, nursing and medical staff. *Acute Pain*, 9(2): 71–75.

Melnyk, B. M. and Fineout-Overholt, E. (eds) (2019). *Evidence-based Practice in Nursing and Healthcare: A guide to best practice*, 4th edn. Philadelphia, PA: Wolters Kluwer Health/Lippincott, Williams & Wilkins.

Nursing and Midwifery Council (NMC) (2018a). *Future Nurse: Standards of proficiency for registered nurses*. London: NMC.

Nursing and Midwifery Council (NMC) (2018d) *Realising Professionalism: Standards for education and training Part 3: Standards for pre-registration nursing programmes*. London: NMC.

Pellegrino, E. D. (1979). The anatomy of clinical judgements. In H. T. Engelhardt, Jr, S. F. Spicker and B. Towers (eds), *Clinical Judgement: A critical appraisal*. Dordrecht: D. Reidel. pp. 169–194.

Rees, C. (2010). Evaluating and appraising evidence to underpin nursing practice. Chapter 7 in K. Holland and C. Rees, *Nursing: Evidence-Based Practice Skills*. Oxford: OUP. pp. 167–196.

Rycroft-Malone, J. and Bucknall, T. (eds) (2010). *Models and Frameworks for Implementing Evidence-based Practice: Linking evidence to action*. Oxford: Wiley-Blackwell.

Schön, D. (1983). *The Reflective Practitioner: How professionals think in action*. New York: Basic Books.

Standing, M. (2017). *Clinical Judgement and Decision Making for Nursing Students*, 3rd edn. Exeter: Learning Matters.

Stewart, E. (2006). Nursing guidelines: Development of catheter care guidelines for Guy's and St Thomas'. *British Journal of Nursing*, 15(8): 420–425.

Thompson, C. (2003). Clinical experience as evidence in evidence-based practice. *Journal of Advanced Nursing*, 43(3): 230–237.

Thompson, C. and Dowding, D. (eds) (2009). *Essential Decision Making and Clinical Judgement for Nurses*. Edinburgh: Churchill Livingstone Elsevier.

Tingle, J. (1990). Eusol and the law. *Nursing Times*, 86(12): 70–72.

Turner, S., D'Lima, D., Hudson, E., Morris, S., Sheringham, J., Swart, N. and Fulop, N. J. (2017). Evidence use in decision-making on introducing innovations: A systematic scoping review with stakeholder feedback. *Implementation Science*, 12: 145.

Walsh, M. and Ford, P. (1994). *Nursing Rituals, Research and Rational Action*. London: Heinemann.

Xu, W., Towers, A. D., Li, P. and Collett, J. (2006). Traditional Chinese medicine in cancer care: Perspectives and experiences of patients and professionals in China. *European Journal of Cancer Care*, 15(4): 397–403.

Further Reading

Rycroft-Malone, J. (2004). 'The PARIHS framework: A framework for guiding and implementing evidence-based practice', *Journal of Nursing Care Quality*, 19(4): 297–304.

Web Resources

Centre for Evidence-Based Medicine at the University of Oxford: www.cebm.net (accessed 15 August 2022).

Evidence-based practice (EBP) – helpful videos explaining what it is and how to make the most of it:

Part 1: www.youtube.com/watch?v=5yReXbAh7xI (accessed 4 June 2022).

Part 2: www.youtube.com/watch?v=ALUPyUZ_L04 (accessed 4 June 2022).

Health Education England – range of resources provided specifically for nurses, midwives and allied health professionals to support them via e-learning regarding the pandemic situation: www.hee.nhs.uk/coronavirus-covid-19/coronavirus-covid-19-information-nurses (accessed 4 June 2022).

Helene Fuld Health Trust National Institute for Evidence-based Practice in Nursing and Healthcare: https://fuld.nursing.osu.edu (accessed 15 August 2022).

Joanna Briggs Institute: https://jbi.global (accessed 15 August 2022).

Royal College of Nursing: *Catheter Care: RCN guidance for nurses* (2021): https://www.rcn.org.uk/-/media/Royal-College-Of-Nursing/Documents/Publications/2021/July/009-915.pdf (accessed 4 June 2022).

'The Study of Nursing Care' series of reports – PDFs of all 14 titles are freely available from the RCN's website, from its library catalogue, special collections: https://rcn.sirsidynix.net.uk/uhtbin/cgisirsi/x/0/0/5?searchdata1=study%20of%20nursing%20care%20project%20reports%7b490%7d (accessed June 4 2022).

4

REFLECTION AND LEARNING FROM DECISION-MAKING

Debbie Roberts

Chapter objectives

The aims of this chapter are to:

- explore how and why experiential learning is a useful tool in the development of decision-making skills in nursing;
- develop some basic skills underpinning reflection;
- explore how to learn from experience using reflection;
- learn how to use frameworks for structured reflection and to guide decision-making actions;
- consider how experiential learning and reflection contribute to decision-making as a qualified nurse.

Introduction

This chapter explores the concept of learning from your experience in clinical practice and is designed to help you to use reflection as a means of learning, both to make decisions in practice and to learn from the decisions that you have made. The use and value of reflective practice will be explored in many of the chapters to come as well: it is considered essential to the development of decision-making skills as a student nurse and for your ongoing personal and professional development once you have qualified as a registered nurse.

The Role of the Future Registered Nurse

Following extensive review of the NMC (2010) regulations governing the education and training of student nurses and the knowledge and skills required of professional qualified nurses to deliver future health care, the NMC (2018a) approved a new set of standards to underpin the future role of the registered nurse. As a result, it was eventually agreed by the professional body in consultation with major stakeholders, such as the NHS, service users and carers, that all pre-registration nursing curricula should be redesigned. Subsequently, they were implemented fully from September 2020 for all new entrants on to programmes at the schools of nursing throughout the UK. This meant that there was an overlap between what was known as the 2010 curriculum (as students beginning their programme on or before 2019 may not complete their undergraduate courses until 2023) and the new 2018 one, with students having to gain competencies (2010) and proficiencies (2018) to achieve registration and their graduate award (see Chapter 1 for further explanation of these outcomes).

The NMC's *Future Nurse: Standards of proficiency for registered nurses* was approved for use by all providers of nurse education in the UK from September 2020. They describe a vision for the role of the nurse in the twenty-first century and, along with the specific details given for achieving this, have established a baseline for the knowledge and skills needed to underpin future programmes of learning (Chapter 2 outlines the other documents that, together with this, complete the educational standards). This includes what would be required from a partnership between universities, schools of nursing and health care services, where students are expected to gain practice experience, supported by both experienced practice supervisors and assessors. It is also expected that learners will be supported by new ways of learning and technology so that they can carry out their future roles.

The NMC states that its vision for future nurses in relation to their role is that they will:

> work in the context of continual change, challenging environments, different
> models of care delivery, shifting demographics, innovation, and rapidly

evolving technologies. Increasing integration of health and social care services will require registered nurses to negotiate boundaries and play a proactive role in interdisciplinary teams. The confidence and ability to think critically, apply knowledge and skills, and provide expert, evidence-based, direct nursing care therefore lies at the centre of all registered nursing practice. (2018a: 3)

This vision really emphasises the need for student nurses to be able to learn through and from their experiences in clinical practice. In addition, they need to be able to make decisions underpinned by an evidence base (Chapter 3) and advanced critical thinking (Chapter 2). Most importantly, nurses need to ensure that they continue to develop their knowledge and skills, to be able to work in ever-changing situations that impact on their specific work context.

As seen in the Preface and other chapters, this last point became very much a reality, with the global pandemic caused by the COVID-19 virus having a huge impact on communities worldwide. It also greatly affected how learning took place in both university and practice settings. As the virus put a halt to the movement of people across countries and in local situations, too, as well as people being unable to mix with others, including student colleagues, families and friends, it meant that knowledge and practice learning had to be delivered in new ways. In the UK, during the height of the pandemic in 2020 and early 2021, exceptionally, certain students (mainly final-year students) became paid workers as well as retaining their learner status. The NMC (2022) issued emergency and recovery standards for nurses' education (see Chapter 14 for more details), due to the need for an increase in the number of health care workers to support a pressured and ongoing depleted workforce. As a result, the NMC had to agree new standards to ensure that student nurses could achieve their registration status. Some of you reading this book may well have experienced this change in student status for a short period of time and had to manage new ways of learning in order to not only keep up with gaining knowledge and skills to achieve in your assignments but also to learn from practice experience by working alongside your practice supervisors and assessors.

What Is Learning from Experience and How Can You Learn from It?

Learning from experience is sometimes referred to as 'experiential learning', because the experience is at the heart of learning. As a student nurse, you will try to make sense of what is happening in the fast-paced environment of clinical practice and will observe, and gradually play a part in, making decisions about nursing interventions and care.

The NMC's standards of proficiency, which have been structured by being grouped into seven areas of nursing, known as 'platforms', state in platform 1 that: 'Being an accountable professional', also reinforces the importance of being able to learn from experience by stating that:

> Registered nurses continually reflect on their practice and keep abreast of new
> and emerging developments in nursing, health and care. (2018a: 7)

To meet this requirement, as a student nurse, you should proactively take responsibility for learning from practice, seeking support and asking for feedback in order to develop your knowledge and skills. The key is to learn from your practice experience and weave in your theoretical knowledge, to enable you to relate theory to your current and future nursing practice.

Learning from our experiences means that we can either use what we have learnt to develop and enhance future experiences or learn from any mistakes or wrong decisions that we have made so as to not make them again. As a student nurse, you may most commonly do the latter, because most of you are learning new knowledge and skills, and in situations in which there is an opportunity for mistakes to be made. Making mistakes can be a difficult and uncomfortable experience, and usually there are consequences of our doing so. Of course, you will have practice supervisors and others supporting you in your practice learning experience, and they are there to help you to identify which are the best decisions to make concerning your own practice. Talking through what your various possible options are with your supervisors when making practice decisions that may have an impact on the safety of patients, for example, is an essential requirement of your learning, and will help you develop confidence in decision-making as you progress through your programme of study.

An example of where a normal practice of washing your hands before undertaking new procedures was seen as an accepted part of a nurse's daily work, and where you had confidence that you knew what you were doing was correct, suddenly became one that not only impacted your clinical learning environment but also your external personal life. For many this required new learning tools to ensure that your skills were in fact up to date; tools that could also be accessed via non face to face contact and from various forms of technology and media.

An editorial by Ng and Or (2020) highlighted one possible approach – that of using a virtual classroom to ensure strong links between the theoretical learning of hand hygiene and the actual clinical training for student nurses, given that university campus sessions had been suspended. This was an innovative response to meeting an immediate need to ensure best practice in hand hygiene by student nurses. Adapting to new ways of working like this, however, requires consideration of what existed previously and learning from various experiences. This is where reflecting on what we know already and what we have experienced is so important.

Reflection is about sense -making and finding solutions to clinical or practice-based experiences. That is what Ng and Or (2020) sought to do when they established a plan for how to continue to teach the practice of hand hygiene safely during the pandemic.

In an Australian study involving seven student nurses, Hanson and McAllister describe reflection as 'learning from mistakes to prevent mistakes' (2017: 92). Their paper provides some interesting general ideas for students about adversity. The research describes the approach of sharing narratives or stories about practice with fellow students (and potentially others) and how hearing stories from a range of other people was helpful in that students could then start to think about how they might react or respond in similar situations.

Learning from other people's experiences in this way is known as 'vicarious learning' and it can be a particularly helpful strategy for student nurses. Hanson and McAllister (2017) explain that students can experience feelings of discomfort or adversity because they may not always be able to deliver care in the way that they have been taught at university. The reality of clinical practice may not always coincide with your prior ideas.

Hanson and McAllister suggest that 'being able to respectfully contribute to the decision-making process was a skill that could be learnt' (2017: 92). The paper presents some powerful data extracts that provide great insights into some of the experiences of this group of respondents and an example is provided of responding to adversity (2017: 92).

Mistakes or errors can also occur during your experiences in clinical practice, but it is hoped that these will not endanger the patients in your care, colleagues or yourself. For most students, learning to engage in or to undertake practice will entail learning a new set of skills that are underpinned by clear rationales and EBP. Normally, many will have the opportunity to learn these skills in the safe environment of what are called 'clinical skills rooms', 'laboratories' or 'clinical simulation rooms', in which both the environment and the scenarios around which the skills are taught replicate those that you might find in clinical placements. Whether it is in clinical practice or one of these rooms, it is important that you take some time to think carefully about how and why you made a mistake and, most importantly of all, how to ensure that you do not make the same mistake again when a similar situation presents itself.

'Reflection' is a commonly used term in nursing for this practice of thinking carefully about why and how things went well or why and how any error has been made, remembering what you did and why. It is one way to learn from experience and improve your knowledge and skills.

According to Thompson, Aitken, Doran and Dowding (2013), around half of all adverse events involve some kind of error, so they point out that it is only right that we examine carefully the nature of nurses' decision-making. Of course, it is also important to remember that nurses and other health care professionals are often required to make decisions when the information available is incomplete or unclear (Thompson et al., 2013). Furthermore, decision-making is not an exact science. There is evidence to suggest that 'when given the same information, and undertaking the same decisions, nurses will make consistently different judgements and decisions' (Thompson et al., 2013: 1721). At this point you may wish to go back and read Chapter 3 and review what constitutes evidence-based practice.

However, it important to stress that learning from experience does not take place only when events have a negative outcome; it is just as important that nurses are able to identify when things went well or an outcome was positive, for the nurses and/or the patients or, more widely, when such things have an impact on others or the total care given to patients. This can help you to ensure that such good practice continues in the future or that it can be the foundation for considering new practices. Work through Activity 4.1 to start reflecting on decisions.

Activity 4.1

1. Think about a recent experience in practice, when a decision you made with the involvement of a patient achieved a positive outcome for that person.
2. Reflect on why you considered that this was also a positive experience for you.
3. What was important about that decision?

Making decisions as a student nurse is part of your learning to become a qualified nurse and learning from these helps you to gain confidence, especially when you discuss them with your supervisors and mentors. This is an important reflection on practice, thinking about what went well or otherwise. Making decisions can be a stressful experience, however, especially if you have not experienced a particular scenario before or you have to make a decision where there is no immediate support from a colleague available. An example could be having to manage a patient's care after a fall in the bathroom and having to prioritise decisions for the immediate care of that patient. This is only one of a myriad of potential scenarios that have an impact on the activities of nurses during a shift. Student and qualified nurses can be exposed to many potentially stressful events and, over time, develop different coping mechanisms to manage them as well as resilience (Ching, Cheung, Hegney and Rees, 2020).

Stress, Coping and Developing Resilience

There are multiple stressors (things that cause us stress) in pre-registration nurse education. The NMC's (2018a) standards include several outcome statements that allude to the fact that being a student nurse is potentially stressful and that, in all care settings and in all areas of practice, you should, as indicated in platform 1: Being an accountable practitioner:

understand the demands of professional practice and demonstrate how to recognise signs of vulnerability in themselves or their colleagues and the action required to minimise risks to health (2018a: 8, platform 1, Outcome Statement 1.5)

demonstrate resilience and emotional intelligence and be capable of explaining the rationale that influences their judgements and decisions in routine, complex and challenging situations (2018a: 9, platform 1, Outcome Statement 1.10)

A literature review by McCarthy, Trace, O'Donovan et al. (2018) outlines some of the stressors and coping mechanisms faced by student nurses. See Activity 4.2 to explore this paper further. Interestingly, the authors reveal that, from the 25 studies reviewed, stressors stemmed from clinical, academic and financial sources, with clinical stress being the most significant one. The fear of making a mistake or causing harm was most frequently reported as a source of clinical stress.

Activity 4.2

1. Access and read the paper by B. McCarthy, A. Trace, M. O'Donovan, C. Brady-Nevin, M. Murphy, M. O'Shea and P. O'Regan (2018), Nursing and midwifery students' stress and coping during their undergraduate education programmes: An integrative review, *Nurse Education Today*, 61: 197-209.
2. After reading the paper, take some time to think about what you would do if you thought that you had made a mistake.
3. Read the content of this chapter again up to this point to help you to consider some options.
4. Initially, of course, you need to determine whether or not you have, in fact, made a mistake. Inform one of your supervisors or mentors to check this and discuss what you believe happened and what your error was.
5. If you did make an error that had an immediate impact on patient or colleague safety, you may need to respond immediately and seek help from others.
6. Following any action and resolution, it will be important to reflect on the whole event with your mentor or supervisor.

To reiterate, if you think that you have made a mistake, you *must* tell your practice supervisor, no matter how difficult that may seem. Once the mistake has been ratified and everyone is clear that a mistake has been the result of a decision that you made, initially you will have to agree that you made a mistake and apologise (perhaps directly to a patient) that this has happened.

You will also need to explain or suggest to your mentor or supervisor how the situation could be remedied and what you have learnt from it as a whole.

Remember to:

- take responsibility for what happened;
- explain how it happened;
- apologise sincerely for your error;
- commit to learning from the mistake so that it will not happen again, along with undertaking some further reading concerning the error itself and all possible outcomes;
- make an accurate record of what took place in the patient's care plan and/or notes, agreeing this with and receiving guidance from your mentor or supervisor, as the information needs to be as accurate as possible, plus, as you are a student, make sure this is countersigned by a qualified nurse;
- if the patient required additional care as a result of your decision, the doctor will also write what treatment was given in the patient's notes.

Making decisions as a student nurse – and, in fact, being a student nurse in both academic and clinical practice settings – can be challenging, so the ability to become and remain resilient is important. Resilience is associated with the ability to keep calm in adverse conditions and manage personal conflict and stress (Cleary, Visentin, West, Lopez and Kornhaber, 2018). Having undertaken an integrative review, Cleary et al. (2018) identified studies that found developing resilience has a positive influence on nursing students. It is associated with the ability to engage successfully with professional practice and maintain well-being. Increasingly, it is also seen to be an attribute of graduates. Although resilience is increasingly cited in nurse education literature, it seems that there is not a common definition of what it is. Programmes to promote the development of resilience among nursing students remain in their infancy (Sanderson and Brewer, 2017).

Reflecting Before, During and After Action

The major study on reflection by Schön (1983) provides us with two main types of reflective activity: reflection *in* action and reflection *on* action.

More recently, it has been suggested that these two forms of reflection originally outlined by Schön are insufficient to account for contemporary experiential learning. Edwards (2017) provides an interesting perspective on the importance of reflection *before* action. Edwards points out that reflecting before action can be useful for thinking about a task in terms of the psychomotor skills required for it, a placement in terms of the service provided or disease trajectories of the patients cared for and preparing for the potential emotional aspects of the situation. By purposefully thinking about the emotions that a practice situation might evoke, and being aware of them, anxiety can be alleviated, and it may help you to feel better prepared. Equally, it can be helpful to reflect on situations that you might encounter in clinical practice for the same reasons. Edwards suggests, for example, that:

> students can begin to pay attention to gain an awareness of, and participate in, early reflection. Reflection-before-action can help to build an awareness of and appreciation for what is going on around them and begin to facilitate students to take notice of practice situations; a mindfulness whereby nurses can become attentive towards their actions prior to them taking place. (2017: 4)

Furthermore, by paying careful attention to reflecting before action, it may be possible for particular experiences to be singled out that otherwise may go unnoticed. Edwards's paper also outlines the importance of the idea of 'noticing', which is something that is explored further in Chapter 11.

Reflecting before action is when reflective activity starts when students begin to explore what is required of them – referred to by van Manen (1991: 102–105) as 'anticipatory reflection' – and may be particularly useful for novices. Complete Activity 4.3 to explore this action in preparation for your next placement.

Activity 4.3

1. A registered nurse has asked you to admit a patient or client to the ward. That means you will have to ask the person a number of questions and fill out the appropriate documentation. You have observed the registered nurse do this several times before, but now she has asked you to take the lead.
2. What do you do?

To answer question two of Activity 4.3, you may have decided to recall some of the previous occasions on which you have observed a patient being admitted to hospital, remembering carefully what the nurse did and the manner in which she asked her questions. You may then have thought about what you are going to say and how you are going to say it. You may even have practised saying it to yourself without speaking it out loud. This is what is known as anticipatory reflection: you make a plan of action concerning events that are yet to happen.

Try to use reflection before action next time you are asked to undertake a relatively new procedure in clinical practice and, if possible, find some quiet space or time before you undertake the task. This might involve going to a physical space or simply taking the time to stop and think about what you have been asked to do. Alternatively, make a decision to tell the person who has asked you to undertake the procedure that you either do not want to undertake this, because you are not completely sure of what to do, or ask them to come with you whilst you undertake the procedure, to ensure that you are doing it correctly. This will be an important decision that you have made, based on the assessment of your own practice skills and knowledge but also on your reflection on previous experience and practice capabilities.

If you do decide to go ahead and undertake the procedure, try to practice what you will say and how you will say it. You may come up with several versions of the same conversation, based on what the patient or client might say to you.

You can even use reflection before action to rehearse psychomotor skills. For example, you may practise your aseptic non-touch technique in the treatment room on the ward or a relevant clinical space. You may wish to double-check the way in which you will unpack any sterile equipment required, using reflection on previous opportunities or encounters to compare the different patient scenarios. Most importantly in such situations check with a practice supervisor, as it is not just about the actual skill itself, but the context and the patients that you may need to consider before proceeding. There may also be knowledge and skills that you draw on which determine your actions and decisions whilst undertaking any nursing intervention, skill or procedure.

Reflecting After Action or on Action

Learning to reflect on the actions taken during or after the event have long been thought to be helpful ways to learn from experience. Activity 4.4 provides an opportunity to look at reflecting during an event in the form of collaborating to make clinical decisions.

Activity 4.4

1. For an example of a reflection from a third-year student nurse relating to collaborative clinical decision-making access and read the following paper:
   L. Griffith and M. Board (2018). Influences on clinical decision-making during a community placement: reflections of a student nurse. *British Journal of Community Nursing*, 23 (12): 606–609.
2. The paper examines the collaborative decision-making in relation to nursing knowledge; and uses Carper's ways of knowing to structure the reflection. This is a unique way of trying to make sense of a clinical situation and use of the framework appears to have helped the student to draw together the various aspects of the nurses' knowledge in use.
3. Try to use the reflective questions posed by Griffith and Board to consider a clinical experience.

Student nurses make an important contribution to the care of patients and clients, helping to ensure that they are cared for in a safe environment. This was particularly true during the COVID-19 pandemic (see Chapter 14 for more on this). In particular, students often bring a new or independent point of view to the clinical environment and are able to see things that perhaps have become so commonplace as to be invisible to the staff permanently working in that area. This means that students are well placed to voice concerns if they think that patient safety is being compromised in some way.

As a student nurse you may witness care that you feel is below the expected standard or you may be placed on a ward where you perceive the learning environment to be poor. In such situations, you need to think about what might constitute an issue of patient safety or a sub optimal learning environment and decide when and how to raise a concern. Doing this can be difficult and may place students in a position of conflict.

Fisher and Kiernan (2019) undertook a small study of 12 student nurses on an adult nursing programme in one Higher Education institution in the UK. The study aimed to provide a better understanding of the factors that influence student nurses to voice concerns (or not) when witnessing sub-optimal care. It revealed four key themes: context of exposure, fear of punitive action, team culture and hierarchy. You can explore these in Activity 4.5.

Activity 4.5

1. Access and read the paper by M. Fisher and M. Kiernan (2019), Student nurses' lived experience of patient safety and raising concerns, *Nurse Education Today*, 77: 1-5.
2. Read the data extracts presented against each theme: context of exposure, fear of punitive action, team culture and hierarchy. For example, consider the following data extract under the theme of 'context of exposure':

   Erm it was the first day of management placement and my mentor, we were doing the medication round and this elderly woman was prescribed erm 15 mg of codeine and we didn't have it on the ward; we only had 30 mg, so my mentor decided she would give the 30 mg and I said to her could she not check why she was only prescribed 15 because 15 is a bit of an unusual dose really: you don't normally see that. And she just said; no, it won't kill her, it'll be fine, and she gave it, and I didn't really know what to do. (2019: 2)

3. Think about your response and whether you have witnessed similar situations in clinical practice. Would you raise a concern? What policy and procedure would you follow to do this? How would you raise a concern in a professional manner?

4. Finally, read and consider this extract from Fisher and Kiernan's paper:

> There was a perception amongst students that they instinctively knew when something was wrong if it was transparent and conspicuous. Other areas of practice that rely perhaps more upon clinical decision-making and professional judgement by the registrant can possibly lead to the student being reluctant to challenge what after all may be perfectly legitimate practice tailored to that individual patient:
>
> 'I'm doubting myself in what I know, but I am still a very junior member of staff compared to other people, so I might get something completely wrong and wouldn't want to look like a fool in front of my peers.' (Participant L, 3rd year female student). (2019: 2)

5. Think about how you will recognise when something is wrong. What would be your priority action?

The study by Fisher and Kiernan (2019) suggests that 'the decision to raise a concern is dependent essentially on moral courage' (2019: 4). Even though the students knew this, and sometimes wanted to act to raise a concern, they remained reluctant to do so, often because they wanted to be accepted by the team and fit in or feared reprisals (Fisher and Kiernan, 2019).

It is important to try to create some purposeful time at the end of every shift or day you spend in clinical practice in order to reflect on the day's events, to learn from them (see Activity 4.6 to help you to do this). This is more than simply thinking things over. It is important to review what happened, what could have happened (if a different approach was taken) and what might happen in the future using different approaches (Rolfe, Jasper and Freshwater, 2011).

Activity 4.6

1. Try to make some decisions about how you intend to find the time and space for regular reflection during your clinical placement.
2. Discuss this with your clinical supervisor and ask how he or she can help you to make this a reality.

It will be a professional development responsibility for you, to ensure that you can use reflection to learn from decision-making in practice. Most module timetables at universities include sessions for reflection on practice, during which students have the opportunity to share with their colleagues' specific examples of clinical decision-making and, through this reflection and sharing, gain possible new insights into their own actions and those of others.

Considering the issues raised and discussed so far, next we can explore some options to take or guide you to become more reflective in your practice.

There are many different models of frameworks for using to reflect on your practice learning. Most of them have key elements, which are identified in the following section. (See the well-known model Boud, Keogh and Walker (1985) in Further Reading section at the end of this chapter.)

(1) Returning to the Experience

Within this stage you are expected to recall salient events without making any judgements. Try to describe the event without missing a single detail, either by writing down what happened (the incident or event) or thinking about the mental process you went through and replay the experience in your mind. As you do this you may uncover some judgements that were made at the time of the event. This involves the use of memory, and, of course, as human beings tend to recall only what we want to recall, so our memories can be flawed. To overcome this, it is a good idea to try to recall the incident soon after the event has taken place, so that events are fresh in your mind. This is particularly relevant when you have been involved in a situation where you are asked to make a statement.

Consider, for example, a situation in which you helped a colleague being threatened by a visitor and the colleague suffered a serious injury. In such a situation, it would be important for you to record exactly what happened, rather than what you thought had happened, so documenting your own and others' actions as soon as possible after the event would be imperative for your account to be as clear as possible in terms of what you saw, what you did and what others did.

Reflecting on the situation later, you may recall some further aspects that escaped you immediately after the event. It is important to make a note of anything else that happened, or you or others did as they come back to you. Examples might be the colour of the assailant's coat or the brand of shoes the person was wearing, which you may not have been able to remember at the time of the incident because everything was happening so quickly.

(2) Attending to Feelings

Within this stage, you will need to focus on your feelings and, in particular, on any negative feelings. It is important to observe the feelings evoked whilst you were going through the experience, because negative feelings about yourself may be a barrier to learning. If you make a mistake, you may feel that you made a wrong decision. Consequently, it is important not to miss out this aspect of reflection. Try doing this in Activity 4.7.

— Activity 4.7 —

1. Reflect on the example of the situation given, under the heading 'Returning to the experience', as if you helped a colleague being threatened by a visitor and the colleague suffered a serious injury.
2. Consider the situation again and determine what kind of feelings might have been involved in the situation described as explained in point 2 (Attending to Feelings).

There would definitely be feelings involved in the scenario in point 1: returning to the experience – as if this had been yourself in that experience. You may, of course, not have considered them at the time – that is, during your 'reflection in action' phase of the incident. You may, for example, have made a decision without pausing to consider the outcome of your intervention, to protect your colleague, but that may have led to a mistake on your part, resulting in an exacerbation of the situation. Alternatively, you may have taken a minute or two to consider alternative options, because you had been in a similar situation previously. This 'reflection on action' opportunity may bring back unhappy or challenging memories, but also, by revisiting prior learning, you would be more confident about your immediate decision-making regarding the patient and the threat to your colleague.

It is important to record all such feelings when undertaking critical reflection on practice and, most importantly, why you had them and what impact they had on your decision-making, both at the time and since the situation was resolved.

(3) Re-evaluating the Experience

The re-evaluation of an experience should not be completed until the first two types of reflection above have been completed. This stage involves re-examining the experience in light of your original intent, associating new knowledge with existing knowledge, and integrating all this into your conceptual framework.

Re-evaluation has four stages, which are also helpful for understanding the complete cycle of reflection and reflective practice:

1. **Association** This stage involves relating new data (or information) to that which is already known. How do these new ideas or new knowledge relate to what you already know? How can you begin to bring some of the ideas together?
2. **Integration** This stage involves seeking relationships among the data. Are there similarities and/or differences between some of the new ideas and things that you already know? Do certain ideas seem to go together?

3. **Validation** This stage involves determining the authenticity of the resulting ideas and feelings. Am I right to feel this way? Is there evidence that other student nurses have had similar experiences? Here, it is important that you consider your experience in relation to those of other student nurses. You might want to access some examples of student nurses' reflections whilst in clinical practice (see the Further reading section at the end of this chapter).

4. **Appropriation** This stage involves making the knowledge you have gathered your own. As a student nurse, you may find that it is a difficult struggle learning some aspects of nursing practice. This is not uncommon, for example, Wenger (1998: 47) describes the concept of practice as including both the explicit and the tacit. That is, it includes what is said and what is left unsaid, what is represented and what is assumed, subtle cues, untold rules of thumb, most of which may never be articulated, yet they are unmistakable signs of membership of the community of practice.

In nursing, there can be many unwritten, implicit rules that you, as a student, need to learn. Reflection is one way to think about some of those unwritten rules, to make sense of clinical practice and to make appropriate decisions in relation to patient care and your own nursing actions. We can see an example of this in Case study 4.1.

CASE STUDY 4.1: A STUDENT'S REFLECTION ON AN EXPERIENCE IN A CLINICAL PLACEMENT

Having settled into the department and familiarised myself with the routine, it was possible for me to contribute as a member of the team, taking on some of the responsibilities and roles. There was a call on the 'standby' phone in the accident and emergency (A&E) department, which stated that a 76-year-old male had been found collapsed on a nearby street by the ambulance crew. He wasn't breathing and there was no sign of a pulse, so they had started cardiopulmonary resuscitation (CPR). It would take them six minutes to reach the department.

The staff who were allocated by the coordinator to be in the resuscitation room started to get their individual equipment ready for the patient's arrival. I stood there and watched in amazement at their efficiency. I could feel my heart pumping faster and I wondered how long the ambulance would be. Those six minutes felt like six seconds.

When the ambulance pulled up outside the department, my mentor, Jane, ran out to meet the paramedics. I followed, not knowing what else to do. The doors opened for me to see an elderly gentleman lying on a stretcher with blood covering his face and chest. It was a shock to see. Jane took over from the paramedics and started CPR. The paramedics pulled the patient into the resuscitation room on the trolley; I ran behind them with adrenaline pumping round my body, wondering what the next step was. This was a new experience for me.

The team was waiting for the patient in the resuscitation room. It started to get noisy in the cubicle: the team leader was phoning for X-rays and electrocardiograms (ECGs); others were trying to find any identification that would tell us who the gentleman was. The patient was still not breathing and had no pulse.

The team leader told me to commence chest compressions. Pressing down firmly and smoothly, I did the compressions. These should be done at a rate of about 80 per minute. I paused whilst the team leader gave the oxygen and I restarted the compressions, both of us working in a rhythm. I was amazed at the depth of concentration I had on the patient, watching his chest rise and fall with the oxygen being pushed into his lungs by the team leader. I was hoping for some signs of life.

My arms were starting to ache, and I could feel the heat from the overhead light beginning to make me sweat and feel hot. I looked up to see the time: I'd been doing my compressions for nearly ten minutes. I thought of having a break. I looked around for someone to take over: there was nobody free. They were all busy carrying out their own tasks for the patient. I could carry on - I wasn't exhausted - but I just felt, at the time, that I needed a rest.

I did wonder how long the team were going to keep on trying and who out of the team would disengage the procedures. It was then that the circulating nurse asked if I was all right. I said 'Yes' straight away, without even thinking, because I didn't want the rest of the team to think I wasn't strong enough mentally or physically. I carried on, trying to be professional. The clock was showing 1.20 p.m.: I'd been doing CPR for 20 minutes. I was hot and sweaty; my arms ached like mad; I'd started to get cramp in my calves: I was exhausted. I wanted to stop now, but I didn't want to ask.

Just then, the team leader asked the team if anyone in the room felt that the procedure should continue. I could hear the team discuss the outcome, which they all felt should be to discontinue treatment. The team leader thanked everyone for doing their best and asked me to step down. My legs were shaking as I stepped down from the bed, and my arms and neck were so stiff.

Physically, I withdrew from the situation, but not mentally. I looked and looked at the patient with sadness, because now it was final: now, he was dead; before, there had been hope. I sat down on a chair and watched the team leave the room. Reflecting then, I was thinking more about his family, knowing that, whilst I knew he was dead, they didn't. I wondered where he was going when he collapsed in the street.

There may be elements of this case study that you can relate to in other chapters throughout the book, so you might want to return to it several times when this happens. At each reading, you might see different aspects of the situation come to the fore as you reflect on it. Consider what you have learnt so far by completing Activity 4.8.

Activity 4.8

1. Can you identify any of the elements of reflection discussed in this chapter in Case study 4.1, a student's reflection on an experience when at a placement in an A&E department?
2. Write down your thoughts and feelings of what you think was happening in the student's experience.

The incident in Case study 4.1 could be referred to as a 'critical incident', or a significant event. This is a term that will be familiar to many of you because it is used to refer to what students have to describe and then critically reflect on to demonstrate practice learning or for a theoretical nursing assignment (see Gimenez (2019) for guidance on how to write such an assignment).

The event was clearly significant for this student. This is evident from the way in which the student articulates what took place: there is a depth to and a great level of detail in the account. We really get a sense of what it was like for the student, physically, mentally and emotionally, during this resuscitation event. The student is able to articulate the feelings and thoughts experienced:

> I could feel my heart pumping faster … Those six minutes felt like six seconds … Jane ran out to meet the paramedics. I followed, not knowing what else to do … I ran behind them with adrenaline pumping round my body … I was amazed at the depth of concentration I had on the patient, watching his chest rise and fall with the oxygen being pushed into his lungs by the team leader. I was hoping for some signs of life. My arms were starting to ache, and I could feel the heat from the overhead light beginning to make me sweat and feel hot.

When starting to reflect on experiences to learn from them, it is important to be able to separate the emotions and feelings from the facts of the event that took place. Complete Activity 4.9 to practice doing this.

Activity 4.9

1. To use experiences in order to learn, it is important to be able to separate the emotions and feelings from the factual event that took place within the activity itself. Re-read Case study 4.1 and consider how these were made visible by the student nurse in their reflection.
2. To help you might also want to print out Case study 4.1 and use a highlighter pen to pick out the emotions and feelings that the student described.

You will also experience significant events of the kind described in Case study 4.1 and, to enable you to learn as much as possible from them, try to write about each one soon afterwards, in as much detail as possible. Write about the feelings you experienced as well, both physical and emotional.

Remember, an event does not have to be a negative experience to be significant. Also, as the student in the case study found, what happened was a learning experience that generated both positive and negative thoughts. Indeed, we can be sure that, in discussions with a practice supervisor or mentor or when the student wrote up the second part of the reflection – which would focus on what was learnt from the experience – many issues would arise. We have only touched on the initial impressions so far, but in Activity 4.10, you can now consider the student's additional learning experiences.

Activity 4.10

1. Read through Case study 4.1 again.
2. Make notes on the major issues you think this student learnt about regarding the various decision-making situations that occurred during the experience.
3. Consider the decisions made by the student and those made by the other members of the multidisciplinary team (MDT).

Following on from Activity 4.10, let us take, for example, the student's description of how (before the patient arrives in the department) the members of the A&E team gather their equipment and otherwise prepare for the arrival of the patient. This could be taken to indicate a very high level of teamwork, everyone knowing what was required of their role in that scenario.

Reflecting on this might lead you to explore decision-making as part of teamwork during resuscitation. The team almost instinctively knew what to do and each member of it was able to be involved in one or more of a number of different activities and/ or processes simultaneously. The individuals in the team would have been observing the multiple cues from the patient and the environment, internally analysing the information or data from those cues and altering their practices as a result in order to influence the delivery of care.

To build on your learning from the case study, using your printout from Activity 4.9, read the case study again and, in a different colour, highlight the cues from the environment, the mentor and team leader that the student described. You can find out more about reading or noticing cues in Chapter 11, which focuses on risk assessment and patient safety.

Also, do you think the scenario demonstrates that this student made links between theoretical knowledge – such as the underpinning knowledge of physiology used – and the decisions made? One example that could indicate this could be when the student observed that 'no pulse and not breathing' led to the decision to undertake and continue cardiopulmonary resuscitation (CPR).

The decision to stop a resuscitation attempt is complex and usually context specific. The focus of attention will move away from the patient and towards team communication (Anderson, Slark and Gott, 2021). In their study of pre-hospital resuscitation decision-making, Anderson, Slark and Gott describe how the decision to stop featured discussion among the crew, bystanders and family (if present). They suggest that 'experienced individuals preferred to seek crew consensus and stage the breaking of bad news to family but did not require family and crew agreement to enact a decision to terminate resuscitation' (2021: 700). Interestingly, the study also shows that less experienced personnel might keep going with a resuscitation attempt if the decision to terminate appeared too hard to make.

Commonly used Models or Frameworks of Reflection

The final part of this chapter provides a brief overview of some new models or frameworks of reflection that you can use to undertake your own reflection on clinical practice in relation to decision-making.

Such models or frameworks can be useful in helping you to learn from decision-making because they provide a structure for your thinking and reflective writing. Some people find structures useful; others find them restrictive and prefer simply to write their ideas down as free text. Whatever your usual preference, you might find it useful when you are starting out thinking about the development of your own decision-making skills to use the models or frameworks to guide you initially. It is important to point out that no single model is best – you may find that you use different models or frameworks to help you to reflect on different incidents or events at different times in your career.

There now follows a description of two models that you could try and use.

1. The Me, My, More, Must Model of Reflection

This model is designed to encourage learners to keep their values at the forefront of their thinking. Learners can then consider the impact of those values prior to having a clinical experience and, more importantly, 'make sense of their values in order to become the professional that they aspire to be' (Wareing, 2017: 271).

Self-awareness is an important aspect of reflection. Wareing (2017) explains the development of values-based practice and its relationship to clinical decision-making, which is based on values as well as facts, as values are fundamental to humankind. He goes on to stress the importance of good communication skills, which are needed to influence clinical decision-making, particularly when patients and or health care staff have legitimate differing perspectives. Prompts are provided to guide you to consider each of the four stages of the model – Me, My, More and Must – when reflecting. Wareing outlines the importance and relevance of each stage of the model to values-based practice.

Activity 4.11

1. Access and read the paper by M. Wareing (2017) Me, my, more, must: A values-based model of reflection, *Reflective Practice*, 18(2): 268-279.
2. The paper provides a full description of this model for reflection. Try to apply it to a recent clinical experience, bringing the 'Me' element of the model to the fore. The aim is to help you as a learner to consider who you are and the impact of your personal values on your reflective activity.

Wareing reminds us that:

> Learning from practice requires a high degree of personal agency including motivation, curiosity and the ability to participate and negotiate a range of learning opportunities whilst encountering different communities of practice. (2017: 275)

2. The Holistic Reflection Model

This model was presented by Bass, Fenwick and Sidebotham (2017), who suggest that contemporary models or frameworks of reflection encourage transformative learning by asking the reflector, or person reflecting, to focus inwardly on personal and professional belief systems. They suggest that learning should be both personal and professional.

The reflector examines their personal assumptions concerning everyday practice. The process should be iterative and move those reflecting forwards in their development, thus resulting in transformative learning.

Bass, Fenwick and Sidebotham present a holistic model of reflection using 'six integrated, interdependent phases designed to promote detailed critical reflection at a deeper personal and holistic level as the learner progresses through the programme' (2017: 231) Figure 4.1).

The authors provide guidance on using the model, with prompts for each section (2017: 232). Importantly, this model is also linked to progression through a programme of study (in this case, midwifery), but the principles could be applied to nursing education generally.

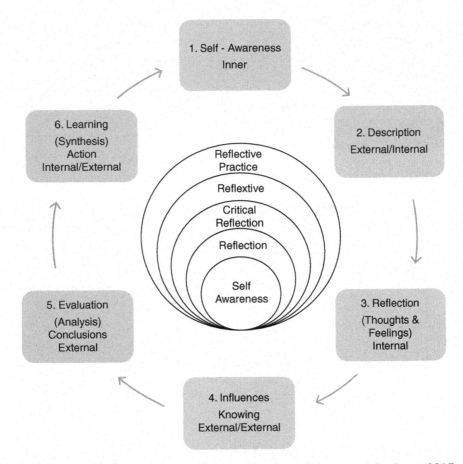

Figure 4.1 The holistic reflection model (Bass, Fenwick and Sidebotham, 2017, reproduced with permission of the authors).

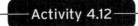Activity 4.12

1. Access the article: J. Bass et al. (2017) Development of a model of holistic reflection to facilitate transformative learning in student midwives, *Women and Birth* 30: 227-235.
2. Read Table 2 from the article: Guidance and prompts for students when using the Holistic Reflection Model and then use these to understand the 'six integrated interdependent phases', namely Phase 1: Self-awareness; Phase 2: Description; Phase 3: Reflection; Phase 4: Knowing; Phase 5: Evaluation and Phase 6: Learning.

Ultimately, the choice of model or framework is very personal, and you might find that different models will suit you at different times as you progress through your course. The examples here have been provided to give you some ideas for how to reflect and the sorts of questions that you can ask yourself to learn from your practice-based experiences.

Conclusion

This chapter has provided you with an overview of the principles of learning from experience and reflection. It has also introduced you to some models or frameworks that can be used to help you to make sense of clinical encounters and, in particular, decision-making.

Like all skills in nursing, and your learning experiences generally, reflection takes practice. In other words, it will require time and effort on your part in order to learn from your experiences. You can reflect on your own or with others, but the most important thing about reflection is that you commit to making future actions better and use it to help refine your decision-making skills.

References

Anderson, N. E., Slark, J. and Gott, M. (2021). Pre-hospital resuscitation decision making: A model of ambulance personnel experiences, preparation and support. *Emergency Medicine Australasia*, 33: 697–702.

Bass, J., Fenwick, J. and Sidebotham, M. (2017). Development of a model of holistic reflection to facilitate transformative learning in student midwives. *Women and Birth*, 30: 227–235.

Ching, S.S.Y., Cheung, K., Hegney, D. and Rees, C.S. (2020). Stressors and coping of nursing students in clinical placement: A qualitative study contextualizing their resilience and burnout. *Nurse Education in Practice*. 42. 102960. https://www.sciencedirect.com/science/article/pii/S1471595318302580?via%3Dihub (accessed 24 May 2022).

Cleary, M., Visentin, D., West, S., Lopez, V. and Kornhaber, R. (2018). Promoting emotional intelligence and resilience in undergraduate nursing students: An integrative review. *Nurse Education Today*, 68: 112–120.

Edwards, S. (2017). Reflecting differently: New dimensions – reflection-before-action and reflection-beyond-action. *International Practice Development Journal*, 7(1): article 2.

Fisher, M. and Kiernan, M. (2019). Student nurses' lived experience of patient safety and raising concerns. *Nurse Education Today*, 77: 1–5.

Gimenez, J. (2019). *Writing for Nursing and Midwifery Students*, 3rd edn. Basingstoke: Palgrave Macmillan.

Griffith, L. and Board, M. (2018). Influences on clinical decision making during a community placement: Reflections of a student nurse. *British Journal of Community Nursing*, 23(12): 606–609.

Hanson, J. and McAllister, M. (2017). Preparation for workplace adversity: Student narratives as a stimulus for learning. *Nurse Education in Practice*, 25: 89–95.

McCarthy, B., Trace, A., O'Donovan, M., Brady-Nevin, C., Murphy, M., O'Shea, M. and O'Regan, P. (2018). Nursing and midwifery students' stress and coping during their undergraduate education programmes: An integrative review. *Nurse Education Today*, 61: 197–209.

Ng, Y-M. and Or, P. L. P. 2020. Guest Editorial: Coronavirus disease (COVID-19) prevention: Virtual classroom education for hand hygiene. *Nurse Education in Practice*. 45: 102782. https://www.ncbi.nlm.nih.gov/pmc/articles/PMC7252133/pdf/main.pdf (accessed 25 May 2022).

Nursing and Midwifery Council (NMC) (2010) *Standards for Pre-registration Nursing Education*. London: NMC.

Nursing and Midwifery Council (NMC) (2018a). *Future Nurse: Standards of proficiency for registered nurses*. London: NMC.

Nursing and Midwifery Council (NMC) (2022). *Current Recovery Programme Standards*. London: NMC.

Rolfe, G., Jasper, M. and Freshwater, D. (2011). *Critical Reflection in Practice: Generating knowledge for care*, 2nd edn. Basingstoke: Palgrave Macmillan.

Sanderson, B. and Brewer, M. (2017). What do we know about student resilience in health professional education?: A scoping review of the literature. *Nurse Education Today*, 58: 65–71.

Schön, D. A. (1983). *The Reflective Practitioner: How professionals think in action*. Guildford: Arena.

Thompson, C., Aitken, L., Doran, D. and Dowding, D. (2013). An agenda for clinical decision making and judgement in nursing research and education. *International Journal of Nursing Studies*, 50: 1720–1726.

Van Manen, M. (1991). *The Tact of Teaching*. New York: State University of New York Press.

Wareing, M. (2016). *Becoming a Learner in the Workplace: A student's guide to practice-based and work-based learning in health and social care*. London: Quay Books.

Wareing, M. (2017). Me, my, more, must: A values-based model of reflection. *Reflective Practice*, 18(2): 268–279.

Wenger, E. (1998). *Communities of Practice. Learning, meaning and identity*. Cambridge University Press.

Further Reading

Barksby, J., Butcher, N. and Whysall, A. (2015). A new model of reflection for clinical practice. *Nursing Times*, 111(34/35): 21–23.

Boud D, Keogh R and Walker D (1985) Promoting Reflection in Learning : a model, Routledge, Oxon.

Patterson, C., Moxham, L., Brighton, R., Taylor, E., Sumskis, S., Perlman, D., Heffernan, T. and Hadfield, L. (2017). Nursing students' reflections on the learning experience of a unique mental health clinical placement. *Nurse Education Today*, 46: 94–98.

Smith, S. and Hunt, J. (2019). Communication skills: Placement reflections of a children's nursing student. *Nursing Children and Young People*, 1: 19–23.

Web Resources

Academic skills, The University of Melbourne: Reflective writing https://www.youtube.com/watch?v=SntBj0FIApw (accessed 6 June, 2022).

5

ETHICAL ISSUES AND DECISION-MAKING IN PRACTICE

Marcia Kirwan

Chapter objectives

The aims of this chapter are to:

- explore decision-making within ethical principles, models and frameworks;
- consider the development of professional and ethical practitioners;
- explore the place of professional values in decision-making;
- demonstrate through case studies how decisions in practice frequently have an ethical element.

Introduction

From the previous chapters, it has been established that decision-making is integral to the nurse's role. In this chapter, we look at how many decisions nurses make require that they determine the 'right thing to do' in a given situation. How the nurse comes to that determination depends on many things, not least of which is adherence to the professional standards laid out in the NMC's (2018e) *The Code: Professional standards of practice and behaviour for nurses, midwives and nursing associates*. Upholding the dignity of the people being cared for, assessing and responding to their individual needs, preferences and concerns, acting in their best interests, and respecting their rights, in terms of privacy and confidentiality, is an expectation on all good nurses. Just as qualified nurses are accountable practitioners, student nurses are expected to demonstrate this through achievement of the NMC's (2018a) *Future Nurse: Standards of proficiency for registered nurses*. Platform 1: Being an accountable practitioner outcomes, for example, require that nurses understand and accept their responsibilities in relation to decision-making, with peoples' values, needs and preferences being kept to the fore, and that they demonstrate courage, transparency and a willingness to challenge perceptions and behaviours that contravene the standards of *The Code*, in themselves and others.

Frequently nurses' decisions around the 'right thing to do' are in response to moral or ethical issues. It is not possible to be prescriptive as to how a nurse should act in response to such questions or dilemmas, so it is useful that guiding principles and frameworks are available to use when such issues occur. Ethical or moral decision-making is never easy and, generally, important issues are at stake. These might include issues such as life, death, suffering, beliefs, values, harm, treatments, interventions – or simply what is the right or wrong thing to do in a given situation. Prioritising the needs and wishes of the person in need of care might require a suspension of the values or beliefs of the nurse. How the nurse responds in such cases is likely to have an impact on the person requiring care in the first instance, but also on the individual nurse, and potentially beyond that person and situation. In contemporary nursing practice, increased workloads and patient acuity, combined with reduced resources and funding, can compound the difficulties nurses face around decision-making. Moral distress can occur when a nurse decides on the right thing to do, but the organisation, systems or other factors make it impossible for the nurse to act in line with that decision. Resilience and courage are frequently required to ensure that nurses can be accountable for their decisions and practice *and* maintain the professional standards required of them in a contemporary health care system. Moral resilience is where ethical decision-making can occur without moral distress as an outcome (Lachman, 2016).

This chapter is concerned with how nurses understand their decision-making role in relation to values, beliefs, relationships, contexts, ethical principles and frameworks.

The nature of ethics is explored as it is applied in the nurse decision-making process. There are activities to reinforce and expand on learning and relevant examples are presented and discussed. The first one to complete is Activity 5.1.

Activity 5.1

1. Access and read the NMC's (2018e) *The Code: Professional standards of practice and behaviour for nurses, midwives and nursing associates* and the NMC's (2018a) *Future Nurse: Standards of proficiency for registered nurses.*
2. Outline the points in each that might be considered to have a link to professional values and ethical practice.
3. As you read through this chapter, consider your answers and determine which ones you would now either add or remove and make a note of the reasons why.
4. Consider how you could achieve proficiency in being accountable for delivering evidence-based care and decisions.

Accountability

Chalmers stated that:

> It is through accountability that nurses can claim to be a profession, and it is through accountability that the profession can continue to support and develop nursing practice for the benefit of patient care. (1995: 33)

This demonstrates that accountability, as a core element of nursing, has, for a long time been linked to the professionalisation of nursing. This remains the case as changes occur in both the role of the nurse and nurse education across many countries. The concept of accountability continues to be a central tenet of how nurses function as professionals within the health service, and this is highlighted in platform 1 of the NMC document entitled *Future Nurse: Standards of proficiency for registered nurses* (NMC, 2018a), which outlines nurses' responsibilities as follows:

> Registered nurses act in the best interests of people, putting them first and providing nursing care that is person-centred, safe and compassionate. They act professionally at all times and use their knowledge and experience to make evidence-based decisions about care. They communicate effectively, are role models for others, and are accountable for their actions. Registered nurses continually reflect on their practice and keep abreast of new and emerging developments in nursing, health and care. (2018a: 7)

Nurses are accountable not simply to their employer and their professional body but also to their patient, who is described by Sellman as 'more-than-ordinarily vulnerable' (2011: 51), and, beyond that, to wider society. Semple and Cable (2003) point out that there is a moral dimension to accountability that means nurses are also accountable to themselves as moral beings. In Ireland, as in other countries, the Nursing and Midwifery Board of Ireland's (NMBI) *Code of Professional Conduct and Ethics for Registered Nurses and Registered Midwives* dictates, for principle 2 (Professional responsibility and accountability), as one of its values, that 'nurses and midwives are professionally responsible and accountable for their practice, attitudes and actions; including inactions and omissions' (2021: 13).

In order to exercise accountability in relation to decision-making, nurses must ensure they are making decisions that are based on up-to-date evidence at all times. Along with that, however, they must know they are acting in the best interests of the patients. The idea that nurses are accountable for 'omissions' in their work is a profound worry for nurses who are practising in contemporary health care systems. Not all decisions are made in a constraint-free environment.

The context in which nurses practice may place limits on their decision-making, where the 'right thing to do' is not an available option, and the reality of practice challenges the nurses' personal values and those of the profession as a whole. This places a further burden on nurses to be accountable for decisions made under such circumstances. The related phenomena of care left undone (Ausserhofer et al., 2014; Lucero et al., 2010; Sochalski, 2004), missed nursing care (Kalisch, 2006; Kalisch et al., 2009) or implicitly rationed nursing care (Schubert et al., 2008) are frequently linked to nurses' decision-making processes. Nurses faced with limited or absent resources, increased workloads, changing patient profiles or lack of leadership may find themselves having to make decisions about which care can be carried out and which remains undone or incomplete (Jones, Hamilton and Murray, 2015).

Such decisions can be linked to poor patient outcomes in the first instance, as patients go without necessary care. Equally, however, the impact on individual nurses is often profound, with moral distress and role conflicts identified as outcomes in such situations (Papastavrou, Panayiota and Georgios, 2014). The inconsistency between the reality of nurses' care provision and the care that they would want to provide, if circumstances would allow, can be a heavy ethical burden for them.

Decision-making in times of reduced resources is often based in prioritising medical interventions such as medications or procedures over other aspects of care for which the effects are seen as less immediate, such as mobilisation, hygiene or psychosocial care. It is unsurprising that nurses feel conflicted or guilty if they are unable to provide the care they deem necessary or be the kinds of nurses that they want to be.

Nonetheless, whatever the setting or challenges, nurses are expected to act responsibly and effectively in all situations and to provide 'reasoned justification' for decisions taken (Thompson et al., 2006: 384). When deciding on the morally correct course of action – or 'the right thing to do' – it is essential that, in addition to giving consideration to the requirements of the profession as outlined in *The Code*, nurses' decision-making comes from an ethical domain of practice.

'Ethics' in nursing is concerned with examining situations and questions in practice, analysing them by considering all angles and courses of action, and helping nurses to arrive at a decision and possible action for which coherent rationales can be provided. Weaver, Morse and Mitcham (2008) recommend that nurses have a sense of 'ethical sensitivity' at times of clinical uncertainty. This requires nurses to be able to bring together experience, knowledge and ethical codes to inform their decision-making. The impact of the COVID-19 global pandemic has given rise to a high level of clinical uncertainty for nurses and other health workers where, for many, there has been conflict in relation to their duty of care. McKenna highlights this conflict:

> A foundation of nursing practice is the duty of care with the attendant obligations to alleviate suffering, restore health and respect the rights and dignity of every patient. However, nurses must balance this duty of care for patients with their duty of care to themselves and their family members. These conflicting duties in a pandemic can cause serious moral and emotional distress. A nurse's duty to care for patients is not absolute. If the COVID-19 virus places nurses at serious risk if they contract it, it is unfair and disproportionate to expect them to undertake such heightened health risks to uphold their duty of care. (2019: 1)

In the initial stages of the pandemic, many student nurses in the UK also had to make personal decisions regarding either taking a break from their programmes of learning in university and practice, due to the inability to pursue studies as normal, or, for many final-year students, being able, through the emergency regulations implemented by the NMC (2020), to undertake their studies full-time in practice as paid members of the clinical workforce. While working as paid members of the workforce the students were still required to achieve the required proficiencies in order to graduate and qualify as nurses. (See the Web resources section at the end of this chapter for the links for the NMC's website for full information.)

Regardless of the circumstances in which student nurses, with the support of their supervisors or mentors, are caring for patients and their families, any decisions made on placement are part of their learning to be accountable as future qualified nurses.

Making decisions that nurses are accountable for as individuals is also influenced by their values, which could, at times, themselves have an impact on their decision-making.

Values

What do we mean by 'values' in the context of ethical decision-making? Fry and Johnstone view a value as:

> A standard or quality that is esteemed, desired, considered important or has worth or merit. Values are expressed by behaviours or standards that a person endorses or tries to maintain. (2008: 210)

All individuals have a set of values, which may stem from their family values or their religious or cultural backgrounds. On becoming a nurse such values will contribute to how individuals act, but socialisation into the profession may add another layer of values. These values are generally adopted from watching others practice nursing. Personal values and professional values may coexist happily for individual nurses, but due to the nature of nursing and health care generally, it is unlikely that this will always remain the case. Frequently, situations can occur where the two sets of values conflict. For example, how a nurse believes things should be done and how things are actually done in practice can differ (Thompson et al., 2006). If such conflict is ongoing, with the nurse's values consistently in conflict with actual practice, this can lead to situations where patient care is compromised and of poor quality. The Francis Inquiry (2013) highlighted incidents where nurses' values were compromised so regularly that it became the norm in one hospital trust.

Values can be both individual and shared (within communities of practice or professions). Equally, the values of an individual nurse and the profession at large may be in conflict with the beliefs and values of a patient. Sometimes patients' beliefs and values can be difficult to understand and, therefore, to support. These are challenges that all nurses face during their careers and it is important to recognise our own values, their origins and their worth, while also acknowledging the values of others (both individual and professional), along with any differences and conflicts. Activities 5.2 and 5.3 provide an opportunity to think about values.

Activity 5.2

1. Identify some personal values which are important to you.
2. Consider where these values may have come from.
3. Have your values changed over time? (As a child, a teenager, a young adult, a student nurse?)
4. Try to remember an incident in practice where your values caused you to question practice.

   - Describe the incident.
   - How did you feel initially?

- Did you voice your concerns? If so, what was the outcome? How did you feel afterwards?
- If you chose not to challenge, why did you make this choice? How did you feel afterwards?
- If a similar situation were to arise again, how would you respond? Why?

5. Read Case study 5.1 and consider what was happening here and to which values you can relate.

CASE STUDY 5.1: EXPERIENCE OF AOIFE, A SECOND YEAR STUDENT NURSE, DURING PRACTICE PLACEMENT

Aoife is a second-year student nurse who was on a morning shift on a general medical ward. She and a staff nurse, Sally, were allocated to care for 14 patients in two six-bed wards and two individual side rooms. Over half their patients required full assistance with washing, dressing, eating and drinking.

Aoife checked in on an 87-year-old female patient in side room 1 at 8.04 a.m. She discovered that the patient, Mrs Matthews, had been incontinent overnight and was in urgent need of attention. She was unable to get out of bed and would need full assistance from two nurses. She had not wanted to call a nurse during the night 'because they are so busy'.

Aoife told Mrs Matthews that she would get help and come back immediately. Aoife informed Sally and suggested that they start inside room 1. Sally responded, 'That's a job for two! If we both go into that room, we will be tied up for 45 minutes at least, which means nobody else gets help with breakfast or a wash. We need to get this lot sorted out here before we go in there.'

Aoife suggested that she call the care assistant from the other side of the ward to help her inside room 1. Sally said, 'Don't do that, they have enough to do at that end. We will get to side room 1, just not immediately.'

Aoife was upset - Mrs Matthews reminded her of her granny at home in Galway - but Sally was her mentor and would be assessing her during her placement.

Aoife and Sally worked fast through breakfasts, mindful of Mrs Matthews. They got back to side room 1 at 8.59 a.m. By then, Mrs Matthews was cold, tearful and had missed breakfast.

Activity 5.3

1. Read Case study 5.1 again and this time consider what was happening in terms of the decision-making that took place.
2. Now consider the following issues:

- The values at play in the scenario.
- The decisions made at each point and the possible reasons behind them.
- The outcomes for student, staff nurse and patient.

- Are the outcomes different for all if?
  - this is a once-off incident
  - this is a regular scenario on this ward?
- What could have been done differently?
- Which NMC (2018a) platforms are relevant here?

Let us now look at some of the issues that you may have considered by reading the case study and completing the activities, plus some possible responses.

Decision-Making Concern for Student Nurse Aoife

A decision was made by the staff nurse that conflicted with Aoife's view of how care should be provided. Aoife felt compelled to comply with the staff nurse's plan and was upset by what happened as a result. The outcome for the individual patient was reported as poor.

Observations

The context in which this student experience occurred is not uncommon. It was a busy general ward with many patients, possibly older people, who need assistance with the activities of daily living. This can result in rationed or delayed care, where nurses make individual pragmatic decisions. It may be that the staff nurse made her decision based on the 'greater good' – helping 12 patients instead of just one. It may be that she made her decision based on experience – the time involved in addressing the needs of one patient would ultimately compromise the care provided to the others.

We do not know if other patients needed immediate help. It may be that the staff nurse resented the student's approach. She may have felt that a more consultative approach would have been more appropriate.

The patient outcome in this case was poor, and the student nurse was upset, but it is likely that the staff nurse also had feelings of regret. Ultimately, she made the decision that resulted in delayed patient care. This may have been a one-off situation, or it may have been the latest in a long list of unsatisfactory care-rationing decisions made by nurses on that ward. How to make the right decision in challenging work environments is of concern to most good nurses. Paying attention to ethical principles in day-to-day decision-making can help nurses to 'do the right thing'.

Let us next consider how ethical principles can help you to develop ethical decision-making.

Ethical principles

Ethical principles, derived from theory, can assist nurses in moral or ethical decision-making processes. These principles can be useful when the values and beliefs of a nurse are in conflict with those of others.

As accountable professionals, nurses must be able to provide a coherent and credible rationale for action or inaction, using a process in which issues are considered and decisions made are explicit and well founded. By paying attention to ethical principles, nurses can examine moral or ethical questions from all viewpoints, consider outcomes and actions, and arrive at 'the right thing to do' through a systematic analysis. Fundamental ethical principles to be considered are:

- respect for persons
- beneficence
- non-maleficence
- justice.

Respect for persons

'Autonomy' relates to respecting the ability of the individual to make their own decisions in their own best interests – that is, a person's right to self-determination (Lachman, 2006). This concept was born out of the work of the classical philosophers Plato and Aristotle and later medieval scholars (Thompson et al., 2006). The philosopher Kant (1724–1804) further defined autonomy as being linked to moral maturity, which is when one can make decisions for oneself as a moral agent.

Autonomy in health care is seen in the explicit commitment to respect individual choices in relation to treatment, non-treatment, privacy, truth-telling and confidentiality. *The Code* addresses the requirement of nurses to respect the autonomy of clients and patients through the statement named: Prioritise People (NMC, 2018e 6):

1. Treat people as individuals and uphold their dignity ...
2. Listen to people and respond to their preferences and concerns ...
3. Make sure that people's physical, social and psychological needs are assessed and responded to ...
4. Act in the best interests of people at all times
5. Respect people's right to privacy and confidentiality ... (2018e: 6)

The *Standards of proficiency for registered nurses* (NMC, 2018a) further explains the responsibilities of the nurse with regard to respecting the autonomy of those in need of nursing care. For platform 1: Being an accountable practitioner, outcome 1.9 is that nurses are expected to:

> understand the need to base all decisions regarding care and interventions on people's needs and preferences, recognising and addressing any personal and external factors that may unduly influence their decisions. (2018a: 8)

This standard acknowledges that there will be times when nurse and patient or client values are in conflict but outlines the nurse's role as one in which the provision of care is person-centred at all times.

Outcome: 1.14 further clarifies this, stating that the role of the nurse is to:

> provide and promote non-discriminatory, person-centred and sensitive care at all times, reflecting on people's values and beliefs, diverse backgrounds, cultural characteristics, language requirements, needs and preferences, taking account of any need for adjustments. (2018a: 9)

It is clear that people have the right to make decisions to engage with or refuse treatment options, and for their choices to be respected. The principle of autonomy focuses on a compassionate and respectful relationship between a caregiver and the person in receipt of care. The NMC *Standards of proficiency for registered nurses* document (2018a) explicitly points out that it is a requirement for nurses to pay attention to differences of culture, values and beliefs, and to ensure that personal values do not infringe on a person's right to self-determination. Truth-telling by nurses in order to facilitate decision-making by patients or clients around their care is also tied into this principle of autonomy. The difficulties here for nurses might be a temptation to unduly influence or coerce where values are in conflict.

Beneficence

'Beneficence' is an ethical principle that is linked to the duty of nurses to ensure that their actions benefit and assist others. It outlines the nurse's obligation to always act in the best interests of the person and contribute to their overall well-being. The challenge of this ethical principle for nurses lies in ensuring that beneficence does not tip over into paternalism.

Beneficence can also be seen as a duty to care (Thompson et al., 2018) that incorporates the roles of advocacy of behalf of clients and persons needing care and protecting the rights of vulnerable people. The risk of straying into paternalistic territory can be significantly reduced when nurses balance the principle of autonomy with beneficence. This ensures that decision-making remains focused on the needs of people and their right to make decisions about their care. This may involve accepting and supporting a choice to refuse treatment, which may conflict with nurses' values and beliefs, but working to alleviate symptoms and preserve dignity.

Non-maleficence

The principle of 'non-maleficence' describes the duty to 'do no harm' (Lachman, 2016). This includes a duty to minimise risk and harm, including physical, psychological or emotional harm. This can be achieved through open and meaningful communication between persons, that is, between caregiver and person needing care, and between team members. It can also be interpreted as a duty to maintain professional standards of care, ensuring up-to-date, evidence-based practice and maintaining competence. Nurses making decisions using this principle should apply a process of shared decision-making in the first instance, along with up-to-date knowledge and experience.

Justice

The principle of 'justice' or fairness has at its core the equal worth of people and respect for the rights of individuals (Lachman, 2016). This includes non-discrimination on the basis of gender, race, religion, age, illness or otherwise. It also implies equity in relation to health care – that all should have equal access to necessary care and resources. While this principle has political and geopolitical implications, it also applies to nurses in direct care provision. Nurses need to make decisions around resource and time allocation and must be careful that these decisions are just and fair. We can now revisit the four principles discussed in Activity 5.4.

Activity 5.4

1. Re-read Case study 5.1 (student nurse Aoife's experience) earlier in this chapter.
2. Examine the decisions that were made in relation to the four principles outlined above.
3. How might these principles have helped the nurses to arrive at different decisions?
4. To explore these important principles relating to student nurses in practice, read Case study 5.2, then answer the questions in Activity 5.5.

CASE STUDY 5.2: ETHICAL PRINCIPLES: THIRD YEAR STUDENT NURSE EMMA'S EXPERIENCE IN PRACTICE

Third-year student nurse, Emma, was on a learning placement in an A&E department of a large general hospital. Over the course of her placement, she had seen several people attending with mental health difficulties – a teenage girl brought in by her parents following a serious self-harm episode, a 35-year-old teacher and father of two suffering from severe depression, a male law student experiencing an acute psychotic episode and a 54-year-old woman experiencing a manic episode following not taking her medication for bipolar disorder. Each of these patients was seen by the mental health liaison nurse in the first instance and, where deemed necessary, by the on-call psychiatrist. Emergency admission to a mental health unit was expedited in two cases and a next day outpatient appointment in two cases.

On one Saturday night at 11 p.m., a very dishevelled homeless man was brought in by ambulance. He was bleeding from a head laceration and had other minor abrasions on his hands and bare feet. The paramedic's report stated that the man had been found wandering on the high street between lanes of traffic in a highly agitated state. He appeared to be hallucinating, with disordered thinking. He spoke very little English and was very resistant to help, providing no details regarding his head laceration.

On arrival at A&E, he was noisy and uncooperative, smelled of alcohol but was not aggressive. Nursing staff told Emma that Piotr was well known to them, 'a frequent attender' with a longstanding psychiatric history. He was known to have a diagnosis of schizophrenia and had several admissions to the psychiatric services. Following those admissions, he had rarely been compliant regarding taking his medications and was known by the homeless services as a long-term rough sleeper. He had no known relatives and was thought to be from eastern Europe.

Emma was present when the consultant and nurse manager discussed Piotr's case. They felt that the priority was to calm him down and suture his head laceration. The mental health liaison nurse was not in the department at weekends, and they felt that there was no point in contacting the on-call psychiatrist as Piotr 'never complies'.

The nurse manager asked Emma to draw up medication as prescribed, to calm Piotr for suturing. Noting that Piotr was barefoot, the nurse manager also asked her to search through the left belongings store for socks and shoes for Piotr and to leave them in his cubicle. She said, 'He normally sleeps it off and then leaves the department, so if we leave some shoes with his belongings, he might take those too.'

Emma was concerned that Piotr may have a serious head injury, but that possibility was not being considered. A head injury could account for his symptoms and behaviour, but staff only saw his 'schizophrenia'. She was concerned that medication to calm him down would further mask a head injury. She felt an interpreter could help with communication and perhaps find out if Piotr had an explanation for the head laceration. When she suggested this to staff, her view was dismissed on the grounds that Piotr was a frequent attender for whom, ultimately, little could be done. Again, she was asked to draw up the medication. It was pointed out that if she was uncomfortable with this, another student would be asked to help. Emma reluctantly drew up the medication and, with three other nurses restraining Piotr in accordance with the hospital policy, administered the medication as directed,

Piotr calmed down, the wound was sutured, he slept for a while and as predicted, later left the department. No neurological observations were noted during his time in A&E. Those who saw him leave said that he remained agitated and was still hallucinating.

Activity 5.5

1. Examine Case study 5.2 in relation to the ethical principles outlined above.
2. Were any of the principles violated?
3. How might adherence to the principles have helped in this case?
4. The professional standards set out in *The Code* (2018e) state that nurses must act in the best interests of patients at all times. Did the student nurse in this case believe that the interests of the patient were kept to the forefront here? Explain your answer.
5. Which standards from platform 1 are in question here?
6. Are any other of the NMC's platforms relevant here?

7. Which alternative courses of action were open to the student in this case?

8. What would you have done? And consider what risks might be associated with your actions?

In the following section is a discussion of these issues as related to Emma's observations of her experience in Case study 5.2 and the issues raised in Activity 5.5.

Decision-Making Concern for Student Nurse Emma

Emma felt that this patient was treated differently from how other patients were being treated. She did not believe that the staff were acting in his best interests. She complied with other nurses' wishes against her better judgement.

Observations

Nursing students in clinical practice can feel vulnerable when situations arise that may be a cause for concern. In this case, the student nurse voiced her concerns to other members of staff, but they were dismissed. Francis (2015) has highlighted that as student nurses are up-to-date educationally, they have an important role to play in bringing care deficits to attention while they are on clinical placements. He suggests that students have yet to be bruised by consistent poor practice and can bring a fresh enthusiasm and compassion to situations, based on contemporary best practice.

It has to be acknowledged that an important aspect of nurse education is socialisation into the profession, which enables students to develop an individual professional identity (Brennan and Timmins, 2012). The socialisation process described by Melia (1987) and latterly by Levett-Jones and Lathlean (2007, 2008, 2009) is an important process, but it is vital that, in their efforts to assimilate, student nurses do not compromise their own values and those of the profession. Levett-Jones and Lathlean (2009: 348) speak about student nurses on placements having a 'precarious sense of belonging', which can influence their decision-making based on fear of rejection or being ostracised. This should not be the case – students should have the moral courage to raise concerns when they feel that members of staff are not acting in the best interests of a patient. Their actions are protected by both professional standards and legislation.

'Moral courage' can be defined as the willingness to do the right thing even if this carries personal risk. It is seen as a means of bridging the gap between personal values and professional responsibilities (Lachman, 2009, 2010). Where students witness unchallenged poor standards of practice when on placements, they often report negative personal feelings and feel negatively towards the profession (Bickhoff, Sinclair and Levett-Jones, 2017).

The Department of Health (2015) states that those involved in the delivery of care have a duty to safeguard patients and a breach of that duty could lead to sanctions by regulatory bodies. Nurses, including student nurses, have a responsibility to voice their concerns. This responsibility is of particular importance when student nurses and midwives are asked to practice beyond their competence, limitations and scope of practice.

To support ethical decision-making in practice, you may find that ethical frameworks help to guide your thinking.

Ethical frameworks

Nurses working in contemporary health care systems – and, therefore, student nurses – are regularly faced with ethical questions in relation to nursing practice and care provision (Mallari and Tariman, 2013). These questions can be about big ethical issues – euthanasia, abortion, advanced directives, assisted suicide – or the more day-to-day issues – of scarcity (and, therefore, allocation) of resources, refusal of treatment, withdrawal or continuation of treatment in cases of a terminal diagnosis, disagreement within teams, consent or concerning the ability to consent (Leuter et al., 2013).

To assist nurses, many ethical frameworks have been developed. Mallari and Tariman (2013) conducted a review of the frameworks used for decision-making in nursing practice. Ten of them were identified in the literature as being used for ethical dilemmas in practice, with international and national codes of ethics for nurses being the most frequently used.

The *ICN Code of Ethics for Nurses* was first established by the International Council of Nurses (ICN) in 1953 and more recently revised in 2021 (see Web resources, ICN, 2021). This international code has been used as a model for national codes of ethics in many countries, including the development of *The Code* in the UK. National codes take into account the contextual and culture-specific aspects of nursing practice in the country concerned and should be updated regularly to reflect changing contexts. In this way, nurses can remain responsive to emerging issues and address changes within society and health care in their nursing practice. Professional nurses must use their country-specific code of practice and ethics, where available, to make decisions within an ethical framework where 'doing the right thing' can be a complex and, often, ambiguous concept. We can consider some of these issues in the context of the UK in Activity 5.6.

Activity 5.6

1. Read the ICN's (2021) *International Code of Ethics for Nurses* (see the Web resources section at the end of this chapter for the link).

2. Map the similarities and overlaps between it and the NMC's (2018e) *The Code: Professional standards of practice and behaviour for nurses, midwives and nursing associates.*

3. Then map how both those documents contribute to the standards for nurses set out in the NMC's (2018a) *Future Nurse: Standards of proficiency for registered nurses.*

The NMC sets and reviews the standards required for professional nurses in the UK in an effort to ensure that members of the public are protected and served appropriately by the profession at large, and that it remains relevant in contemporary health care systems. The proficiencies outlined in the recent publication entitled *Future Nurse: Standards of proficiency for registered nurses* (NMC, 2018a) outline what can be expected of a nurse today.

To explore some of the issues related to both professional and personal safety and accountability, consider the issues in Case study 5.3 and answer the questions that follow in Activity 5.7. Any issue that arises where you are unsure of the response can be shared with your personal tutor or academic supervisor.

CASE STUDY 5.3: FINAL YEAR STUDENT NURSE: PERSONAL AND PROFESSIONAL SAFETY AND ACCOUNTABILITY

Molly, a final-year student nurse, was working in the trauma ward of a university hospital. A 22-year-old male patient, Andrew, was admitted following a road traffic incident in which he sustained bilateral leg fractures.

Molly admitted Andrew to the ward and prepared him for theatre. Over the next few days, she looked after him post-operatively. When he followed her on Instagram, she was surprised, but, without much thought, she followed him back and they also followed each other on Snapchat.

When Molly was off duty over the weekend, she posted updates on both platforms regularly and chatted with Andrew and other Instagram and Snapchat friends. Andrew took screenshots of some of her photos and sent them on to his college friends as evidence of the 'hot nurses' who were caring for him.

On Sunday afternoon, while his friends were visiting, the ward manager administered Andrew's IV antibiotics. While chatting to Andrew and his visitors, she became aware of an ongoing Snapchat conversation between Molly and Andrew and heard reference to 'hot nurses'.

On Monday, when Molly returned to work, she was allocated to a different group of patients that did not include Andrew. After handover, the ward manager asked to speak with her privately.

The ward manager was very angry, and Molly was taken aback when she realised that the ward manager knew about her social media connection with a patient. She suddenly became aware that this might be inappropriate. The ward manager indicated that Molly's school of nursing would need to be made aware of the incident. Molly was deeply upset that this might have an impact on her progression to registration as a qualified nurse.

Activity 5.7

1. Think about Molly's decision-making, described in Case study 5.3.
2. Do you think that her actions were appropriate?
3. Are there any risks involved here? For whom?
4. Consider the NMC guidelines for nurses on social media use.
5. Consider context in relation to decision-making.
6. Consider the nurse–patient relationship.
7. Consider how many of the NMC platforms are relevant here.

Decision-Making Concerns for Student Nurse Molly

Molly applied her personal approach to social media connections to the context of her professional life. This resulted in a blurring of the boundaries between nurse and patient, as well as compromising her professionalism.

Observations

Social media usage is ubiquitous in today's world and has become an essential tool for maintaining personal and professional connections. Meeting new people, however casually, frequently results in a social media connection. In the incident in Case study 5.3, Molly followed Andrew on Instagram without much thought, as she might have done if she had met him socially. In doing so, however, she violated the normal nurse–patient boundaries.

Scruth et al. (2015: 10) point out the 'speed and ease' of social media, which means potential consequences and outcomes are not necessarily included in decision-making'. The NMC's *Guidance on Using Social Media Responsibly* (which should be read in conjunction with *The Code*) states:

> Nurses, midwives and nursing associates should not use social networks to build or pursue relationships with patients and service users as this can blur important professional boundaries. (2018e: 5)

The standards of a nurses' personal social media usage should not be applied within a professional context. It was inappropriate for Molly to allow a patient to follow her on social media in the first place, but by following him, too, she changed the direction of their relationship. *The Code* outlines that all forms of social media must be used responsibly, and to do otherwise may jeopardise the ability of students to join the register. This includes the building or pursuing of relationships with patients through social media. The NMC's *Guidance* on using Social Media Responsibly (NMC, n.d.) also points out that nurses should be aware that patients may access social media profiles without the nurses' knowledge, so great care should be taken generally by nurses in how they present themselves on their social media sites. The personal consequences can be serious, but, equally, this can have an impact on how the profession is viewed by the public.

To further your understanding of various types of decision-making needed in practice, consider those facing Louise, a newly qualified nurse, in Case study 5.4, then complete Activity 5.8. In the case study, we see how Louise's values could have an impact on shared decision-making.

▬▬▬ CASE STUDY 5.4: THE IMPACT OF ▬▬▬ VALUES ON SHARED DECISION-MAKING: THE EXPERIENCE OF LOUISE, A NEWLY QUALIFIED NURSE

Louise was caring for a 14-year-old girl who had been admitted recently. The girl, Beth, had come from school to A&E with acute abdominal pain. Initially, acute appendicitis was considered, and this was communicated to her parents by phone. They had been in Dublin on holiday but were now on their way home. Beth had stayed in the family home with her 17-year-old sister. Following the call to Beth's parents in Dublin, appendicitis was excluded by A&E staff and Beth was diagnosed with an ectopic pregnancy. She was admitted to a surgical ward by Louise and was prepared for surgery.

It was likely that Beth's parents would arrive while she was in the operating theatre. Beth and her sister did not want their parents to know about the pregnancy and had decided to tell them that she had an appendectomy. They asked Louise to tell their parents this when they arrived as they would be angry and appalled if they knew the truth.

Louise could see that both girls were very distressed and anxious about their parents' reaction. She knew that it was unlikely the surgeons would be free to meet with the parents after surgery as they had further cases, so she was certain she would be the first point of contact for the anxious parents.

Louise was conflicted about how she should respond, but valued telling the truth and candour, both professionally and personally. She knew that she could avoid providing details to the parents by saying the surgeons would speak to them tomorrow. She could just reassure them that the surgery went well, and Beth would be fine. However, she knew that the girls' secret would be revealed eventually and wondered if she could help by speaking to the parents first. She decided that when the parents arrived, she would take them to the family room and tell them the truth about their daughter's condition. She felt that they had a right to know, and she could help them to accept the situation before they saw their daughter. She was confident that this was the right thing to do, and it was in keeping with her professional standards. She felt that she could empathise with the parents and daughters equally and was ideally placed to help them through this difficult time. Louise was aware that she was growing in confidence as a newly qualified staff nurse, so this was a situation where she could demonstrate her professional competence.

Activity 5.8

1. What do you think is happening in this case study?
2. Why do you think Louise has made this decision?
3. What are the possible outcomes?
4. Is Louise's decision in the best interests of her patient?
5. Examine Louise's actions in light of the NMC's (2018a) platform 1.
6. Are any other of the platforms relevant here?
7. How might the patient feel? How might the parents feel?
8. How might you have acted in these circumstances?
9. Consider truth telling and candour as standards in nursing.

Decision-Making Concerns for Staff Nurse Louise

Louise was a newly qualified – and, therefore, relatively inexperienced – nurse, who made a decision based on her personal value system. It was one that she felt would be in the best interests of the patient and her family.

Observations

In her efforts to help the patient, and therefore do good overall, Louise's actions could be interpreted as paternalistic. She, correctly, felt strongly that telling the truth and candour are core nursing values. However, this case is not straightforward.

The patient in this case can be described as 'more than ordinarily vulnerable' (Sellman, 2011). The consequences of Louise's decision could be serious for all family members. What the right thing to do is not clear.

Louise was not comfortable colluding with the patient and her sister by lying to their parents, and she should have made that clear to both of them. Furthermore, rather than act alone, Louise could have consulted with more senior colleagues about this issue.

Nurses must demonstrate ethical sensitivity when faced with difficult decisions. Also, when considering context in decision-making, this should also include level of experience. As a more junior nurse in terms of experience, Louise should have taken her lack of experience into account, considered her scope of practice and sought guidance from others. *The Code* directs that a nurse should 'ask for help from a suitably qualified and experienced professional to carry out any action or procedure that is beyond the limits of your competence' (2018e: 13).

Louise's competence in general as a young nurse is not in question here, but her competence regarding handling this ethical dilemma may be. This was likely to be the first time Louise found herself in this position, so she should have stopped to consider her competence to arrive at the right decision. Competence is not constant– nurses may be fully competent in many areas of practice, but still find themselves in a situation where they consider themselves inexperienced or lacking in competence. It is at this point that a nurse must be confident enough to ask for help or guidance (NMBI, 2021). The family dynamics were not considered either. Louise failed to consider the impact of her intended actions.

The Code requires that nurses recognise the limits of their competence, and endeavour to examine any potential risks to patients. Louise did not pay due attention to these requirements.

Following your reading and reflection on all the case studies in this chapter (see Chapter 4 for models of reflection to help you do this), consider the prompts in Box 5.1 and how these can be helpful when you need to make choices or a decision in learning situations that arise in practice.

Box 5.1

Prompts to Aid Ethical or Moral Decision-Making

- Values
- Context
- Level of experience
- Relationships
- Professional standards
- Ethical principles
- Tell the truth
- Raise concerns
- Courage
- Resilience

To ensure that you know what to consider when you have to make decisions in your nursing or practice that have an ethical dimension, you will find a number of helpful points to consider in the checklist in Box 5.2.

Box 5.2

Observation Points to Aid Ethical Decision-Making

- Pay attention to a person's right to self-determination and to make decisions concerning their own treatment and care.
- Accept that your values may differ from those of the person you are caring for.
- Accept that your values may differ from those of other members of the team.
- Ensure that the person's wishes are foremost in all decision-making.
- Engage in shared decision-making whenever possible.
- Ensure that you communicate all relevant information effectively and appropriately to the person that you are providing care for.
- Ensure that you recognise and acknowledge biases.
- Ensure that you protect people from harm or potential harm and maintain safety at all times.
- Ensure that your knowledge is up-to-date and evidence-based.
- Ensure that you acknowledge your level of experience or any lack of experience.
- Ensure that you recognise the unique vulnerabilities of all parties in any situation.
- Pay attention to ethical principles, standards for practice and relevant guidelines.
- Be able to provide rationales for actions or for not taking actions based on the standards, guidelines and ethical principles.

Conclusion

In this chapter we have looked at the nature of ethical or moral decision-making in health care. We have seen how values and ethical principles might influence our thinking regarding doing the right thing when ethical or moral issues arise in our clinical practice. By means of everyday scenarios, we have learnt that ethical or moral decision-making is not simply confined to the 'big issues' but can and does occur in relation to the simplest nursing tasks. The intent behind each scenario was to ask you to think about decision-making in terms of what is 'the right thing to do'. Nurses, by virtue of their close proximity to patients, their inherent compassion and their professional regulations, may find themselves having to decide on 'the right thing to do' within a constrained context. A context can be the environment in which care is delivered, patients' wishes, personal and professional values, levels of experience or the availability or use of resources. During the pandemic, the context of care, both in hospitals and community settings, had a major impact on the agency of nurses as accountable practitioners and as individuals. It also posed challenges to how nurses practice, how they think about their practice and how they make decisions in practice.

As the case studies demonstrated, attention must be paid to context, but also to possible outcomes as a result of decision-making. Outcomes for the patient are of paramount importance, but outcomes for family, society, the nurse or the nursing profession must also be considered.

References

Ausserhofer, D., Zander, B., Busse, R., Schubert, M., De Geest, S. et al. (2014). Prevalence, patterns and predictors of nursing care left undone in European hospitals: Results from the multicountry cross-sectional RN4CAST study. *BMJ Quality & Safety*, 23(2): 126–135.

Bickhoff, L., Sinclair, P. M. and Levett-Jones, T. (2017). Moral courage in undergraduate nursing students: A literature review. *Collegian*, 24: 71–83.

Brennan, D. and Timmins, F. (2012). Changing institutional identities of the student nurse. *Nurse Education Today*, 32(7): 747–751.

Chalmers, H. (1995). Accountability in nursing models and the nursing process. I R. Watson, R. (ed.), *Accountability in Nursing Practice*. London: Chapman Hall. pp. 33–48.

Department of Health (2015). *Safeguarding Policy*. London: The Stationery Office.

Francis, R. (2013). *Report of the Mid Staffordshire NHS Foundation Trust Public Inquiry* (Volume 1–3). London: The Stationery Office.

Francis, R. (2015). *Freedom to Speak Up: An independent review into creating an open and honest reporting culture in the NHS*. London: The Stationery Office.

Fry, S. T. and Johnstone, M. (2008). *Ethics in Nursing Practice: A Guide to Ethical decision-making*. Oxford: Blackwell Publishing.

Jones, T. L., Hamilton, P. and Murray, N. (2015). Unfinished nursing care: State of the science. *International Journal of Nursing Studies*, 52(6): 1121–1137.

Kalisch, B. (2006). Missed nursing care: A qualitative study. *Journal of Nursing Care Quality*, 21(4): 306–313.

Kalisch, B., Landstrom, K. and William, B. K. (2009). A comparison of patient care units with high versus low levels of missed nursing care. *Health Care Management*, 37(4): 320–328.

Lachman, V. D. (2009). *Ethical Challenges in Healthcare: Developing your moral compass*. New York: Springer.

Lachman, V. D. (2010). Strategies necessary for moral courage. *The Online Journal of Issues in Nursing*, 15(3).

Lachman, V. D. (2016). Moral resilience: Managing and preventing moral distress and moral residue. *MEDSURG Nursing*, 25(2): 121–124.

Leuter, C., Petrucci, C., Mattei, A., Tabassi, G. and Lancia, L. (2013). Ethical difficulties in nursing, educational needs and attitudes about using ethics resources. *Nursing Ethics*, 20(3): 348–358.

Levett-Jones, T. and Lathlean, J. (2007). Belongingness: A montage of nursing students' stories of their clinical placement experiences. *Contemporary Nurse*, 24: 162–174.

Levett-Jones, T. and Lathlean, J. (2008). Belongingness: A prerequisite for nursing students' clinical learning. *Nurse Education in Practice*, 8: 103–111.

Levett-Jones, T. and Lathlean, J. (2009). 'Don't rock the boat': Nursing students' experiences of conformity and compliance. *Nurse Education Today*, 29: 342–349.

Lucero, R. J., Lake, E. T. and Aiken, L. H. (2010). Nursing care quality and adverse events in US hospitals. *Journal of Clinical Nursing*, 19: 2185–2195.

Mallari, M. G. D. and Tariman, J. D. (2013). Ethical frameworks for decision-making in nursing practice and research: An integrative literature review. *Journal of Nursing Practice Applications and Reviews of Research*, 7(1): 50–57.

McKenna, H. (2019). COVID-19: Ethical issues for nurses. *International Journal of Nursing Studies*, 110(2): 103673.

Melia, C. (1987). *The Occupational Socialization of Nurses*. London: Tavistock.

Nursing and Midwifery Council (NMC) (n.d.). *Guidance on using Social Media Responsibly*. London: NMC.

Nursing and Midwifery Council (NMC) (2018a). *Future Nurse: Standards of proficiency for registered nurses*. London: NMC.

Nursing and Midwifery Council (NMC) (2018e). *The Code: Professional standards of practice and behaviour for nurses, midwives and nursing associates*. London: NMC.

Nursing and Midwifery Council (NMC) (2022). *Current Recovery Programme Standards*. London: NMC.

Nursing and Midwifery Board of Ireland (NMBI) (2021). *Code of Professional Conduct and Ethics for Registered Nurses and Registered Midwives*. Dublin: NMBI.

Papastavrou, E., Panayiota, A. and Georgios, E. (2014). The hidden ethical element of nursing care rationing. *Nursing Ethics*, 21(5): 583–593.

Schubert, M., Glass, T. R., Clarke, S. P., Aiken, L. H., Schaffert-Witvliet, B., Slone, D. M. and De Geest, S. (2008). Rationing of nursing care and its relationship to patient outcomes: The Swiss extension of the International Hospital Outcomes Study. *International Journal for Quality in Healthcare*, 20(4): 227–237.

Scruth, E. A., Pugh, D. M., Adams, C. L. and Foss-Durant, A. M. (2015). Electronic and social media: The legal and ethical issues for healthcare. *Clinical Nurse Specialist*, 29(1): 8–11.

Sellman, D. (2011). *What Makes a Good Nurse: Why the virtues are important for nurses*. London: Jessica Kingsley.

Semple, M. and Cable, S. (2003) The new code of professional conduct. *Nursing Standard*, 17(23): 40–48.

Sochalski, J. (2004). Is more better?: The relationship between nurse staffing and the quality of nursing care in hospitals. *Medical Care*, 42(2): 67–73.

Thompson, I. E., Melia, K., Boyd, K. M. and Horsburgh, D. (2006). *Nursing Ethics*, 5th edn. Edinburgh: Churchill Livingstone.

Weaver, K., Morse, J. and Mitcham, C. (2008). Ethical sensitivity in professional practice: Concept analysis. *Journal of Advanced Nursing*, 62(5): 607–618.

Further Reading

Ball, J. E., Murrells, T., Rafferty, A. M, Morrow, E. and Griffiths, P. (2014). Care left undone during nursing shifts: Associations with workload and perceived quality of care. *BMJ Quality & Safety*, 23(2): 116–125.

Robinson, S. and Doody, O. (2021). *Nursing and Healthcare Ethics*, 6th edn. Edinburgh: Elsevier Health.

Romero-García, M., Delgado-Hito, P., Gálvez-Herrer, Antonio Ángel-Sesmero, M. J., Raquel Velasco-Sanz, T., Benito-Aracil, L. and Heras-La Calle, G. (2022). Moral distress, emotional impact and coping in intensive care unit staff during the outbreak of COVID-19. *Intensive and Critical Care Nursing*, 103206.

White, S., Tait, D. and Scammell, J. (2021). Nursing students' evolving professional values: Capturing their journey through co-operative inquiry. *Nurse Education in Practice*, 54: 103117.

Web Resources

Nursing and Midwifery Council (NMC): www.nmc.org.uk (accessed 15 August 2022).

Information for students and educators: Coronavirus (COVID-19): Information and advice: www.nmc.org.uk/news/coronavirus/information-for-students-and-educators (accessed 10 July 2022).

Current Recovery Programme Standards (updated January 2022): https://www.nmc.org.uk/globalassets/sitedocuments/education-standards/current-recovery-programme-standards.pdf (accessed 10 July 2022).

NMC Guidance on the use of social media. Accessed on 10/7/2022 via: https://www.nmc.org.uk/globalassets/sitedocuments/nmc-publications/social-media-guidance.pdf (accessed 15 August 2022).

Nursing and Midwifery Board of Ireland NMBI - the regulatory body for nursing and midwifery in Ireland: www.nmbi.ie (accessed 15 August 2022).

The International Council of Nurses (2021) *The ICN Code of Ethics for Nurses*: www.icn.ch/system/files/2021-10/ICN_Code-of-Ethics_EN_Web_0.pdf (accessed 21 June 2022).

6

COMMUNICATION SKILLS AND DECISION-MAKING IN PRACTICE

Jenni Templeman and Karen Holland

Chapter objectives

The aims of this chapter are to:

- explore a range of communication strategies as they relate to decision-making;
- explore how communication can influence how we relate to others through our interpersonal skills;

- use case studies to explore how student nurses can meet the NMC's (2018a) proficiencies in relation to communication and communication skills;
- explore how effective communication skills are essential in decision-making situations in nursing practice.

Introduction

This chapter explores the various aspects of communication and how these relate to our own interpersonal skills when communicating with others. The effectiveness of our communication – that is, how good we are at passing on information and ensuring that another person understands what we are trying to say – has a direct effect on both our own decision-making skills and the decisions made by those around us.

We have all come across health care professionals who have a good 'bedside manner' and those who do not. Historically, this term has been used to describe those who can communicate effectively and relate to patients as human beings. It is very important that, through the words we use, the person listening is able to understand what we mean. In nursing and health care generally, there is an increasing emphasis on communication as a means of building therapeutic relationships with both patients and their relatives.

It is important to note here that the global pandemic due to COVID-19 meant that there was a significant change in how communication had to be arranged between these groups, often in very distressing circumstances. Patients had to be hospitalised, some for long periods, without any face-to-face contact with family and others close to them. When communication was possible, it had to be undertaken via phone or the Internet, with the support of nurses and other members of the health care teams caring for patients in hospital settings. In community settings, especially nursing and care homes, the situation was similar. There have been poignant images of family members at the windows of their relatives' rooms at care homes in the press and on television. In addition, communication between health professionals and patients has been affected by the wearing of masks of various kinds and other protective clothing, depending on the severity of the physical needs of the patients, with battling the effects of the virus on their bodies being the priority. Talking to patients who were on ventilators in intensive care units during the various peaks of the virus contagion was also a challenge.

Communication using new technologies, and the ease of access to these by the wider community, extends far beyond patients' reliance on others for information about their health and well-being. It now encompasses the building of a more interpersonal form of communication, in which patients can be viewed as 'the expert' in their conversations with nurses and doctors, an increased awareness of cultural influences and the use of social networking sites, as well as the numerous Internet sites now available, offering possible diagnoses and treatment options for the general public.

For those patients who have been hospitalised as a result of serious side effects of the virus, however, this engagement has been problematic. Only after they were discharged from hospital were they perceived as 'experts' on its impact on their health and lives, with many appearing on various social media platforms and in the press, advising people about their symptoms and, in the majority of cases, for everyone to adhere to government guidance and to stay as safe as possible.

Making decisions about patients' health and, often, whether or not to accept those made on their behalf by others, is a real challenge for health professionals when communicating with patients and their families. In normal circumstances, it is part of a nurse's role to make decisions *with* patients and their families, not *for* them, and to understand the importance of learning how to how engage and communicate well with people. This is clearly evident in the fact that the NMC's (2018a) *Future Nurse: Standards of proficiency for registered nurses* now includes a set of proficiencies (across seven key areas of practice – called 'platforms' – see Chapter 1) with outcomes, from which it is evident that, to achieve them, there is an implicit recognition that it is essential to communicate effectively and appropriately. In addition, this document includes two Annexes with Annexe A specifically stating what communication and relationship management skills 'a newly registered nurse must be able to demonstrate in order to meet the proficiency outcomes' (NMC, 2018a: 27). It further states that:

> Effective communication is central to the provision of safe and compassionate person-centred care. Registered nurses in all fields of nursing practice must be able to demonstrate the ability to communicate and manage relationships with people of all ages with a range of mental, physical, cognitive and behavioural health challenges.

> This is because a diverse range of communication and relationship management skills is required to ensure that individuals, their families and carers are actively involved in and understand care decisions. These skills are vital when making accurate, culturally aware assessments of care needs and ensuring that the needs, priorities, expertise and preferences of people are always valued and taken into account. (NMC, 2018a: 27)

These skills are relevant to nurses in all fields of practice and also apply to all care settings. Regardless of the environment in which student nurses may find themselves undertaking a learning placement, then, achieving effective communication with others, as well as demonstrating the skills required to do so, have to be achieved as part of their registration as a qualified nurse. Effective communication and understanding patterns of communication and behaviour are central, core elements of nursing practice.

Let us look at some examples of these in Box 6.1 and then complete Activity 6.1.

Box 6.1

Annexe A, Section 3: Evidence-Based, Best Practice Communication Skills and Approaches for Providing Therapeutic Interventions (NMC 2018a: 27/28)

At the point of registration, the registered nurse will be able to safely demonstrate the following skills.

1.1   underpinning communication skills for assessing, planning, providing and managing best practice, evidence-based nursing care

1.2   actively listen, recognise and respond to verbal and non-verbal cues

1.3   use prompts and positive verbal and non-verbal reinforcement

1.4   use appropriate non-verbal communication including touch, eye contact and personal space

1.5   make appropriate use of open and closed questioning

1.6   use caring conversation techniques

1.7   check understanding and use clarification techniques

1.8   be aware of own unconscious bias in communication encounters

1.9   write accurate, clear, legible records and documentation

1.10 confidently and clearly present and share verbal and written reports with individuals and groups

1.11 analyse and clearly record and share digital information and data

1.12 provide clear verbal, digital or written information and instructions when delegating or handing over responsibility for care

1.13 recognise the need for, and facilitate access to, translator services and material. (2018a: 28)

Activity 6.1

1. You can see that the stem of the main overarching outcome to be achieved with regard to communication skills to be used in patient care includes the phrase 'evidence-based'. To achieve proficiency in the skills listed in Annexe A, Section 1, as a student nurse, you are expected not only to carry them out but also to know why you are doing so, underpinned by your knowledge of the evidence available to ensure best practice.

2. Imagine that your practice assessor is asking you to tell them what this evidence is that you, as a future registered nurse, are expected to adhere to, both from the NMC's (2018e) *The Code: Professional standards of practice and behaviour for nurses, midwives and nursing associates* and from any other literature you are aware of that you can use to inform your response.

3. As a goal agreed with your personal (academic) tutor, choose three of these specific skills and make a record in your ongoing reflective diary of how you have achieved them in your practice as a student nurse, together with the evidence base underpinning best practice in those areas.

Some of you may also be completing specific communication-related modules. The information you gather for Activity 6.1 may help you in writing an essay for one of those parts of your studies too. An example could be reflecting on the overarching skills related to assessing, planning, providing and managing care for a specific patient or client you met during your placement. You would need to offer, for example, an understanding of the needs of individuals from different cultures, especially in relation to their being able to communicate verbally with you in either English or their own main language. Also your ability to communicate with different people in a care context will depend on your understanding of how they view non-verbal communication, such as touch and personal space (Holland, 2020), or the importance of asking about their cultural or spiritual beliefs based on your own reading and evidence to underpin your assessment (see the Further reading section at the end of this chapter and Case study 6.4 for more information regarding communicating with patients when English is not their first language).

Communication Skills: A General Overview

In the course of our development as human beings, one of the first skills that we learned was to communicate ideas through the medium of language. This we developed and refined from mere sounds to form commonly understood words and phrases (Bach and Grant, 2010). Over time, our methods of communication, in written and spoken form, have become increasingly sophisticated. In the present day, we have highly advanced technologies and networks at our disposal, such as digital forms of communication, the Internet, workplace intranet and social networking sites (Webb, 2011).

There are so many different facets of communication involved in clinical practice today that it would be impossible to define them all, but we can consider some of the more general ones. For example, Balzer-Riley considers that 'Communication involves the reciprocal process in which messages are sent and received between two or more people' (2004: 6), whilst Hargie and Dickson suggest that 'interpersonal communication can be thought of as a process that is transactional, purposeful, multi-dimensional, irreversible and (possibly) inevitable' (2004: 41).

Nursing involves the need for good communication skills that have a therapeutic effect on the delivery of good care. That is because nurses who can communicate at an emotional level are seen as warm, caring and empathetic (Webb, 2011). Those who possess such qualities instil trust and confidence in others which can foster care related conversations. Opening up dialogue in this way enables patients to be actively involved in their care and choice of treatment options, including self-care at the point of being discharged from health or social care services.

Research consistently suggests that when nurses provide a good environment, use therapeutic communication and give accurate information, patients experience positive health benefits, such as reduced pain and lowered blood pressure (Kwekkeboom, 1997; Webb, 2011). The patient profile in current nursing practice is a complex blend of both acute and chronic illness, with an emphasis on patient choice, self-care, individual patient preferences and incorporating their values and expectations with regard to treatment options.

Both written and spoken forms of communication are important ways to transmit vital information about patient issues in nursing. It is through effective and good communication, and the development of therapeutic relationships between nurses and patients, that nurses can identify their unique individual needs (Foy and Timmins, 2004; Sharples and Elcock, 2011). Patients need to be listened to, to feel that their concerns are being addressed, be supported and to feel understood within this therapeutic relationship (Gilbert and Leahy, 2007). Some nurses appear to have a natural ability to communicate with people, whilst others have to learn and master this skill. Being able to communicate verbally with people, for example – regardless of how easy or difficult you may find it at first – is something you can work on and develop over the course of your learning, both on placement and at university. To gain proficiency the evidence-base underpinning how and why you do this is an essential requirement.

It is also important to remember that students will have some learning in common regardless of their eventual field of nursing practice; but application of skills is required for everyone. Experiencing a different placement during your course of study will bring you into contact with different people, including other team colleagues who also have to be communicated with, but also different people at different times of the day or night. The context in which you communicate with people is as important as how you communicate with them. Complete Activity 6.2 to reflect on some of the learning experiences you have had during placements.

Activity 6.2

1. Consider your learning experience in *one* recent practice placement.
2. What was the main mode of communication in that placement?
3. What kinds of communication skills did you use? (See the skills in Box 6.1 at the beginning of this chapter.)
4. What impact did the environment that you were in have on communication in general?
5. What do you think were your challenges?

A possible example of a recent placement could be a busy A&E department or a secure mental health unit. Even the names of these placement areas will already give you an idea of the overall environment in which you will be expected to further develop your ability to communicate effectively, with patients and people generally – patients' families, members of the multidisciplinary team and other professionals. In addition, each placement will have its own system of non-verbal communication, such as documentation, nursing language and terminology to be learnt, as well as a myriad of other skills that are needed to translate what you know about therapeutic intervention skills into action (NMC, 2018a: 29).

We can now look at various forms of communication in order for you to start building up your evidence base (see also Chapter 3, on the key skills of evidence-based decision-making).

Verbal Communication

We use verbal communication in every aspect of our daily lives, so it is surprising that we are not experts in this particular skill. As we have seen, communication lies at the heart of nursing and, together with interpersonal and decision-making skills, it underpins all phases of clinical practice, for both student and qualified nurses. Communication and interpersonal skills are inseparable from the care and compassion that we give to our patients. *Effective* communication is a continuous thread and theme throughout nursing, and, together with the interpersonal skills, fosters quality and competent caring (Sharples and Elcock, 2011).

Communication (both verbal and written) is a prerequisite to competent nursing practice because it is a way to transmit vital information about patients in terms of both the care given to them and documenting the findings. For example, nurses use verbal communication in important ways on a daily basis but, often, this information is misunderstood. Miscommunication of patient information occurs, which may lead to health errors and can be detrimental to patient care. These mistakes are sometimes evident in the adherence to times for administering medication (see Tiwary et al., 2019).

Within any health care setting, students need to adjust to different clinical placement environments, each with its own particular jargon and specialist language. Also, in the specialised area of theatre, voices are often muffled as a result of the face masks that need to be worn. The nursing and medical personnel also speak in their 'theatre' jargon, which may be misinterpreted and not understood. This specialised jargon and language is apparent in each of the specialty disciplines within healthcare practice. This concept of new or unfamiliar language and terminology within health care is often different from the language that students use in their off-duty time (Holland, 2020).

During your professional development, even as a qualified nurse, you may experience a lack of communication confidence following a distressing and challenging situation communicating with a patient, which may lead to a certain degree of stress and anxiety. However, one of the best ways to improve your verbal communication skills is to develop your listening skills (Sharples and Elcock, 2011).

Active Listening

To develop your listening skills, you will need to develop your *active listening* skills, because the reason that you speak is either to pass on information to other people or listen to what they have to say. Miscommunication will occur if the information that you pass on is not clear or clearly understood.

Hearing is part of active listening, as is the recognition of non-verbal communication, often referred to as 'body language' (McCabe and Timmins, 2013). Always check that information has been clearly delivered in your communications with patients and colleagues. When either speaking or listening, check whether or not the person you are talking to can actually hear you or is able to talk back to you. For example, communicating and listening actively with someone who is hard of hearing and wears hearing aids or has had a stroke impacting their speech, is very different to talking with someone who has no such challenges.

Active listening also means that you are paying attention to what is being said and how it is being said (Sharples and Elcock, 2011). Eye contact, head-nodding and facial expressions are body postures and gestures that may give you an indication of whether your communication is clear, and if you are being understood. In clinical practice, a nurse may ask the patient if they have understood what has been explained, because active listening is a deliberate commitment to engage fully with everyone – colleagues, patients and staff (Foy and Timmins, 2004).

Another aspect of active listening is being able to remain silent and allow the other person to speak. Nurses sometimes have difficulty doing this, especially when breaking bad news, as their instinct is to want to keep reassuring the person receiving the bad news. We can see the importance of listening to people on the phone, for example, in organisations such as the Samaritans who are a 'listening service'. Unlike nurses however those engaged voluntarily in listening to phone calls or engaging in responding to 'live' texts, do not engage in therapeutic engagement with the caller. See Box 6.2 for the key aspects of active listening for nurses.

Box 6.2

Active Listening as a Nurse

Active listening involves:

- Looking directly at people when you are speaking and when they are speaking to you.
- Not interrupting people when they are speaking.

- Observing others' body language and taking note of what they say.
- Reflecting your feelings in your body language and facial expression.
- Observing people for feedback on your communication.

Developing Communication Skills: Scenario-based Learning

So far, we have considered the main types of communication skill required as a nurse and how you might approach the interpersonal aspects of communication. Now we will explore some possible scenarios that you may come across in practice placements and elsewhere in your learning experience.

To ensure that you are fully aware of all aspects of your professional accountability, personal knowledge and development, access and read *The Code* (NMC, 2018e), which also includes guidance on record-keeping, and the Nursing and Midwifery Council (NMC) *Standards of proficiency for registered nurses* (NMC, 2018a) including Annexe A: Communication skills. Use these to help you to consider how learning from the case studies can help you to achieve the required communication proficiencies.

Now consider Case study 6.1 and then undertake Activity 6.3 that relates specifically to the content of the case study.

CASE STUDY 6.1: COMMUNICATING WITH A DYING PERSON

An 80-year-old man, recently diagnosed with terminal cancer, is admitted to the oncology ward for pain management. Jo, a third-year student nurse, is conducting his admission in a friendly, yet professional, manner. The patient says to Jo, 'I want to die at home in my own surroundings, not in hospital. I know I'm going to die soon.'

Jo is a little taken aback by this statement but remembers what she has been taught about active listening skills and showing warmth, empathy and friendliness towards patients, who put their trust in a nurse. Jo draws the curtains around the patient's bed to maintain privacy and moves a chair closer to the patient. She holds his hand and asks him if he would like to talk about his feelings related to what he has just said. Jo maintains eye contact with the patient and makes sure that her facial expressions and gestures reflect her interest in and understanding of what the patient is saying. Jo's professional and friendly manner has developed into a trusting and respectful therapeutic relationship between herself and the patient. The patient asks Jo a few questions that she cannot answer, so she suggests that the patient ask her practice supervisor, who is a qualified palliative care nurse, and the doctor.

After their discussion, Jo tells the patient that she has documented his request in his care plan and that, with his permission, she will discuss his request with her mentor and supervisor first. Jo and her supervisor then arrange a meeting between the doctor and the patient to enable him to discuss his concerns and his request to die at home. The patient had given his permission for Jo to discuss his request and concerns with her mentor or supervisor.

──── Activity 6.3 ────

Identify the main communication issues identified in Case study 6.1.

1. Do you think that Jo's active listening skills were effective?
2. Did Jo adhere to the NMC's *The Code* (2018e) with regard to confidentiality and disclosure?
3. In what other ways could Jo support the patient with regard to seeking more information?
4. Do you think that holding a patient's hand could be therapeutic?
5. Would you feel comfortable talking to a patient about dying and death?
6. What evidence and knowledge could be helpful to you if you were in a similar situation to Jo's?
7. Consider your responses in relation to achieving the major proficiency set out in Box 6.1: Annexe A, Section 3: Evidence-based, best practice communication skills and approaches for providing therapeutic interventions (2018a: 29) and then access the NMC Standards and outcomes for platform 1: Professional accountability, to determine how the communication skills in Box 6.3 will help you to become proficient.

──── Box 6.3 ────

Platform 1: Being an accountable professional

Registered nurses act in the best interests of people, putting them first and providing nursing care that is person-centred, safe and compassionate. They act professionally at all times and use their knowledge and experience to make evidence-based decisions about care. They communicate effectively, are role models for others, and are accountable for their actions. Registered nurses continually reflect on their practice and keep abreast of new and emerging developments in nursing, health and care. (NMC, 2018a: 7)

From this we can see, for example, that evidence-based decisions about care are central to achieving proficiency, as is communicating effectively. To provide person-centred, safe and compassionate care also requires you to use 'caring conversation techniques', as well as actively listening and ensuring that any verbal and non-verbal communication actions are in keeping with *The Code* (NMC, 2018e) and professional accountability.

Written Communication

During your course of study, there are numerous opportunities for you to learn about written communication and how to document aspects of both patient care and your own personal and professional development. Student nurses learn how to document patients' notes, records, charts and nursing care plans, under the supervision and guidance of a practice supervisor or other appropriate health care personnel. There are legal and ethical reasons why student nurses are guided by their practice supervisors who are registered nurses when completing documentation with regards to patient care. The student nurse's documentation and record-keeping are always reviewed and countersigned by a qualified nurse. Once qualified, the nurse is professionally accountable and responsible for their acts and omissions regarding documentation and record-keeping according to the laws of the country and the NMC (2018e: 10: section related to record-keeping and documentation).

As a student nurse, you will have numerous opportunities to practice your verbal skills independently but will not have had the same opportunities for independently practising record-keeping, that is, without your decisions being countersigned as appropriate. (See the Web resources section at the end of this chapter for a link to an example of a Practice Assessment Record and Evaluation tool, which is used in partnership with its practice placement partners.)

Once you are qualified as a registered nurse, your literacy (or written word) will be judged as being a key part of your ability to deliver high-quality care, as evidenced by concrete skills, such as your charting, record-keeping and writing abilities and, of course, patient assessment and documenting care (Anders, Douglas and Harrigan, 1995; Learner, 2006; Sharples and Elcock, 2011). To explore this issue of documentation as communication, consider Case study 6.2 and complete Activity 6.4 which focuses especially on decision-making.

■■■■■■■ CASE STUDY 6.2: DOCUMENTING ■■■■■■■ PATIENT OBSERVATIONS

Anna is a first-year student nurse who commenced her nursing programme six months ago. She is working on the surgical ward at an NHS Trust hospital in the UK. After talking to her main practice supervisor about previous experience in practice and what she has learnt in the clinical simulation sessions at university, he has delegated to Anna taking and recording the patients' four-hourly physiological observations in a six-bed area of the ward. This activity involves taking each patient's temperature, respiratory rate, blood pressure, pulse rate, level of consciousness and urinary output, then recording the findings on the modified early warning scoring (MEWS) chart.

Mr Robin is an older person in bed five in this small ward area. He underwent abdominal surgery two days ago and still has an intravenous infusion and urinary catheter in situ, a nasogastric tube on free drainage and a large abdominal wound.

Anna introduces herself to him and requests permission to conduct the observations. She makes sure that Mr Robin is comfortable before proceeding. She notices that he seems to be drowsier than he was earlier when she first met him after starting her shift. Prior to and after taking his observations, Anna checks his name, age and patient number on both the chart and his armband.

Whilst documenting the observations on the MEWS chart, Anna notices that the patient's MEWS scoring at 7, thus indicating deterioration in the patients' condition. Also, a small volume of urine in his catheter bag is also rather dark and concentrated. Anna remembers that a score of 3 is normal for the MEWS assessment, as she was taught this at university and by one of her practice supervisors on the ward.

Anna makes Mr Robin comfortable, reassures him after taking his observations and hurries off to report the MEWS chart findings to a qualified member of staff on her team.

Activity 6.4

1. Identify the main communication and decision-making issues in Case study 6.2.
2. Do you think that Anna responded correctly, reporting the patient's observations immediately?
3. Was her behaviour towards the patient professional?
4. Did she act within her scope of practice as a student nurse according to *The Code* (NMC, 2018e)?
5. The registered nurse she reported her findings to immediately reviewed the patient and contacted the hospital's critical care outreach team, because the patient's condition could deteriorate rapidly and put his health in danger. The outreach nurse assessed Mr Robin and prescribed additional intravenous fluids for him and hourly observations.
6. Why do you think the outreach nurse prescribed additional fluids and hourly observations? How did she arrive at those decisions from the verbal and non-verbal communication with the student and the registered nurse? (See the Web resources section at the end of this chapter for a link to a booklet by the National Institute for Health and Care Excellence (NICE) (2018) for critical care outreach teams.)

Issues to Consider Regarding Communication

Anna's named practice supervisor thanked her for responding so swiftly and acting in an intelligent and efficient way. In addition, she thanked her for both reporting her observations and findings and reassuring Mr Robin.

Anna and her supervisor worked together to update Mr Robin's care plan and ensured that the changes advised by the outreach staff were documented in the doctor's notes. The doctor in charge was also informed about this and the change to the patient's care.

As this event was part of Anna's learning experience whilst on placement, her nominated practice supervisor documented her actions in Anna's placement document. At university, Anna's personal academic tutor congratulated her on the excellent final report she had been given from the placement. Anna had based one of her written reflections on practice for her ongoing learning portfolio on this event. This enabled Anna and her personal tutor to discuss the situation in more detail – in particular, the fact that what she recorded not only showed how she had undertaken observations and recorded them but also how she was learning to make a link between physiological observations and decision-making, resulting in prompt action to ensure the safety of the patient in her care (see also Chapter 12 for more on decision-making in complex situations). Documenting and recording care can be via paper-based or computer-based care-planning tools. In Anna's case, initially, all the recordings and observations were made in writing on the official charts used to document them.

We can also begin to see the way in which Anna documents her actions and the patient's situation in practice. She has clearly showed communication between her and her personal tutor as well as ensuring that she has completed a written reflection record for her learning portfolio. She can come back to this record in the future when she is more experienced as a student nurse, to compare similar learning situations.

You may already have records of your own experiences, similar to Anna's, that you can refer to and, using your chosen reflective tool (see Chapter 4 for examples), can reflect on a recent written example in your practice reflection documentation and compare it with past examples of written documentation (so for example, you can compare your documentation from the first year to that produced during your second and/or third years). Has your documentation and writing ability changed and improved?

You may require additional support with writing nursing documentation, and it is important that you discuss this with your personal tutor and share your specific learning needs with your practice supervisors and assessors.

Reflection and improving your reflective practice are important for this and generally but also for evidence given during the NMC's revalidation process to maintain your registration at intervals after you have qualified. This process was updated in 2021 (see the Web resources section at the end of this chapter for a link).

From the example of Anna's experience in Case study 6.2, we can see that communication of different kinds is linked inextricably with decision-making. Anna also showed us, by reporting her findings to her practice supervisor immediately, that she made her decision within the limits of her own competence and, therefore, the NMC's (2018a) *Standards of proficiency* according to her stage of progression on the course.

Communicating Through Social Networking Sites

Communication and making decisions are not restricted to clinical decisions, however. Increasingly, NHS Trusts, for example, offer us an insight into what care is available within individual, local NHS Trusts but also how well they are doing in terms of patient care. In addition, many organisations now use a variety of modes of communication to offer information to both staff and patients. (See the Web resources section at the end of this chapter for a link to example policies and how various social media modes can be used.)

The development and use of social networking sites, plus the facility provided by instant messaging, have expanded exponentially in recent years. Estimates of its usage from a number of online sites reported that this was around 2.45 billion active users per month in the third quarter of 2019, with Facebook the biggest social network in the world. In 2021, this figure for active users per month had increased to 2.91 million (Statista, 2021). Naturally, use has also increased among those working as nurses, midwives, health visitors and so on and, in turn, the NMC has had to rule on an increasing number of cases of inappropriate use of social media, resulting in some of those involved being disciplined and even removed from the register. (See the Web resources at the end of this chapter for a link to access the NMC's website for information on all cases its panels have heard, including those specifically related to social media behaviour.)

What is important is that the NMC shares the reporting of these serious cases via their website, making the cases visible to the public and to student nurses alike. In this way, the NMC is demonstrating its primary function to protect the public as decisions regarding fitness to practice are transparent. The cases also highlight the behaviours and standards expected of professional registrants.

Regarding social media specifically, it is not just about the part that social media plays in the behaviour of the nurses concerned but also how a series of events involving its use can result in nurses being reported for a fitness to practice issue.

To become more familiar with *The Code* (NMC, 2018e) for professional practice in relation to social media complete Activity 6.5.

Activity 6.5

1. Access and read the NMC's (n.d.) *Guidance on using Social Media Responsibly* (see the Web resources at the end of this chapter for the link).
2. Note the key issues related to the use of social media.
3. Consider the impact of these issues on the role of different health and social care professionals in a specific environment related to your own field of practice – that is, adult, learning disability, mental health or children and young people's nursing.
4. Search for codes of conduct in relation to social media in different countries and determine what the key similarities are between them all, in terms of their impact on how nurses should communicate with people in their care (see the Web resources section at the end of the chapter for the link to Australia's as an example).

Communication and Social Media for Student Nurses

We recognise the importance of the growing area of uncertainty for many student nurses in how to safely use social networking within their role as a student nurse and also ensure that use of any kind of social media interaction in a personal capacity does not impact on their current practice.

We wish to approach the issues from a communication and decision-making perspective. In this way, we hope to reaffirm the expectations that professional bodies worldwide, such as the NMC in the UK, have of all nurses regarding social media and professional behaviour.

With the development of instant messaging, social networking platforms and other forms of online communication, we can transmit and receive information almost instantaneously. What we divulge may be visible on personal websites and blogs, discussion boards and in emails. This also applies to all kinds of content shared online, whether in the form of text, photographs, other images, videos or audio files. Increasingly, organisations, too, have come to rely on instant messaging to transmit information to large numbers of people. The NMC and most universities also engage with students in this way, as do many other professional bodies with their members worldwide.

On a more practical, day-to-day level, we, as health care professionals, use the media to communicate with our peers, family and others, so it is essential that we use them responsibly to ensure that those communications abide by our professional code of conduct. This, of course, also applies to students and qualified nurses and midwives working in other parts of the world as it does to those working in the UK.

Unfortunately, many student nurses have needed to be disciplined on the basis of their fitness to practice because of issues arising as a consequence of an ill thought through comment, the posting of an inappropriate photograph on a social networking site or an inappropriate text to a 'friend'. The instantaneous nature of these networking sites leaves little time for us to reflect as we are swept along in the spontaneity of the moment when we send messages to others. The key has been pressed before we have time to reconsider if it was the right thing to do!

Now read Case study 6.3, as cited in Chadwick (2013), which is called 'a cautionary tale'. To add to your understanding of communication and social media in relation to professional accountability, access the NMC's (2020.) *Caring with Confidence: The Code in action* and watch the related short animation resources on the use of social media, as well as other key themes focused on upholding *The Code* (see the Web resources section at the end of this chapter for the links).

■■■■■■■ CASE STUDY 6.3: SHARING VIEWS THROUGH ■■■■■■■ SOCIAL MEDIA: A CAUTIONARY TALE

A student, unhappy with the way in which a lecturer delivered one of the teaching sessions in the university, posted a very derogatory review of the session on her Facebook site, including the lecturer's name and which university it was, and which course she was undertaking as well as what she thought personally about this lecturer. The outcome was of course that a colleague of the lecturer became aware of this public-facing message and escalated the incident to become a disciplinary matter, in which the student nurse's fitness to practice as a nurse was called into question. Her decision to write such a comment because she was angry about the session and the lecturer's teaching was no excuse, because there are formal mechanisms in most universities such as staff-student committees, that she might have used to explore these kinds of issues. In this case, the student decided for herself that she did not to want to be a nurse because of all the 'stupid rules' and she chose to leave the course before any disciplinary action could be taken (Chadwick, 2013: 95).

Now complete Activity 6.6 regarding the use of and access to your personal social networking site.

Activity 6.6

1. What are the privacy settings of one of your social networking sites?
2. Have you ever decided to accept someone on social media whom you did not know personally as a friend?
3. Are your friends real or virtual?
4. Access and watch again the short animation mentioned before Case Study 6.3 in relation to the social media section of the NMC's *Caring with Confidence: The Code in action* to reaffirm your understanding of the pitfalls to avoid.

The NMC (2019) clearly identifies that a health professional's behaviour in the 'real world' and that on social networking sites should be considered subject to the same professional acceptable standard, and that the same rules of conduct apply to both. The ever-increasing usage of social networking sites and the reliance on this form of rapid communication may result in this becoming an established method of communication between organisations and students, for example when their virtual online learning site is out of action and an urgent message is required to inform students of a change in their timetable. However, whilst the social norms of conduct and behaviour continue to evolve, the levels of acceptability in professional behaviours are a constant and should always be adhered to. See the following box for a list of some examples of the inappropriate use of social networking sites.

Box 6.4

Examples of Inappropriate Use of Social Networking Sites

(From the NMC's *Guide to Social media use* (2019: 3); see the Web resources for the link to the full guidance document)

- Posting inappropriate comments about colleagues or patients.
- Use of social networking sites to bully or intimidate colleagues.
- Pursuing personal relationships with patients or service users.
- Posting or distributing sexually explicit material.
- Using social networking sites in any way that is unlawful.
- Posting manipulated photos that are intended to mock individuals.

From this we can see that it is essential to maintain effective professional communications at all times for all media. To ensure that you are fully aware of your personal and professional responsibilities regarding social media and being a student, undertake Activity 6.7.

Activity 6.7

1. What specific guidance does your university set out regarding the use of social media, professional practice as a student nurse and any disciplinary processes?
2. Make a point of accessing and reading this, making a note of what is specified in your student portfolio or adding a link to it if you have an e-portfolio.

You also need to be aware of the myths surrounding what is acceptable in communication, particularly when using social networking sites, blogs or instant messaging (see Box 6.5 for examples).

Box 6.5

Myths about Social Networking Communications

- It is misguided to believe that any communications about work-related issues – including conversations about patients, complaints about colleagues or a clinical area – are private and anonymous.
- It is misguided to believe that any communications via social networking sites, blogs or instant messaging are private and can only be accessed by the intended recipients. Once a message has been posted, it can be disseminated to others easily.

- It is misguided to believe that sharing of patient information with another person is harmless, even if that private information is disclosed only to the intended recipient. This may still be a breach of confidentiality if the patient has not given permission for that information to be shared.
- It is misguided to believe that you may communicate with patients and service users, even if they are no longer in your care.

Communication and Decision-Making

Communication and decision-making are closely interwoven in nurses' daily clinical practice. Decision-making improves as nurses gain more experience of nursing different patients with different health issues and incorporate intuition and evidence-based research as sources of knowledge and information.

According to Thompson and Dowding (2002), clinical decision-making may be defined as choosing between alternatives. It is a process that, as nurses, we undertake on a daily basis when we make judgements about the care that we provide to our patients. It involves observation, critical thinking, evaluating the evidence, applying knowledge, problem solving, reflection and clinical judgement (Standing, 2010). As nurses gain experience, the process of clinical decision-making becomes easier.

Decision-making is a complex activity that also requires knowledge, intuition, and evidence-based practice based on robust research findings (see Chapter 1). The inexperienced or novice nurse is guided in clinical practice by the various protocols, guidelines, policies, and care pathways that can be used to make decisions, but as the nurse gains more experience, decision-making becomes more intuitive. This is a process of both personal and professional development, which, with time, empowers our clinical practice and sharpens our decision-making skills. The student nurse is continually learning these skills through observing more experienced staff making decisions within clinical practice. Evidence-based practice is a process by which nurses and other healthcare practitioners make clinical decisions using the best available research evidence, their clinical expertise, and patient preferences (Thompson, 2003). (See Chapter 3 for EBP and decision-making.)

Decision-making as a process helps the nurse to select the best course of action that optimises a patient's health and minimises any harm (Standing, 2010). The nurse is professionally accountable for accurately assessing a patient's needs using the appropriate sources of information and planning nursing interventions that address problems (Standing, 2010). These NMC (2018a) decision-making proficiencies will be evaluated throughout the student nurse's programme of learning, as will the achievement of competencies to be achieved by those students following the curriculum set for the earlier NMC Standards (NMC, 2010b). (See Chapter 1 for further information.)

In current nursing practice, shared decision-making with the service user is at the hub of patient-centred care and in keeping with nursing values (Sharples and Elcock, 2011). The aim of the UK government's White Paper *Equity and Excellence: Liberating the NHS* (Department of Health, 2010), when it was published, was to empower patients to share in decisions about their care. Today, patients have a wealth of information at their disposal, via the Internet, social media and so on, and are much more informed about their health and well-being needs than in the past (O'Grady and Jahad, 2010). It can be seen that the plan to empower patients in shared decision-making in their care is happening in practice and is having positive effects (see the Web resources section at the end of this chapter for a link to NHS England's guidance on this subject).

Patients can now gain permission to access their own personal medical records at their GP practices (see the Web resources section at the end of the chapter for a link to the NHS's website). This development shows the intention that care should be shared whenever possible between the patient and the professional, and this includes shared decision-making. To do this, individuals need to be able to access their own care details. A House of Commons Library Briefing Paper (Parkin and Loft, 2020) details all aspects of access, sharing and confidentiality with regard to patient health records, as well as issues related to COVID-19. Issues related to tracking and tracing people who may have the virus and other types of people-tracking information for those who have been deemed to have priority for vaccines for example are also discussed. It is important that nurses understand some of the background to current issues impacting patients' lives and in turn help them to make shared decisions about their care.

As a student nurse or newly qualified nurse, you may feel that you do not have the experience and knowledge to support patients in the decision-making process, but you should encourage them to become involved in their treatment and intervention options (Sharples and Elcock, 2011). Additionally, nurses should include patients in decision-making about nursing interventions and lifestyle choices, as well as be an advocate in situations where other health care professionals are not offering patients the opportunity for shared decision-making (Sharples and Elcock, 2011).

Student nurses and newly qualified nurses are supported by practice supervisors, mentors and preceptors in those clinical situations that require decision-making. Effective communication between nurses and nurses, nurses and other health care workers and nurses and patients is an essential skill that will be required of you as a qualified nurse.

Now consider Case study 6.4, which explores shared decision-making and communication, and undertake Activity 6.8 that relates to it.

CASE STUDY 6.4: SHARED DECISION-MAKING: PLANNING FUTURE CARE

A 30-year-old man is being assessed in A&E by Michael, a newly qualified nurse. As he is still in his period of preceptorship, his preceptor has agreed (as part of Michael's ongoing professional development) to observe him manage the care of this patient, assisting as directed by Michael, and give him feedback afterwards.

The patient complains that he has not felt very well for a couple of days and has not taken any of his normal insulin that day. He says that he had a big breakfast of sugared cereal, though, but he says he has not eaten anything since because he wasn't feeling very well, and he needed more insulin. He has a high blood glucose level and is displaying signs of uncontrolled diabetes. In broken English, he informs Michael that he is an insulin-dependent diabetic, comes from Poland and has been working in the UK for two months.

After taking his history, it is clear that the patient has difficulties speaking and understanding English, as well as being unable to tell the staff the complete history of his diabetes. Michael, after discussion with his preceptor, contacts the hospital's Polish interpreter to assist him in communicating with the patient.

Michael realises that, to help the patient achieve a state of well-being and control of his diabetes, the patient will require acute medical intervention, diabetic education regarding his medication, a referral to the hospital's diabetic dietician and follow-up outpatient appointments. This will involve a collaborative team effort involving Michael, the specialist diabetic nurse, the interpreter, the dietician and the attending doctor in A&E.

Given the patient's immediate needs, the team decides to admit him to help him with controlling his diabetes, check why he hasn't been feeling very well and set up further management, involving a multidisciplinary approach to support the patient on discharge.

Activity 6.8

1. Identify the main issues in Case study 6.4, then answer the following questions.
2. Do you think that a multidisciplinary approach will help the patient to achieve well-being on discharge from hospital?
3. Was Michael's decision in assessing the patient's priority needs effective in this scenario?
4. What were the most important communication issues faced by Michael and the patient?
5. Reflect on the decision-making process adopted by Michael and consider a clinical decision that you have made recently. What was the decision about? What judgements led you to make this decision?
6. Focus on the communication aspect of each clinical decision-making situation.
7. You might wish to make a note of these questions and your responses to support your own achievement of shared decision-making.

Communication and Therapeutic Relationships

Communication is an essential component of nursing care that contributes to the attainment of an effective therapeutic relationship with patients. McMahon defines a 'therapeutic relationship' as one that can be seen to be:

> achieving beneficial outcomes for the patient's problems, using interventions that acknowledge and complement the work of other therapists and with due regard for the goals and individuality of the patient. (1998: 10)

These goals may include learning to deal with a newly diagnosed life-limiting illness or beginning a long-term self-administered medication programme.

Woskot (2006) argues that the efficacy of a therapeutic relationship may directly affect the outcomes. It is important to the success of the patient's journey that the nurse is able to demonstrate empathy and support, give information well and facilitate the development of a therapeutic relationship with the patient.

The ultimate aim of nurses using therapeutic communication skills is to provide a sense of well-being for patients, making them feel relaxed and secure (McCabe and Timmins, 2013). This therapeutic relationship should encourage patient-centred communication in which the patient is respected as an individual and has control over the care that they receive. Wright (2021) explores therapeutic relationships in both nursing theory and practice and includes a number of reflective activities to consider to support learning. She reaffirms the importance of effective communication skills to support therapeutic relationships and achieving the outcomes of NMC (2018a) proficiencies.

Self-awareness is a critical feature in the development of therapeutic relationships. Nurses should be aware of their position or stance within the nurse–patient relationship and how they, as nurses, are perceived by others. Self-awareness is a significant tool for improving nurse–patient interaction and so is integrated into nurse education programmes. Being self-aware as a nurse is also essential for the successful implementation of the therapeutic relationship and is important for their professional and personal development (McCabe and Timmins, 2013).

Bach and Grant (2010) state that acknowledgement of our own values, attitudes and beliefs as nurses is necessary to ensure that we become sensitive to complex situations. Indeed, prejudice, language, stereotyping and being judgemental are significant barriers to a therapeutic relationship and the subsequent associated decision-making. Therapeutic communication results in a focused and purposeful relationship between a nurse and the patient that helps the nurse to assess, plan, implement, and evaluate the care needed by a patient in a safe and competent manner (McCabe and Timmins, 2013). Roper, Logan and Tierney (2001) emphasise the need for patient participation and patient-centred care in nursing. Their model allows for the specific assessment of an individual's needs and the importance of an interpersonal relationship between a patient and a nurse.

The NMC Standards (NMC, 2018a) and proficiencies stress the importance of appropriate behaviour between nurses and patients, and stipulate that all nurses must use therapeutic principles to engage, maintain, and, where appropriate, disengage from professional caring relationships. They must also always respect professional boundaries. Consider Case study 6.5 regarding the issue of respecting professional boundaries, then complete Activity 6.9 that relates to it.

CASE STUDY 6.5: MAINTAINING PROFESSIONAL BOUNDARIES

Josh, a mature student, aged 40, is a second-year nurse who accompanies his practice supervisor, a psychiatric community nurse, to assess a 36-year-old woman with a diagnosis of psychosis.

The patient has been compliant with her present medication and is maintaining her autonomy and independence. She enjoys talking to Josh, because he reminds her of a previous partner, and she mentions that she feels relaxed and at ease discussing her problems and fears with him.

On this particular day, Josh informs her that his placement is nearing completion in a few days. He reassures her that it has been a pleasure meeting her and wishes her well for the future. She is visibly upset that she will no longer see Josh and asks him if he would visit her on his days off. Josh agrees to do this without discussing it with his mentor or practice supervisor, who had stepped out of the room to check on another patient so is unaware of the exchange.

Activity 6.9

Identify the main issues in Case study 6.5 and make a note of these.

1. Will Josh be failing to maintain his professional boundary if he visits the patient at home?
2. Has Josh upheld professional standards of practice and adhered to *The Code*?
3. There are issues of personal safety that may arise as a result of visiting the patient and the possibility of encountering her friends and family. To what potential risks could Josh be exposed?
4. How should Josh have ended this therapeutic relationship?

To consider the issues arising in Case study 6.5, you will need to be knowledgeable about the NMC's current standards and guidance relating to verbal and written communication and accurate record-keeping, as well as relationships with others.

If you are ever in doubt about making the right decision in any situation, it is imperative that you seek guidance from more experienced colleagues, your personal tutor or your practice supervisor. Who you choose will depend on the kind of decision that is required.

Decision-making is an acquired skill, which is developed and refined through experience, and as you gain more practice, your confidence in making decisions will increase. If following a curriculum based on the NMC 2010a standards. you will be expected to achieve all the generic and field-specific competencies detailed in the NMC's (2010a) *Standards for Pre-registration Nursing Education* (especially relevant in this case is 'Domain 2: Communication and interpersonal skills', 2010a: 15–16) or alternatively attaining the proficiencies stated in all seven platforms of the NMC's (2018a) *Standards of proficiency for registered nurses*. Developing your decision-making skills when communicating with people, and in other contexts, is essential for your successful attainment of these NMC outcomes.

Reflecting on your communicating and interpersonal skills and experiences will facilitate the development of an increasing confidence in your ability to manage the complex decision-making situations required of a qualified nurse. This will benefit not only you but also, ultimately, the patients and clients in your care.

Conclusion

Throughout your learning experiences as a student nurse, you will learn to identify appropriate communication strategies to deliver safe and effective patient care, as well as those required to work together with your colleagues and other professionals in both practice and university environments.

To develop your communication skills, you will need to assess and reflect on the effectiveness of your interpersonal skills. This chapter has offered a number of learning activities, resources and evidence of good practice to help you achieve successful outcomes to becoming a future qualified nurse.

References

Anders, H., Douglas, D. and Harrigan, R. (1995). Competencies of new registered nurses: A survey of deans and health care agencies in the state of Hawaii. *Nursing Connections*, 8(3): 5–16.

Bach, S. and Grant, A. (2010). *Communication and Interpersonal Skills in Nursing*, 2nd edn. Exeter: Learning Matters.

Balzer-Riley, J. (2004). *Communication in Nursing*. St Louis, MO: Mosby.

Benner, P. (1984). *From Novice to Expert: Excellence and power in clinical nursing practice*. Menlo Park, CA: Addison-Wesley.

Department of Health (2010). *Equity and Excellence: Liberating the NHS*. White Paper. London: The Stationery Office.

Foy, C. and Timmins, F. (2004). Improving communication in day surgery settings. *Nursing Standard*, 19(7): 37–42.

Gilbert, P. and Leahy, R. (eds) (2007). *The Therapeutic Relationship in the Cognitive Behavioural Psychotherapies*. Abingdon: Routledge.

Hargie, O. and Dickson, D. (2004). *Skilled Interpersonal Communication: Research, theory and practice*. Abingdon: Routledge.

Holland, K., Roxburgh, M., Johnson, M., Topping, K., Watson, R., Lauder, W. and Porter, L. (2010). Fitness for practice in nursing and midwifery education in Scotland, United Kingdom. *Journal of Clinical Nursing*, 19(3–4): 461–469.

Holland, K. (2020). *Anthropology of Nursing: Exploring cultural concepts in practice*. Abingdon: Routledge.

Kwekkeboom, K. (1997). The placebo effect in symptom management. *Oncological Nursing Forum*, 24(8): 1393–1399.

Learner, S. (2006). Fears for literacy and numeracy as new nurses fail basic tests. *Nursing Standard*, 20(49): 10.

McCabe, C. and Timmins, F. (2013). *Communication Skills for Nursing Practice*, 2nd edn. Basingstoke: Palgrave Macmillan.

McMahon, R. (1998). Therapeutic nursing: Theory, issues and practice. In R. McMahon and A. Pearson (eds), *Nursing as Therapy*, 2nd edn. Cheltenham: Nelson Thornes. pp. 1–25.

Miller, E. and Nambiar-Greenwood, G. (2011). The nurse–patient relationship. In L. Webb (ed.), *Nursing: Communication skills in practice*. Oxford: Oxford University Press. pp. 30–32.

National Institute for Health and Care Excellence (NICE) (2018). Chapter 27 Critical Care Outreach Teams: Emergency and acute medical care in over 16s: service delivery and organisation. NICE guideline 94. London: NICE.

Nursing and Midwifery Council (NMC) (n.d.). *Guidance on using Social Media Responsibly*. London: NMC.

Nursing and Midwifery Council (NMC) (2009). *Record Keeping: Guidance for nurses and midwives*. London: NMC.

Nursing and Midwifery Council (NMC) (2010a). *Standards for Pre-registration Nursing Education*. London: NMC.

Nursing and Midwifery Council (NMC) (2010b). *Guidance on Professional Conduct: For nursing and midwifery students*. London: NMC.

Nursing and Midwifery Council (NMC) (2018a). *Future Nurse: Standards of proficiency for registered nurses*. London: NMC.

Nursing and Midwifery Council (NMC) (2018e). *The Code: Professional standards of practice and behaviour for nurses, midwives and nursing associates*. London: NMC.

Office for National Statistics (ONS) (2011). *Statistical bulletin: Internet access: Households and individuals, 2011*. London: ONS.

O'Grady, L. and Jahad, A. (2010). Shifting from shared to collaborative decision making: A change in thinking and doing. *Journal of Participatory Medicine*, 2: e13.

Parkin, E. and Loft, P. (2020). *Patient Health Records: Access, sharing and confidentiality.* Briefing Paper No. 07103. London: House of Commons Library.

Roper, N., Logan, W. W. and Tierney, A. J. (2001). *The Roper Logan Tierney Model of Nursing Based on Activities of Living.* Edinburgh: Churchill Livingstone.

Sharples, K. and Elcock, K. (2011). *Preceptorship for Newly Registered Nurses.* Exeter: Learning Matters.

Standing, M. (2010). *Clinical Judgement and Decision Making in Nursing and Inter-Professional Healthcare.* Buckingham: Open University Press.

Thompson, C. (2003). Clinical experience as evidence in evidence-based practice. *Journal of Advanced Nursing,* 43(3): 230–237.

Thompson, C. and Dowding, D. (2002). *Clinical Decision Making and Judgement in Nursing.* Edinburgh: Churchill Livingstone.

Tiwary, A., Rimal, A., Paudyal, B., Sigdel, K. R. and Bsnyat, B. (2019). Poor communication by health care professionals may lead to life-threatening complications: Examples from two case reports. Version 1. *Welcome Open Research,* 4: 7.

Webb, L. (ed.) (2011). *Nursing: Communication skills in practice.* Oxford: Oxford University Press.

Woskot, V. (2006). *Egan's Skilled Helper Model: Developments and application in counselling.* Abingdon: Routledge.

Wright, K. M. (2021). Exploring the therapeutic relationship in nursing theory and practice. *Mental Health Practice,* 24(5): 34–41.

Further Reading

Brown, A. (2020). Will COVID-19 affect the delivery of compassionate nursing care? *Nursing Times,* 116(10): 32–35 (includes a journal club handout and decision-making and communication aspects of care).

Burnard, P. and Gill, P. (2008). *Culture, Communication and Nursing.* Harlow: Pearson Education.

Holland, K. (2017). *Cultural Awareness in Nursing and Health Care: An introductory text.* Abingdon: Routledge.

Holland, K. and Jenkins, J. (eds) (2019). *Applying the Roper, Logan Tierney Model in Practice,* 3rd edn. Edinburgh: Blackwell Science.

Ulenaers, D., Grosemans, J., Schrooten, W. and Bergs, J. (2021). Clinical placement experience of nursing students during the COVID-19 pandemic: A cross-sectional study. *Nurse Education Today,* 99: 104746.

Web Resources

Australia's guidance for social media – Nursing and Midwifery Board, *Social media: How to meet your obligations under the national law*: https://www.ahpra.gov.au/Resources/Social-media-guidance.aspx (accessed 21 June 2022).

Care Quality Commission (England) – guidance for providers of health and social care: www.cqc.org.uk/guidance-providers/adult-social-care/culturally-appropriate-care (accessed 21 June 2022).

National Institute for Health and Care Excellence (NICE) (2018), *Chapter 27 Critical Care Outreach Teams: Emergency and acute medical care in over 16s: service delivery and organisation*, NICE guideline 94: www.nice.org.uk/guidance/ng94/evidence/27critical-care-outreach-teams-pdf-172397464640 (accessed 21 June 2022).

NHS: Medical records access: www.nhs.uk/using-the-nhs/about-the-nhs/how-to-access-your-health-records (accessed 21 June 2022).

NHS England (n.d) Shared decision making to improve health outcomes: www.england.nhs.uk/shared-decision-making/why-is-shared-decision-making-important/shared-decision-making-to-improve-health-outcomes (accessed 21 June 2022).

NHS (2013) *Social Media and Attributed Digital Content Policy* – an example of a policy and how various social media modes can be used: https://www.england.nhs.uk/wp-content/uploads/2018/04/social-media-policy.pdf (accessed 21 June 2022).

NMC (n.d.) *Caring with Confidence: The Code in action* – and watch the related short animations on the use of social media using the second link below: www.nmc.org.uk/standards/code/code-in-action (accessed 28 January 2022) www.nmc.org.uk/standards/code/code-in-action/social-media (accessed 21 June 2022).

NMC (n.d.) *Guidance on using Social Media Responsibly*: www.nmc.org.uk/globalassets/sitedocuments/nmc-publications/social-media-guidance.pdf (accessed 11 July 2022).

NMC Revalidation information: www.nmc.org.uk/revalidation (accessed 28 January 2022).

www.nmc.org.uk/news/coronavirus/information-for-nurses-midwives-and-nursing-associates/revalidation (accessed 21 June 2022).

NMC (2010b) *Standards for Pre-registration Nursing Education*: www.nmc.org.uk/globalassets/sitedocuments/standards/nmc-standards-for-pre-registration-nursing-education.pdf (accessed 21 June 2022).

Office for National Statistics (ONS) (2011) *Statistical bulletin: Internet access: Households and individuals*, 2011: webarchive.nationalarchives.gov.uk/ukgwa/20160106221558/http://www.ons.gov.uk/ons/rel/rdit2/internet-access—households-and-individuals/2011/stb-internet-access-2011.html (accessed 28 January 2022).

Parliamentary and Health Service Ombudsman in the UK – oversees the complaints system: www.ombudsman.org.uk (accessed 21 June 2022).

Practice Assessment Record and Evaluation (PARE) tool, University of Chester: https://onlinepare.net/files/guides/PARE.Placement.Educator.Guide.v1.0.pdf (accessed 21 June 2022).

RCN Advice and guidance on COVID-19, with many examples of challenges to communication: www.rcn.org.uk/covid-19 (accessed 21 June 2022).

RCN End-of-life care and well-being for nurses and midwives, with access to the end-of-life programme and several other key resources: www.rcn.org.uk/professional-development/professional-services/end-of-life-care-and-wellbeing-for-the-nursing-and-midwifery-workforce (accessed 21 June 2022).

RCN Student nurses' area, with advice guides on various areas about which you may have questions: www.rcn.org.uk/get-help/rcn-advice/student-nurses (accessed 21 June 2022).

Royal College of Nursing (RCN) Social Media Guidance 2019: file:///Users/catherineholland/Downloads/Social-media-policy-2019.pdf (accessed 21 June 2022).

PART 2

DECISION-MAKING IN PRACTICE

This part of the book will focus specifically on the four fields of practice in which student nurses will be undertaking their practice learning and exercising their decision-making skills to register as a qualified nurse. Students follow a generic path to achieving the Nursing and Midwifery Council proficiencies, and at the same time follow a pathway of learning in their chosen field. This encompasses an evidence-based approach to decision making and an in-depth underpinning knowledge of specific health and ill health challenges that they are expected to achieve.

The chapters are of value to any student nurse regardless of the pathway of learning they undertake, as those patients, clients and their families they encounter have to be considered in an holistic way. The series of 'learning activities' to be found across all the four chapters can be used to support achievement of learning outcomes and a broad understanding of decision-making in the various fields of practice. It must be noted however that within these broad fields, there are specialised learning environments, and students are encouraged to develop a broader knowledge base in order to engage in evidence-based decision-making.

Each of the chapters are written by colleagues with experience and expertise in these fields and offer an insight into the reality of making decisions.

7

DECISION-MAKING IN MENTAL HEALTH NURSING

Tony Warne and Gareth Holland

Chapter objectives

The aims of this chapter are to:

- explore a number of interrelated issues in the provision of effective mental health care;
- explore how relationships between nurses, service users, carers and other members of the mental health care profession are used to provide effective mental health care;
- explore, through the use of case studies, how decision-making is undertaken in mental health nursing practice;
- enable student nurses to learn how and why effective decision-making is essential to developing and maintaining therapeutic relationships.

Introduction

The chapter first explores the issues involved in how and why mental health nurses come to learn about the decisions they need to make in their clinical practice, and why these are crucial to establishing and maintaining therapeutic relationships. It must be noted that various terms will be used throughout this chapter that refer to individuals requiring care and support from nurses – namely, 'patients', 'service users' and 'clients.'

We also explore some of the challenges and tensions that can arise when there is a difference between what the professional and the service user might feel is the right decision. Reference is made to the prevailing mental health legislation in the UK and, in particular, the legislation around care being provided possibly against an individual's wishes and while they are living in the community. If you are not living or studying in the UK, you should seek out the relevant legislation that applies to your country. You might want to see where the similarities and differences are between that and the UK legislation.

The chapter concludes with a discussion of how the mental health nurse can ensure that inclusive and informed decision-making leads to safe, secure and effective mental health care. By means of the case studies and the discussion, it will enable you, as the student nurse, to learn how different kinds of decision-making can influence the outcomes of care and help you to work towards achieving the Nursing and Midwifery Council's (NMC) (2018a) *Future Nurse: Standards of proficiency for registered nurses*.

It is important to note that while the case studies have a basis in real-life examples of decision-making situations, all names have been changed and contexts not identified, in keeping with the NMC's (2018e) *The Code: Professional standards of practice and behaviour for nurses, midwives and nursing associates*.

Mental Health Nurse Education, Practice and Research

Mental health nurse education, practice, and research have long championed innovative approaches to improving our understanding of the impact – on individuals, the communities in which they live and wider society – of the decisions made and actions taken in the name of therapeutic endeavour. However, improved understanding does not always lead to better decisions being taken by those who have this knowledge.

Many mental health nurses have experienced similar difficulties and challenges in developing their own practice and the teams within which they work. Sometimes, these difficulties have been very complex. For example, like other areas of nursing, in mental health nursing there has long been a theory–practice debate. This debate centres on the argument that the classroom is dominated by theoretical knowledge, with practical knowledge being the domain of clinical practice, and there is rarely any connection between these two different, but related, knowledge areas (Freshwater and Stickley, 2004; Greenway et al., 2019). For many mental health nurses, however, there has also been an ongoing theory–theory debate (Michie et al., 2016), which like others, has challenged the ways in which mental health nurses have carried out their practice.

Preparing for Mental Health Nursing

While some students might relish these debates and discussions, for others they can be uncomfortable, challenging their self-confidence as people and as aspiring professionals (Warne and McAndrew, 2010; Frogeli, Rudman and Gustavsson, 2019). From an educational perspective, it has been argued that contemporary approaches to the educational preparation of mental health nurses requires radical rethinking (Durcan et al., 2017).

It should be possible to think about concepts of 'preparedness' as being both educational and emotional precepts. In this way, the technical and theoretical knowledge required for practice and the attitudes and emotions that influence the individual in practice will become more effectively aligned. It is possible that you will have only thought about this when you have experienced these two aspects not being aligned. Let us think about 'preparedness' as it relates to your own experience in Activity 7.1.

Activity 7.1

Think back to your very first clinical placement and recall how you felt.

1. How prepared did you feel for that particular area of practice?
2. How did you feel when thinking about starting that first shift?
3. Take a moment to think back and reflect on those two aspects. Consider what you would have liked to have known about the practice area and how knowing that might have made you feel.

If you have not yet undertaken your first placement experience, think about what you have been told it is like or what you have discovered. What are your feelings about how prepared you think you are for that first day? You may wish to write about this as part of your ongoing learning experience and share with your personal tutor.

This first activity should help you to think about a concept of preparedness that acknowledges the interrelated and entangling space between 'knowledge' and 'knowing'. Just as theoretical knowledge is implicit in delivering good practice, knowing also forms part of our ability to deal with our interpersonal relationships within the context of our external world (Lakeman et al., 2013). Gaztambide-Fernández and Arráiz Matute (2017) note the difference between these two concepts:

- *knowledge* is described as a conscious secondary process relating to the information residing in our minds.
- *knowing* is an unconscious primary process that influences the way in which we use knowledge.
- *knowing* is also a product of our upbringing and background, which encompasses our beliefs and values, and is culturally and socially bounded.

Consider these two concepts as you complete Activity 7.2.

Activity 7.2

1. Consider how knowledge of mental health nursing is required to enable you to make decisions that relate to you personally and those concerning patients or service users who you will meet in practice.
2. Discuss your answers with your practice or academic supervisor at your next supervision meeting.
3. If you are undertaking a mental health nursing placement, but you are, in fact, following another field of practice learning pathway (for example, adult nursing) are there any differences between this learning pathway and the expected knowledge of mental health nursing that will impact on your experience in that placement?
4. Consider what knowledge you will need to have to be able to contribute to decision-making in that mental health specific placement.

Think about how the generic proficiency and the examples of outcomes to be achieved, set out in platform 1 of the NMC's *Future Nurse: Standards of proficiency for registered nurses* (see Box 7.1) can be used in a different field of practice from your own. Use your deliberations to discuss with your practice supervisor what you wish to focus on achieving during the placement and determine your learning plan.

Box 7.1

Platform 1: Being an accountable professional: The generic proficiency and examples of outcomes to be achieved

Registered nurses act in the best interests of people, putting them first and providing nursing care that is person-centred, safe and compassionate. They act professionally at all times and use their knowledge and experience to make evidence-based decisions about care. They communicate effectively, are role models for others, and are accountable for their actions. Registered nurses continually reflect on their practice and keep abreast of new and emerging developments in nursing, health and care.

1. **Outcomes:**

The outcomes set out below reflect the proficiencies for accountable professional practice that must be applied across the standards of proficiency for registered nurses, as described in platforms 2-7, in all care settings and areas of practice.

At the point of registration, the registered nurse will be able to:

1.2   understand and apply relevant legal, regulatory and governance requirements, policies, and ethical frameworks, including any mandatory reporting duties, to all areas of practice, differentiating where appropriate between the devolved legislatures of the United Kingdom

1.5   understand the demands of professional practice and demonstrate how to recognise signs of vulnerability in themselves or their colleagues and the action required to minimise risks to health

1.9   understand the need to base all decisions regarding care and interventions on people's needs and preferences, recognising and addressing any personal and external factors that may unduly influence their decisions

1.10 demonstrate resilience and emotional intelligence and be capable of explaining the rationale that influences their judgements and decisions in routine, complex and challenging situations

1.11 communicate effectively using a range of skills and strategies with colleagues and people at all stages of life and with a range of mental, physical, cognitive and behavioural health challenges

1.12 demonstrate the skills and abilities required to support people at all stages of life who are emotionally or physically vulnerable

1.13 demonstrate the skills and abilities required to develop, manage and maintain appropriate relationships with people, their families, carers and colleagues

1.14 provide and promote non-discriminatory, person-centred and sensitive care at all times, reflecting on people's values and beliefs, diverse backgrounds, cultural characteristics, language requirements, needs and preferences, taking account of any need for adjustments

1.18 demonstrate the knowledge and confidence to contribute effectively and proactively in an interdisciplinary team

1.20 safely demonstrate evidence-based practice in all skills and procedures stated in Annexes A and B. (2018a: 7-9)

In relation to mental health nursing practice, however, it is the mental health nurse's attitude to 'knowledge' and their aptitude for 'knowing' that will allow them to explore and make sense of their own and other people's experiences, feelings, needs and motives. The ability to 'know me' in order to better learn how to 'understand you' is the crux of the therapeutic relationship and is central to the notion of providing 'holistic care' (Kornhaber et al., 2016; Warne and McAndrew, 2010). We will consider this in the context of decision-making, but it is important, first, that you understand what we mean by a 'therapeutic relationship'.

The Therapeutic Relationship

The therapeutic relationship is central to effective mental health nursing. Such relationships require the individual nurse to be attentive, able to hear the patient's story and, at the same time, provide safety by containing the story and the expressed personal philosophy or inherent beliefs and values of both the patient and the nurse. It has been suggested, however, that for some individuals the processes of self-examination and interpretation necessary to establish and maintain effective therapeutic relationships might be threatening and confusing (Smith, 2017; Warne and McAndrew, 2007).

Many nurses, particularly those at the beginning of their professional careers, strive to possess *all* the knowledge and skills required to be a competent and effective nurse.

However, perhaps it is that we *do not yet know* those things that might be important in terms of becoming and being an effective mental health nurse. For example, novice nurses complete their education and training possessing countless skills and much relevant theoretical knowledge. Yet what many of these newly qualified professionals lack is the knowing required to ensure that such knowledge is used in a meaningful way in relation to the unique individuals with whom they will be working. Recognising this uniqueness reflects another strand of knowledge that might also be useful to consider – that is, patient experience knowledge – and with this the emotionality of the interpersonal space that this knowledge can create between the nurse and patient (Figure 7.1).

While models of decision-making mostly favour a rationalist view of evidence, it has sometimes been argued that service user experience is a 'third strand' of evidence (Rycroft-Malone, 2004). However, while acknowledging service user experience and evidence derived from qualitative studies may be acknowledged, this is often qualified with the rider that the 'best' evidence is drawn from quantitative methods, and a consequent emphasis on standardisation techniques.

Sometimes there can be much resistance, therefore, to acknowledging and valuing patient experience knowledge and this can be difficult to overcome (Gault et al., 2013). We argue here that, in achieving effective decision-making in mental health care, being able to embrace the choices and preferences of service users is something that every nurse needs to try consciously to build into their approach to providing care. Complete Activity 7.3 to reflect on this aspect of mental health nursing.

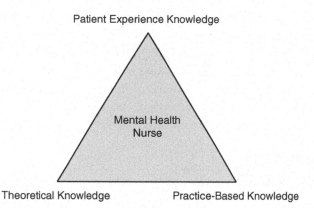

Figure 7.1 caption area:

Patient Experience Knowledge

Mental Health Nurse

Theoretical Knowledge   Practice-Based Knowledge

Figure 7.1 The three major sources of knowledge for mental health nurses.

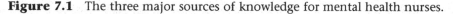

Activity 7.3

Think about a situation that you have experienced in which your practice supervisor discussed with a service user how they wanted to be involved in their own care.

1. What decisions did the service user make?
2. What knowledge did the service user have to support their knowing how to make that decision?
3. Discuss with your practice supervisor how they felt in enabling the service user to make decisions about their own care.

This represents a change in mental health nursing practice – from making decisions *for* service users (patients) to making them *with* them – and reflects the approach of 'no decision about me without me' (Coulter and Collins, 2011).

Making Decisions: Partnerships Between the Nurse and the Patient

In thinking about how to achieve a greater sense of partnership between nurse and patient, the shift required is from decisions based on professional values towards those based on patient values (Coulter, 2010). In many international settings, mental health policy, legislative and professional practice trends have revealed that a more deter-mined approach is being taken towards increasing patient and public involvement within the democratic process of design, delivery and evaluation of mental health services (Gluyas, 2015; Happell, Pinikahana and Roper, 2003; Happell et al., 2019).

Ultimately, many patients will decide for themselves what they will or will not do regarding any treatment offered or provided and exercising this choice will have an impact on the successful outcomes of any particular treatment, the experience of any untoward side effects of treatment and an individual's sense of overall well-being. How patients make decisions is not always well understood, although the interest in patient decision-making within mental health care reflects the general increase in interest in patient-centred interventions that focus on the patients' perspective in health care (McMillan et al., 2013). To consider some of the issues related to service user involvement in making decisions about their own care, undertake Activity 7.4.

Activity 7.4

1. For a good example of how the major change in mental health nursing practice (that is, the 'paradigm shift') has occurred, access and then read the article by T. Warne and S. McAndrew (2007), Passive patient or engaged expert?: Using a Ptolemaic approach to enhance mental health nurse education and practice, *International Journal of Mental Health Nursing*, 16(4): 224-229.
2. While this is not a recently published paper, its exploration of the reasons why so many of us - when we become service users - are content for others to make decisions on our behalf, is still valid. Take some time to think about the last shift in which you were working (and learning) on placement.
3. Can you identify three things that were said or done by nursing colleagues that might, unintentionally, have disempowered service users?

Much has been said in earlier chapters about decision-making theories and how they may be applied in health care. Indeed, much has been written about clinical decision-making and its relationship with information-processing theory and social judgement theory (Soane et al., 2015). Until more recently, in health care settings, much of this work has focused on medical decision-making. Shared decision-making, therefore, represents a radical divergence from the traditional model of the health care professional as paternalistic authority. In mental health care, such approaches usually involve several interrelated elements of decision-making (Chong, Aslani and Chen, 2013; Happell et al., 2019), which we shall now consider in turn.

1. Information

In this context, what we mean by 'information' is all that is required in order to make a particular decision. What this information consists of can differ depending on who has the information, how it is to be used or prioritised and who is processing the information when making a decision. For example, the doctor might use information represented by the signs and symptoms observed when deciding on treatment options. If those treatment options include, say, prescribing medication, then the likely known efficacy of the particular drug will be noted, the usual prescribing range consulted and, if relevant, reactions to any other medications also being taken might be considered. While we may know it, we may or may not disclose other information, such as the probabilities of risks, benefits and lifestyle changes associated with taking a particular medication. In mental health, it is often these considerations that form the basis for decision-making around compliance and not the information on therapeutic value, for example (Haddad, Brain and Scott, 2014).

2. Values

It's clear that different values reflect the importance that people place on information for decision-making, as well as on various aspects of their experience and other factors in the broader context of their encounters with mental health care services (Byrne, Happell and Reid-Searl, 2017; Woodbridge and Fulford, 2003).

In the formal clinical decision-making situation (prescribing medication, for example), quantitative estimates of values are drawn upon that act as proxies for the desired end point of health and well-being, and these are used to balance out any negative aspects of treatments. For example, patients with depression often place high importance (value) on feeling better but may also value avoiding adverse side effects of medication. The relative strength of these values can significantly impact patient preferences for treatment options, subsequently affecting the choices that patients make about treatments (MacDonald-Wilson et al., 2013).

3. Decision-making Context

At any one time, it will be the context within which these relative values are explored that will influence an individual's decision-making within the broader context of their life, and sometimes this can be a powerful influence on the choices that they make.

'Context', as used here, refers to the various aspects of an individual's day-to-day life and functioning, the health care system's structure and process, as well as the broader sociocultural milieu that shapes people's experiences. In the example of a service user being prescribed medication for a mental health problem, therefore, as well as information on the therapeutic value and relative value on quality of life, other considerations may include the perceived social stigma associated with both seeking help and complying with professional mental health service interventions.

4. Preferences

As the service user considers these sometimes-competing strands of information, it is almost inevitable that, in some circumstances, the decision-making choices will be ranked in order of preference. Preferences represent a relatively greater liking of one alternative as compared to (an)other alternative(s).

Using an extreme example from a non-mental health care setting, but chosen because it is a situation that, clearly, will have an impact on individuals' physical and mental health and well-being, consider the decisions that some patients diagnosed with cancer have to make. For the individual, it might be a choice between surgery, radiotherapy or accepting no treatment. In mental health, even with the advent of new neuroleptic drugs, there is evidence to suggest that service users often feel that the choice of treatment for those with serious mental illnesses, is not really a choice (Malla, Joober and Garcia, 2015).

These four elements of decision-making – information, values, context and preferences – should be as important for mental health nurses as they are for service users (Happell et al., 2019). Recognition of the importance of the four elements is crucial if we are to develop an approach that sees mental health professionals being able and willing to provide information to service users in a way that puts their needs first (Roberts and Kim, 2016). Activity 7.5 provides an opportunity to consider these issues further.

Activity 7.5

1. Consider what a nurse might need to ensure is included in an approach to the assessment and review of long-term medication with service users that promotes their preferences.
2. What difficulties do you think might be involved for the:

    *   service user
    *   mental health nurse
    *   other members of the mental health team?

3. What do you consider to be the differences between patient-centredness and service user involvement and participation in shared decision-making processes?

Decision-Making in Practice

In many circumstances in which nurses work with colleagues from other disciplines to provide mental health care services, it is often the mental health nurse who will be in a prime position to ensure that shared decision-making routinely forms part of the care-giving approach (Pathare and Shields, 2012). It is nurses who usually have the greatest contact with service users. It is this consistency in the provision of care that requires the mental health nurse to develop expert communication and interpersonal relationship skills (Kornhaber et al., 2016).

One area of mental health nursing practice in which this can be seen is in the assessment and monitoring of services users' progress against agreed treatment or care plans to ensure that these remain optimal. Warne and McAndrew (2010) noted that, in these situations, it is possible that some mental health nurses approach such assessments with a well-developed intuitive 'feel' for what may be going on yet will remain constrained by the limitations imposed by their training and an uncritical acceptance of empirically based evidence. Indeed, it has long been noted that most health care professionals do not make clinical decisions based simply on intuition (Hogarth, 2010). However, in many therapeutic situations, in which the mental health nurse's ability to communicate and develop relationships are paramount, a fundamental conflict may arise between the need to respond immediately to service user needs and the considered, systematic processes demanded by 'science'.

Schön (1983), in his famous work on the reflective practitioner, argued that practitioners do not always operate using a technical rational basis, and do not routinely or consciously draw on all the separate forms and pieces of information available to them every time they are faced with the need to make a decision in clinical practice. Indeed, sometimes other considerations come into play, as Case study 7.1 illustrates.

CASE STUDY 7.1: DECISION-MAKING AS A NEWLY QUALIFIED NURSE

I can remember when I was working on my first shift as the only qualified member of staff on the ward, approximately a month into my preceptorship period. I was working with two support workers, neither of whom were regular ward staff, but who were experienced colleagues. The ward was unsettled when two patients, Paul and Michael, began fighting at the end of the bedroom corridor. I had no idea what had caused the fight, but immediately ran towards the situation, pulling my personal alarm for the first time as I did so.

The fight was stopped without any serious injury to either of the patients, but Paul began to make a number of threats to harm himself and Michael if he wasn't immediately moved off the ward.

Paul had a diagnosis of borderline personality disorder (BPD) and a history of prolific and extreme self-harm, and I felt that these threats were potentially genuine. Following a discussion with the senior (and very experienced) nurse who had attended the ward in her role as the duty manager, the decision was made to place Paul on one-to-one observation.

As a result, no further violent incidents took place. However, the following day, I was informed by my ward manager that, according to the unit policy, patients shouldn't be placed on one-to-one observation as a result of a threat of self-harm.

While I believe that the decision I made prevented any further violence between these two patients, with hindsight I don't believe that it was the right one. In the heat of the moment, I relied on the advice of senior nurses, because of my lack of knowledge of the policies of the unit in which I was working and a lack of awareness of what might be considered appropriate management of someone with a BPD diagnosis.

Of course, at that time, I was also not very confident in my own skills as a newly qualified nurse.

Decision-Making Issues to Consider in Case Study 7.1

The nurse in this situation was inexperienced and was facing being in the position of the only qualified nurse on duty at the time. The first decision taken was to deal with the situation before it escalated and what would be the correct procedure to follow. The nurse ran to the situation, communicating via a personal alarm that assistance was required. The immediate problem was dealt with, and the potentially difficult situation was contained.

However, as the stabilised situation changed, the nurse was faced with having to make decisions that were outside of their knowledge and experience. Again, understanding the need to gain advice, the nurse relied on the judgement of a very senior and experienced nurse to take the decision to care for one of the service users involved on a one-to-one basis, thus reducing the risk of further harm occurring to either service user or anyone else.

So far, it would be possible to argue that the 'correct' decisions had been taken. It was only the following morning that an alternative way forward was revealed. Partly, this was described as being due to 'unit policy', but such a policy would have been developed from an evidence base and best practice experience. For this nurse, at that time, however, all that was unknown. Interestingly, perhaps, when the nurse had a chance to reflect, they thought that this had not been the right or best decision.

It was clear that, in this case, the nurse was unable to respond to the wider problem, and their decision-making was focused on the one or two aspects that could be dealt with using the information and knowledge available at the time. Arguably, this is not unusual. Many nurses continue to reject a task-orientated approach to care in favour of a more holistic approach and rely on empirically based evidence to shape nursing.

Campbell et al. (2018) note that every experienced nurse will be able to recall situations in which they have drawn on their tacit knowledge and experience to respond immediately to the needs of a situation without necessarily considering whether or not this would have led to the best decision being made.

The newly qualified nurse's post-decision-making action was to reflect on the situation in order to learn from the whole experience. As seen in Chapter 4, the value of revisiting the scenario as a whole enabled them to consider the actions of everyone involved, as well as the feedback given by the ward manager.

It is clear from Case study 7.1 and its possible outcomes that, for mental health nurses, learning to negotiate appropriate care within complex environments necessitates a deep understanding of the process of decision-making. Models may differ in terms of their theoretical position but will often share the same drive towards the making of decisions that are based on sound reasoning, transparency and evidence. As can be seen from Case study 7.1, for both nurses and service users, there might be inconsistencies in the value placed on different sources of evidence. Variations exist that can create ethical and practice dilemmas for mental health nurses attempting to work in non-coercive, person-centred ways while also being cognizant of the evidence underpinning care (Ryan et al., 2014) (see Chapter 3 for additional information on the contribution of evidence-based practice to decision-making).

Case study 7.2 allows us to explore some more of these practice dilemmas.

CASE STUDY 7.2: MANAGING A DIFFICULT SITUATION

During my first experience of night duty as a qualified nurse, I worked every shift as the only qualified member of staff on the ward, and I found the patient group extremely challenging.

One patient in particular had been involved in a number of incidents. Tom was an 18-year-old male with a history of violent assaults on staff and other patients, a tendency to acquire and use weapons in these assaults and, on a previous admission, he had taken another patient hostage.

Shortly after the ward's bedtime, Tom and another patient had refused to go to bed, preferring to pace around the day area in an attempt to intimidate staff. Despite numerous requests from myself and support workers to go to bed, the patients refused. At one point, Tom walked to his bedroom and returned almost immediately with his fists clenched. His body language was extremely aggressive, and I noticed that he had something sticking out of his fist. I asked him what he had in his hand. He said, 'Nothing' and continued to walk towards me in a very intimidating manner. I asked him again and told him to open his fingers, which he did, revealing a very sharp, three-inch screw, which fell out of his hand and under the (locked) door of the kitchen.

With the immediate danger managed, I asked Tom to sit and talk with me - in an attempt to de-escalate the situation without the need to activate my alarm - which he did. He became noticeably calmer during our conversation (although I can't remember what we talked about) and eventually retired to bed. I felt happy with the decision that I had made because no one had been injured or harmed in any way.

During the handover in the morning, however, my colleagues on the early shift were appalled that I had neither pulled my alarm nor placed Tom in seclusion. I was made to feel as though I'd placed everyone I work with in extreme danger as a result of this decision, which was confirmed when, later that day, unable to sleep, I phoned the ward to speak with my manager. The ward manager confirmed that I should have activated my alarm and secluded Tom, and the nursing team on the early shift had made the decision to seclude Tom as a precaution while they reassessed the risk that he posed to staff and patients.

I had made the decision partly on an instinctive reliance on my communication and emerging nursing skills, and partly because I believe that, had I pulled my alarm and a response team attended the ward, this would have caused a much more dangerous situation in that Tom would have felt threatened or challenged and would have been likely to react with violence. However, once the immediate danger had been dealt with, I believe that I should have attempted to manage the long-term risks that Tom posed by determining if he had further weapons or had genuinely intended to cause someone harm.

Approximately two months later, we received information from another patient that Tom had acquired a metal pen, which he was hiding in his bedroom and sharpening in order to

'stab up' a member of staff. In light of the feedback regarding my earlier decision on managing Tom, I arranged to have his bedroom searched and, on finding said pen and because of
Tom's inability to deny that he would harm someone with it, I and the other qualified nurse
on shift made the decision to seclude Tom to manage his pronounced risk to others. (The
decision this time was a shared one, made with another colleague and also influenced by the
previous experience of needing to check a decision that I considered the right one to make.)

However, following this decision, we were informed by the manager that this was not
a decision that we should have made, because it was not entirely in line with our policies
regarding the use of seclusion and the risk was not sufficient to justify it. Making decisions
in practice is complex, but in each of these situations the main issue was the prevention of
risk of self-harm and harm to others, which was the outcome in both situations.

Issues to Consider Regarding the Nurse's Decision-Making in Case Study 7.2

What Case study 7.2 brings to light is the argument that the stages of the decision-
making process can be deconstructed and, in doing so, decision-making behaviour
can be improved (Ryan et al., 2014). While there is general agreement that a decision
involves a retrievable store of organised knowledge arising from prior experience, with
consequent options and choices (Dowie, 1993), when used in the context of mental
health nursing, much of the literature emphasises professionals' options and choices
– their using of their 'expertise' – rather than collaborating with the end user. In Case
study 7.2, such collaboration was not possible, but a solution presented itself, which
the nurse decided to action rather than risk a different, but possibly expected, response.

While mental health nurses should be making 'good' decisions based on sound and
reliable evidence, what constitutes 'good' in mental health practice often remains subject to the preferences of the various professional stakeholders involved in an individual's care and treatment. Likewise, it has been noted that relying on the available 'best
evidence' can have limited utility due to the ambiguity of decision-making applied to
individualised, person-centred approaches to care (Entwistle, Cribb and Watt, 2012).
However, Rolfe (2006) argued that such practice ambiguity can be addressed by clinically active staff using reflection as the vehicle for producing contextualised evidence.

Person-centredness shifts health care away from an exclusive focus on symptoms
and physiological outcomes because service users often value functional outcomes
and their quality of life more highly than they value control of the illness (Noble and
Douglas, 2004; Ryan et al., 2014). In shared decision-making, therefore, the mental
health nurse strives to become a consultant to the service user, helping to provide
information, to discuss options, to clarify values and preferences, and to support the
service user's autonomy.

In Case study 7.3, we can see how a qualified nurse develops Benner's (1984) intuitive approach to decision-making (see Chapter 1).

CASE STUDY 7.3: BECOMING MORE EXPERIENCED IN DECISION-MAKING

While working a night shift, I was asked to provide cover for another acute ward that had no qualified nurse available at the beginning of the shift. Because of the close proximity of the other ward, I was aware of the significant clinical issues that it was experiencing. Although I'd finished my preceptorship a couple of months before, suddenly being placed on another ward forces you to try to establish rapport with new individuals – it is something that any nurse should be prepared for when qualified.

One of the patients on the ward, Carl, had been diagnosed as having no treatable mental illness and was awaiting a transfer back to prison. Carl was a young man with a history of violence, drug abuse and prolific self-harm when faced with stress. Also, Carl had been involved in tattooing himself and other patients on the ward, which posed a significant risk of infection and some safeguarding issues. Staff had been unable to ascertain how he was doing this and were faced with hostility and occasionally violence whenever they attempted to intervene. Carl's argument was that, because he had no mental illness, then how could staff in a hospital justifiably restrict his actions. He used the act of tattooing himself as a coping strategy, albeit a poor one, to avoid acts of deliberate self-harm.

On this particular night, I spent a long time engaging with Carl during one-to-one sessions, because he was experiencing stress as a result of arguing with his girlfriend on the phone and I felt that I had established the foundation of rapport with him. He remained awake throughout the night and, at around 4 a.m., he was found, by staff doing routine checks, to be tattooing his forearm in his bedroom. I approached Carl and spent some time talking with him in his bedroom. He was using a safety pin, which he had acquired from some clothing brought in for another patient, and he had used a contraband lighter to sterilise it. He appeared quite agitated and said that he would assault any member of staff who attempted to prevent him from tattooing himself, and that he would also seriously self-harm if restrictions were put in place to prevent him from acting as he chose.

I returned to the nursing office to discuss the issue with the staff with whom I was working, who were unsure and looked to me to make a decision, as nurse in charge. I weighed up the situation and decided to take a course of action that I believed would resolve the issue without causing unnecessary distress to the patient and without causing risk to staff. I spoke with Carl again and told him that I would allow him to finish tattooing his arm only if he agreed that, when he had finished doing so, he handed in the safety pin and allowed me to clean the site. He agreed and, a short time later, approached me and happily complied with my requests.

This decision was a complex one because I had to consider a number of factors. What would have been my reasons for intervening, had I chosen to do so? This patient had been diagnosed as illness-free and would undoubtedly have deliberately harmed himself significantly, and potentially my colleagues, if we had attempted to restrain him. I believe that it would have caused him great distress to be restrained, particularly when his actions were affecting only himself and he had not posed a risk to others. I was also viewing it in terms of 'safe self-harm', in that he was already at high risk of blood-borne viruses (BBVs) as a result of previous tattoos and years of intravenous (IV) drug use. In allowing me to clean the wound and handing in the pin, Carl allowed me to manage further risk, thereby increasing the safety of the ward. But perhaps most importantly, I made the decision with the patient's wishes and well-being at the centre of my rationale.

At times since qualification as a nurse, these two factors have often appeared to be mutually exclusive and very hard to reconcile. I'd have been entirely justified (not to mention covered by policy) if I'd chosen to restrain Carl, to strip his room of further items that could be used to self-harm and then to manage a volatile, angry, and potentially violent, man accordingly.

However, I wanted to see him as a person, one who was perfectly capable of deciding what to do with his own body and who deserved the opportunity to make these choices. I was worried that I could have been accused of being 'soft' by colleagues, of giving a challenging patient exactly what he wanted in order to avoid conflict, but I'd never wanted to create difficult situations simply based on policy. While they are necessary and at times protective, policies can sometimes provide shelter for bad decisions – or even a lack of decision-making – while confidence, experience and instinct are often far more reliable and flexible. So much nursing education teaches (or attempts to teach) mental health nurses to consider each patient as an individual and I tried to do so here. Rather than managing the situation by forcing Carl to act in the manner that I felt was appropriate, I managed the person, thus allowing him to manage the situation himself, to maintain his dignity and (relative) freedom and to live his life.

Issues to Consider Regarding the Nurse's Decision-Making in Case Study 7.3

What this situation illustrates is that decision-making in clinical practice often relies on an approach that is sometimes described as being intuitive, drawing on prior expertise (Benner, 1984). It has been argued that adopting such an approach can lead to poor decision-making, resulting in unsatisfactory outcomes for all concerned (Elwyn et al., 2010).

Case study 7.3 illustrates that perhaps not all decisions can be found easily in textbooks. This nurse was faced with someone who, on the face of it, had a legitimate claim to be left alone to do what he wanted to do, albeit there were possibly some personal risks involved. There are several issues that have become entangled in this case.

The patient was awaiting transport back to prison because it had been decided he did not have a mental illness that might have been contributing to his criminal behaviour. Although there can be a connection between mental illness and criminal behaviour, this is not always the case. The National Confidential Inquiry into Suicide and Homicide by People with Mental Illness's (2016) *Making Mental Health Care Safer* report and review of 20 years' data, shows that approximately 11 homicides a year in England are committed by people who have a mental illness. In England there are around 725 murders each year. Given these figures, there is insufficient evidence to support the sensationalised stories in the media that people with mental health problems present a danger to the community.

Returning to Case study 7.3, when the patient had been challenged previously by ward staff about his behaviour, he had often responded with hostility and sometimes violence. The nurse had limited resources available and other patients on the ward to keep safe.

The patient was a long-term illicit drug user and had self-tattooed before. On this occasion, he was using an implement that could not be considered sterile, increasing the risk to his own health and well-being and, possibly, that of others around him.

Finally, the nurse in charge was aware of the ward's policy on how to deal with potentially disruptive and violent behaviour and was also aware that other colleagues may challenge the decisions that they had taken on the basis that non-conformity with the norms might make it difficult for others to make decisions in the future.

As the nurse observed, the decision was a complex one. Complete Activity 7.6 to give further consideration to professional decision-making challenges such as those in Case study 7.3.

Activity 7.6

1. Consider what you might have done in the situation presented in Case study 7.3. What ethical issues do you think might arise from looking after someone in a mental health service who does not have a recognisable diagnosis?
2. Which concern do you think was the most important one to take into account when making a decision: the personal safety of the patient and staff; the right to behave in the way in which the patient wanted to; or ensuring that the health of the patient was not compromised by the amateur tattooing?
3. Should limited resources ever be part of a professional decision-making process? If so, what ethical dilemmas may this give rise to?

In Case study 7.3, the nurse drew on a number of interpersonal factors in their decision-making. These appear to have been kindness, genuineness, civility and respect. Effective nurse–patient communication is at the heart of shared decision-making. Effective communication will enable, as in this case, the patient's perspective and contextual factors that may have an impact on the quality of the interaction with the nurse to be taken into account (Nadzam, 2009; NMC, 2018a; Roter, 2003).

Arguably, however, being an effective communicator requires something beyond developing and utilising an effective interpersonal style. It also requires the nurse to harness the insight available from the way in which their beliefs and assumptions, developed from previous experiences, influence the judgements and choices that they make within the decision-making process of care delivery (NMC, 2018e).

The key to effective involvement in decision-making is the relationships established between the patient and the mental health nurse. These are likely to be relationships that are supportive, and which reinforce the feeling of being heard and a sense of being valued as equals. While Case study 7.3 illustrates that the relationship does not have to be explicitly therapeutic to also be effective within mental health care, and indicates that patients do not find it helpful to be told what to do or think, or to have their actions judged. What is valued is help and support that can strengthen their pre-existing coping strategies, and recognises their expertise (Warne and McAndrew, 2007).

Warne and McAndrew (2010) argued that, in therapeutic practice, the most help-ful decisions are those that strengthen existing coping strategies rather than those that weaken them. Achieving effective nurse–patient participation in shared decision-making will also facilitate decisions taken to be transparent and open to scrutiny. While such an approach will benefit the patient, such transparency will also help a nurse to deal with anxieties such as those expressed by the nurse in Case study 7.3 regarding the judgements that their colleagues might make about the decisions they took in resolving the particular decision (Raynor and Warne, 2015).

Conforming to organisational norms has been the subject of much work, from the famous psychological studies carried out by American psychologist Milgram (1963) to the more contemporary studies that have looked at why people conform to organi-sational norms (Nightingale, 2018; Smith et al., 2007). For the newly qualified and appointed mental health nurse, there is great ontological security to be gained in conforming. They avoid harm and stress, by means of the protection of the group. Equally, however, the group can be oppressive and harmful to those who do not con-form (Warne and McAndrew, 2010).

We do not know how the nurse's colleagues in Case study 7.3 responded. We can see, however, from reading the reflection, that they looked to the qualified nurse recounting the experience as the 'nurse in charge' – to make the final decision. It is hoped, however, that the nurse's explanation for pursuing a shared approach to decision-making and, in this example, for achieving a positive outcome would have been a persuasive one, and the nurse's decision would have been accepted as the best one to have taken in that set of circumstances.

Conclusion

A greater emphasis has been placed on involving patients in the decisions made about their treatment and care. Collaborative or shared decision-making in professional practice reflects a shift in focus from professional values towards the values of service users. Patients can be experts as a result of their experiences and their experience of their mental health problems must be seen as unique, whatever the general consensus may be on a particular diagnosis or condition. The challenge for mental health nurses is to develop and nurture the organisational and professional norms that embrace and harness the values of patient participation at the level of individual care and decision-making.

References

Benner, P. (1984) *From Novice to Expert: excellence and power in clinical nursing practice.* Menlo Park, CA: Addison-Wesley.

Byrne, L., Happell, B. and Reid-Searl, K. (2017). Risky business: Lived experience mental health practice, nurses as potential allies. *International Journal of Mental Health Nursing,* 26: 285–292.

Campbell, K., Massey, D., Broadbent, M. and Clarke, K. (2018). Factors influencing clinical decision making used by mental health nurses to provide provisional diagnosis: A scoping review. *International Journal of Mental Health Nursing,* 28(2): 407–424.

Chong, W., Aslani, P. and Chen, T. (2013). Shared decision-making and interprofessional collaboration in mental healthcare: A qualitative study exploring perceptions of barriers and facilitators. *Journal of Interprofessional Care,* 27: 373–379.

Coulter, A. (2010). Do patients want a choice, and does it work? *British Medical Journal,* 341: 4989.

Coulter, A. and Collins, A. (2011). *Making Shared Decision-making a Reality: No decision about me, without me.* London: King's Fund.

Dowie, J. (1993). Clinical decision analysis: Background and introduction. In H. Llewelyn and A. Hopkins (eds) *Analysing How we Reach Clinical Decisions.* London: Royal College of Physicians of London.

Durcan, G., Stubbs, J., Appleton, S. and Bell, A. (2017). *The Future of the Mental Health Workforce.* London: Centre for Mental Health. pp. 4–44.

Elwyn, G., Frosch, D., Volandes, A., Edwards, A. and Montori, V. (2010). Investing in deliberation: A definition and classification of decision support interventions for people facing difficult health decisions. *Medical Decision Making,* 30(6): 701–711.

Entwistle, V., Cribb, A. and Watt, I. (2012). Shared decision-making: Enhancing the clinical relevance. *Journal of the Royal Society of Medicine,* 105(10): 416–421.

Freshwater, D. and Stickley, T. (2004). The heart of art: Emotional intelligence in nurse education. *Nursing Inquiry,* 11(2): 91–98.

Frogeli, E., Rudman, A. and Gustavsson, P. (2019). The relationship between task mastery, role clarity, social acceptance, and stress: An intensive longitudinal study with a sample of newly registered nurses. *International Journal of Nursing Studies,* 91: 60–69.

Gault, I., Gallagher, A. and Chambers, M. (2013). Perspectives on medicine adherence in service users and carers with experience of legally sanctioned detention and medication: A qualitative study. *Patient Preference and Adherence,* 7: 787–799.

Gaztambide-Fernández, R. and Arráiz Matute, A. (2017). On knowledge and knowing. *Curriculum Inquiry,* 47(2): 147–150.

Gluyas, H. (2015). Patient-centred care: Improving healthcare outcomes. *Nursing Standard,* 30(4): 50–59.

Greenway, K., Butt, G. and Walthall, H. (2019). What is a theory-practice gap?: An exploration of the concept. *Nurse Education in Practice,* 34: 1–6.

Haddad, P., Brain, C. and Scott, J. (2014). Nonadherence with antipsychotic medication in schizophrenia: Challenges and management strategies. *Patient Related Outcome Measures*, 5: 43–62.

Happell, B., Pinikahana, J. and Roper, C. (2003). Changing attitudes: The role of a consumer academic in the education of postgraduate psychiatric nursing students. *Archives of Psychiatric Nursing*, 17(2): 67–76.

Happell, B., Platania-Phung, C., Bocking, J., Ewart, S. B., Scholz, B. and Stanton, R. (2019). Consumers at the centre: Interprofessional solutions for meeting mental health consumers physical health needs. *Journal of Interprofessional Care*, 33: 226–234.

Hogarth, R. (2010). Intuition: A challenge for psychological research on decision making. *Psychological Inquiry*, 21: 338–353.

Kornhaber, R., Walsh, K., Duff, J. and Walker, K. (2016). Enhancing adult therapeutic interpersonal relationships in the acute health care setting: An integrative review. *Journal of Multidisciplinary Healthcare*, 9: 537–546.

Lakeman, R., McAndrew, S., McGabghann, L. and Warne, T. (2013). That was helpful, no one has talked to me about that before: Valuing the therapeutics of research participation. *International Journal of Mental Health Nursing*, 22: 76–84.

MacDonald-Wilson, K., Deegan, P., Hutchison, S., Parrotta, N. and Schuster, J. (2013). Integrating personal medicine into service delivery: Empowering people in recovery. *Psychiatric Rehabilitation Journal*, 36(4): 258–263.

McMillan, S., Kendall, E., Sav, A., King, M., Whitty, J., Kelly, F. and Wheeler, A. (2013). Patient-centred approaches to health care: A systematic review of randomized controlled trials. *Medical Care Research and Review*. 70(6): 567–596.

Malla, A., Joober, R. and Garcia, A. (2015). 'Mental illness is like any other medical illness': A critical examination of the statement and its impact on patient care and society. *Journal of Psychiatry and Neurosciences*, 40(3): 147–150.

Michie, S., Carey, R., Johnston, M., Rothman, A. J., Kelly, M., Davidson, K. and de Bruin, M. (2016). From theory-inspired to theory-based interventions: A protocol for developing and testing a methodology for linking behaviour change techniques to theoretical mechanisms of action. *Annals of Behavioural Medicine*, 52(6): 501–512.

Milgram, S. (1963). Behavioural study of obedience. *Journal of Abnormal and Social Psychology*, 67(4): 371–378.

Nadzam, D. (2009). Nurses' role in communication and patient safety. *Journal of Nursing Quality*, 24(3): 184–188.

National Confidential Inquiry into Suicide and Homicide by People with Mental Illness. (2016). *Making Mental Health Safer: Annual report and 20-year review*. Manchester: University of Manchester.

Nightingale, A. (2018). Developing the organisational culture in a healthcare setting. *Nursing Standard*, 32(21): 5363.

Noble, L. and Douglas, B. (2004). What users and relatives want from mental health. *Current Opinion in Psychiatry*, 17(4): 289–296.

Nursing and Midwifery Council (NMC) (2018a). *Future Nurse: Standards of proficiency for registered nurses*. London: NMC.

Nursing and Midwifery Council (NMC) (2018e) *The Code: Professional standards of practice and behaviour for nurses, midwives and nursing associates*. London: NMC.

Pathare, S. and Shields, L. S. (2012). Supported decision-making for persons with mental illness: A review. *Public Health Reviews*, 34(2): 1–40.

Raynor, G. and Warne, T., (2015). Interpersonal processes and self-injury: A qualitative study using Bricolage. *Journal of Psychiatric and Mental Health Nursing*, 23(1): 54–65.

Roberts, L. W. and Kim, J. P. (2016). Are individuals living with mental illness and their preferred alternative decision-makers attuned and aligned in their attitudes regarding treatment decisions? *Journal of Psychiatric Research*, 78: 42–47.

Rolfe, G. (2006). Judgements without rules: Towards a postmodern ironist concept of research validity. *Nursing Inquiry*. 13(1): 7–15.

Roter, D. L. (2003). Observations on methodological and measurement challenges in the assessment of communication during medical exchanges. *Patient Education and Counselling*, 50(1): 17–21.

Ryan, M., Kinghorn. P., Entwistle, V. A. and Francis, J. J. (2014). Valuing patients' experiences of healthcare processes: Towards broader applications of existing methods. *Social Science and Medicine*, 106: 194–203.

Rycroft-Malone, J. (2004). Research implementation: Evidence, context and facilitation – the PARIHS framework. In B. McCormack, K. Manley and R. Garbett (eds), *Practice Development in Nursing*. Oxford: Blackwell. pp. 118–147.

Schön, D. (1983). *The Reflective Practitioner: How professionals think in action*. New York: Basic Books.

Smith, J. R., Hogg, M. A., Martin, R. and Terry, D. J. (2007). Uncertainty and the influence of group norms in the attitude–behaviour relationship. *British Journal of Social Psychology*, 46(4): 769–792.

Smith, J. (2017). Building and maintaining the therapeutic relationship. In J. Smith, *Psychotherapy: A practical guide*. Cham, Switzerland: Springer, Cham. pp. 125–139.

Soane, E., Schubert, J., Herbert, L., Lunn, R. and Pollard, S. (2015). The relationship between information processing style and information seeking, and its moderation by affect and perceived usefulness: Analysis vs. procrastination. *Personality and Individual Differences*, 72: 72–78.

Warne, T. and McAndrew, S. (2007). Passive patient or engaged expert?: Using a Ptolemaic approach to enhance nurse education and practice. *International Journal of Mental Health Nursing*, 16(4): 224–229.

Warne, T. and McAndrew, S. (2010). Learning at the edges of knowing and not knowing. In T. Warne and S. McAndrew (eds), *Creative Approaches to Health and Social Care Education*. Basingstoke: Palgrave. pp. 232–239.

Woodbridge, K. and Fulford, B. (2003). Good practice?: Values-based practice in mental health. *Mental Health Practice*, 7(2): 30–34.

Further Reading

Best, S., Koski, A., Walsh, L. and Vuokila-Oikkonen, P. (2019). Enabling mental health student nurses to work co-productively. *Journal of Mental Health Training, Education and Practice*, 14(6): 411–422.

Conlon, D., Raeburn, T. and Wand, T. (2021). Decision-making processes of a nurse working in mental health, regarding disclosure of confidential personal health information of a patient assessed as posing a risk. *Collegian*, 28: 261–267.

Ewart, S. B., Scholz, B. and Stanton, R. (2019). Consumers at the centre: Interprofessional solutions for meeting mental health consumers physical health needs. *Journal of Interprofessional Care*, 33: 226–234.

Happell, B., Platania-Phung, C., Bocking, J., Campbell, K., Massey, D., Broadbent, M. and Clarke, K.-A. (2019). Factors influencing clinical decision making used by mental health nurses to provide provisional diagnosis: A scoping review. *International Journal of Mental Health Nursing*, 28: 407–424.

Health Education England (2020). *Mental Health Nursing: Competence and career framework*. London: Health Education England.

Tee, S., Lathlean, J., Herbert, L., Coldham, T., East, B. and Johnson, T.-J. (2007). User participation in mental health nurse decision making: A cooperative enquiry. *Journal of Advanced Nursing*, 60(2): 135–145.

Warne, T., McAndrew, S. and Jones, F. (2015). Assessment: The key to effective practice. In M. Chambers (ed.), *Psychiatric and Mental Health Nursing,* 3rd edn. Boca Raton, FL: CRC Press, Taylor & Francis.

Wright, K. M. (2021). Exploring the therapeutic relationship in nursing theory and practice. *Mental Health Practice*, 24(5): 34–41.

Wrycraft, N. (ed.) (2009). *An Introduction to Mental Health Nursing*. Buckingham: Open University Press.

Further Reading: Decision-making Experiences during the COVID-19 Pandemic

Foye, U., Dalton-Locke, C., Harju-Seppänen, J., Lane, R., Beames, L., Juan, N. V., Johnson, S. and Simpson, A. (2021). How has COVID-19 affected mental health nurses and the delivery of mental health nursing care in the UK?: Results of a mixed-methods study. *Journal of Psychiatric and Mental Health Nursing*, 28(2): 126–137.

Godbold, R., Whiting, L., Adams, C., Naidu, Y. and Pattison, N. (2021) The experiences of student nurses in a pandemic: A qualitative study. *Nurse Education in Practice*, 56: 103186.

Liberati, E., Richards, N., Willars, J., Scott, D., Boydell, N., Parker, J., Pinfold, V., Martin, G., Dixon-Woods, M. and Jones, P. B. (2021). A qualitative study of experiences of NHS mental healthcare workers during the COVID-19 pandemic. *BMC Psychiatry*, 21: 250.

Web Resources

Health Education England (2020), *Mental Health Nursing: Competence and career framework*: www.hee.nhs.uk/sites/default/files/documents/HEE%20Mental%20Health%20Nursing%20Career%20and%20Competence%20Framework.pdf (accessed 21 June 2022).

Mental Health Foundation – its website has links to many publications and resources, including a literature review on mental health capacity and the Mental Health Capacity Act 2005, which is focused on decision-making with individuals in a variety of the kinds of situations in which it is relevant: www.mentalhealth.org.uk (accessed 22 June 2022).

Substance Abuse and Mental Health Services Administration (SAMSHA) – this American organisation's website includes numerous resources that support shared decision-making with service users, which, although set in the context of the USA health care system, contains key concepts transferable to situations in the UK: www.samhsa.gov (accessed 22 June 2022).

8

DECISION-MAKING IN CHILDREN'S AND YOUNG PEOPLE'S NURSING PRACTICE

Angela Darvill and Natalie Robinson

Chapter objectives

The aims of this chapter are to:

- consider decision-making in the context of children's and young people's nursing;
- offer examples of decision-making in action through reflection and clinical case studies;
- consider how decision-making can be developed to achieve the proficiencies required by the Nursing and Midwifery Council (NMC);
- discuss the importance of communicating effectively with children, young people and their families to ensure that they can participate and be involved in decision-making.

Introduction

The purpose of this chapter is to address decision-making in the field of children's and young people's nursing practice in relation to the proficiencies outlined in the Nursing and Midwifery Council's (NMC) (2018a) *Standards of proficiency for registered nurses*. In order to explore these proficiencies, we will consider case scenarios from practice, and links will be made between the various examples and proficiencies. Whilst the chapter is specifically describing scenarios from the Children and Young People field of nursing, it can be read and used by students from all four fields of nursing practice.

The chapter will begin with an introduction to decision-making in the field of children's and young people's nursing, followed by the introduction of case scenarios and activities. Key aspects from the scenarios will be related to the NMC's (2018a) standards. The chapter will also include a discussion of the key elements required to make decisions in clinical practice. The evidence base for many of the decisions seen in the scenarios is interwoven throughout the narrative, thus enabling you to see how they link together in nursing practice.

Decision-Making in Children's and Young People's Nursing

The decision-making process for nurses working in this field is complex and requires that they work alongside the child and family to negotiate roles and promote care that is child and family centred (Corlett and Twycross, 2006). Such shared decision-making is at the heart of NHS improvement plans, and a key component in ensuring that care is patient centred. This is emphasised by Coulter and Collins (2011), in *Making Shared Decision-making a Reality: No decision about me, without me*, a report published by the King's Fund, which highlights that shared decision-making is seen as crucial by the professional regulatory bodies, and that health care professionals have a responsibility to share information and make decisions alongside patients. In the field of children and young people's nursing, there is also a need to ensure that any care delivery is child centred.

There is currently a great focus on the provision of healthcare for children and young people, with a need to improve health outcomes. The Royal College of Paediatrics and Child Health's (RCPCH) (2017a) report, *State of Child Health,* collated data from across the UK's four nations that give great insight into child health outcomes in the UK. The report's key findings are that progress is being made to improve the health of children and young people in the UK, however, progress is slow, and inequality hugely affects their health and well-being. The report was updated in England in 2020, with an additional update regarding child health during the COVID-19 pandemic. (See the Web resources section at the end of this chapter for links to the *State of Child Health* report and other reporting by the RCPCH of the impact of COVID-19 on child health services.)

All these reports and updates offer a valuable insight into changing patterns of care and the impact on the normal workforce in child health care. To overcome the perceived inequality and slow progress of changes, the *NHS Long Term Plan* (2019) had already laid out plans to promote a transformation of children's and young people's health services (see the Web resources section at the end of this chapter for the link).

The aim of the plan is to tackle health inequalities, put a focus on prevention rather than cure and help children and young people to navigate the often difficult transition into adulthood. At the heart of this, the *NHS Long Term Plan* recognises that children and young people represent a third of the population and their health determines the NHS's future. To improve the health of children and young people, we must work alongside them to prioritise, plan and implement their care. However, children and young people themselves have highlighted that, despite wanting to be involved in discussions and decisions about their health, they often don't feel that communication with health professionals is effective and adults working in children's health services do not always communicate effectively and appropriately with them (RCPCH, 2017a). This may be due to the instinct of adults to protect children from the distress and burden of decision-making, but that can be a barrier to including children in the process (Coyne and Harder, 2011). The further development and implementation of the NHS plans have been adversely affected by the COVID-19 pandemic.

To think about how you can be involved in supporting children and young people in decision-making consider Activity 8.1.

Activity 8.1

1. Consider how your assessors and supervisors in clinical practice involve children and young people in decisions about their care. Think about how you may negotiate these situations once you are qualified.

2. To help you with this exercise, access and read I. Coyne and M. Harder (2011), Children's participation in decision-making: Balancing protection with shared decision-making using a situational perspective, *Journal of Child Healthcare*, 15(4): 312–319.
3. Discuss with your supervisors how they can help you achieve ONE major goal of taking part in shared decision-making with a child, or a young person and their family.
4. Think about the potential barriers to enabling children to be part of the decision-making process in practice and how, as professionals, we can overcome these.

You may have identified the following barriers:

- adults and health care professionals considering that children and young people need protection;
- children and young people needing protection as they are unwell;
- parents and families answering questions on behalf of their children.

As a health care professional, you should ensure that children and young people are viewed as individuals who need and want to be involved, to participate in their care and have a right to a say. However, for them to be able to do so, they need to be provided with opportunities to learn how to participate in decision-making. Good practice involves developing trusting relationships with children, and ensuring their participation requires knowledge, confidence and imagination (Ehrich et al., 2015). As a child's maturity and understanding increases so their involvement in decisions about their health care should increase. At the same time, parental rights to make health care decisions about or on behalf of their child should decrease.

Decision-making is a key component of the NMC's (2018a) standards of proficiency for all fields of nursing: it is embedded in all seven platforms. Student nurses are required to work towards these standards and demonstrate proficiency at the point of registration.

Decision-making is a difficult process and requires health professionals to think critically, problem-solve and reflect on their practice experience, as well as implement scientific evidence-based practice and their knowledge of ethical values and professional accountability (Highe, 2018). Furthermore, it requires nurses to have the right knowledge, skills and values to think critically, apply evidence, draw on their experience and consider people's needs and preferences (NMC, 2018a).

Although this decision-making process is complex, as noted, at the point of registration, nurses are required to demonstrate proficiency in this area, applied to their specific field of practice (NMC, 2018a). For children and young person's nurses, this may mean negotiating not only the needs and preferences of the child or young person but also their parents or caregivers and wider family.

Despite the positive impact shared decision-making has on the outcomes for children, young people and their families, due to the complexity of the process, current evidence shows that it is not always achieved (Corlett and Twycross, 2006; Coyne and Gallagher, 2011).

Involving children and young people in decisions concerning their care requires nurses to ensure that information is delivered appropriately and at the right level, so that they can understand and actively participate. To promote this, nurses must seek to understand the children's and young people's perspective and not always assume that decisions made about their care by others are expressed in terms of their needs and wants (Söderbäck, Coyne and Harder, 2011).

Nurses also need to be able to adapt their communication to suit the developmental needs of children and young people in their care (Shapcott, 2018). The nurse should use methods of communication appropriate to each child's age and stage of development. With maturity a child's understanding and autonomy increase, influencing the involvement in their personal care decisions (Coyne and Livesley, 2010). The NMC's 2018a *Standards of proficiency for registered nurses*: Annexe A, states:

> Evidence-based, best practice communication skills and approaches for providing therapeutic interventions also apply to all registered nurses, but the level of expertise and knowledge required will vary depending on the chosen field of practice. Registered nurses must be able to demonstrate these skills to an appropriate level for their intended field(s) of practice. (2018a: 27)

Therefore, even though you may not be studying children's nursing, you will still have to be able to demonstrate that you have effective communication across the lifespan. The skills outlined will be applied in varying levels of complexity depending on your chosen field of practice.

To consider effective communication as a children's nurse complete Activity 8.2.

Activity 8.2

1. Access and read the Introduction to Annexe A in the NMC's *Standards of proficiency* (2018a: 27), on communication and relationship management skills, which applies to all four fields of practice.
2. Consider how a student nurse who is learning to become a children and young people's nurse could gain experience, knowledge and skills during their clinical placements in the following:

   3.1 motivational interview techniques
   3.2 solution focused therapies

3.3 reminiscence therapies

3.4 talking therapies

3.5 de-escalation strategies and techniques

3.6 cognitive behavioural therapy techniques

3.7 play therapy

3.8 distraction and diversion strategies

3.9 positive behaviour support approaches (2018a: 29: (see Annexe A: Section 3 – Evidence-based, best practice communication skills and approaches for providing therapeutic interventions)

3. Discuss your goal for *one* of these with your practice supervisor during your next placement, focusing on how they can offer learning experiences and demonstrate decision-making opportunities in this area.

Health care professionals want to provide care in children's and young people's best interests and to do so in ways that allow them to voice their preferences, be listened to, be heard at a level commensurate with their competence, experience, age and ability and their evolving capacity to understand – they know that this is of crucial importance (Alderson, 2017). Good practice involves developing trusting relationships with children, and ensuring their participation requires knowledge, confidence and imagination (Ehrich et al., 2015).

Decision-Making in Children and Young People's Nursing Practice: Legal, Ethical and Professional Standards

Children's and young people's right to participate in decision-making is underpinned by the UN Convention on the Rights of the Child 1989 and (for the United Kingdom) the Children Act 1989.

The Children Act 1989 states that the welfare of the child is paramount. Health care professionals should have regard for the ascertainable wishes and feelings of the child in the light of their age and understanding. The child who can form their own views has the right to express those views freely in all matters affecting them, with the views of the child being given due weight in accordance with their age and level of maturity (UN Convention, 1989).

You may think that health care professionals can make decisions about the care of children just with their parents, without involving the child, believing that children would not understand what is going on: that is not correct. It is important to help children to understand, through age-appropriate language and communication strategies so that they can be involved.

Children want to be involved in decisions about their care, and the benefits for them are that they feel prepared and less anxious, plus it promotes satisfaction with their health care (Coyne and Gallagher, 2011; Coyne et al., 2014; Törnqvist et al., 2015). According to Alderson et al. (2006), children can, and should, make informed decisions about their health care, so that it is in their best interests, and health care professionals should adopt an individualised approach to involving children in decision-making. The individual approach should be based on a child's wants and needs to participate and be involved (Alderson, 2017).

Health care professionals also want to provide care that is in the child's best interests and to ensure that they voice their preferences, are listened to, are heard at a level commensurate with their competence, experience, age, ability and their evolving capacity to understand, which is of crucial importance (Alderson, 2017). It has been suggested that children's participation in decision-making in relation to their health is more dependent on parents' and health professionals' attitudes than on their actual competence (Mårtenson and Fägerskiöld, 2008). Aside from the issue of age and attitudes related to children's competence, some health care professionals seem to believe that children's participation depends on a general assumption about the level of children's competence, and it being defined as a rational subject. This can result in the underestimation of an individual child's competence to understand a situation or information given (Coyne, 2006).

Activity 8.3 will enable you to focus on a child or young person's involvement in their own care and decision-making.

Activity 8.3

Reflect on a recent situation from clinical practice in which you were involved that required the involvement of a child or young person and make a note of the main decision-making issues.

1. How was information regarding health care shared with the child or young person?
2. How did you and other health care professionals communicate with the child or young person?
3. Were the child or young person's needs and preferences considered?

The next part of this chapter will follow a scenario that highlights some of the complexities of decision-making in children's and young people's nursing. The scenario is a fictitious one based on the immediate admission of a child to an assessment unit. It is designed to enable you to link the theory of decision-making and in particular the NMC's (2018a) standards and proficiencies. Several activities have been included to guide you through the decision-making process at key stages in her care.

Scenario 1(a): Decision-making in Practice

A five-year-old girl called Katie is admitted to a children's assessment unit. Katie is accompanied by her mother and younger sibling. Katie has been admitted through open access, as she has a life-limiting illness. She has developmental delay, learning difficulties and complex health needs, including a tracheostomy, and is fed enterally via a gastrostomy tube. Katie's mother has brought her into the assessment unit with symptoms of increased difficulty breathing and episodes of decreased oxygen levels overnight.

Decision-making practices involving children and young people with life-limiting illnesses and complex needs are often multifaceted and so require the children and young people's nurse to consider the child's needs and parental needs alongside legal and ethical considerations. The number of children with life-limiting illnesses is increasing, due to advances in health care technology and disease management (Gormley-Flemming and Campbell, 2011; Popejoy, 2015). As a result of this, there is a great expectation of optimal health and increased life expectancy, and this can make decision-making in child health complex (Gormley-Flemming and Campbell, 2011).

Complete Activity 8.4 and consider the overall care of Katie. It may also help you to identify areas where you need to gain further knowledge and skills during your placement learning.

Activity 8.4

1. Consider what information you would need to gather about Katie in Scenario 1 as part of the assessment process.
2. Consider what measurements and observations are required, what information you would need and how you would gather that information.
3. How will this information inform your clinical decision-making?

You may have considered the following things:

- gathering a set of clinical observations and undertaking a systematic assessment of Katie;
- the use of paediatric early warning scores to identify signs of deterioration (an example is the paediatric early warning score and system (PEW System); (see Web resources for further information);
- taking a full medical history from Katie's mother;
- identifying Katie's preferred communication methods and developmental abilities;

- identifying Katie's normal parameters associated with her overall health challenges, from the history taking, clinical knowledge and reading the medical and nursing notes.

The NMC has set out clear statements of proficiency in platform 3 of the Standards, Assessing needs and planning care (NMC, 2018a: 14/15) and you may wish to reconsider some of these that apply to the care of Katie (Scenario 1) at this point:

> 3.1 demonstrate and apply knowledge of human development from conception to death when undertaking full and accurate person-centred nursing assessments and developing appropriate care plans

> 3.2 demonstrate and apply knowledge of body systems and homeostasis, human anatomy and physiology, biology, genomics, pharmacology and social and behavioural sciences when undertaking full and accurate person-centred nursing assessments and developing appropriate care plans

> 3.15 demonstrate the ability to work in partnership with people, families and carers to continuously monitor, evaluate and reassess the effectiveness of all agreed nursing care plans and care, sharing decision-making and readjusting agreed goals, documenting progress and decisions made. (2018a: 14–15)

Assessment is an essential criterion in the decision-making process. Nurses conduct a thorough assessment of their patients and then make decisions based on the information they have gathered. For example, the nursing assessment may prompt nurses to implement an aspect of nursing care, request a medical review or think about planning for discharge. It is important that, during the assessment process, decision-making practices include the recognition of serious illness.

The Royal College of Paediatrics and Child Health's (RCPCH) (2017b) *Standards for Short-stay Paediatric Assessment Units (SSPAU)* state that children should have a standardised assessment within 15 minutes of their arrival, with regular paediatric early warning scores taken and recorded following this and, where appropriate, an escalation of treatment and care. The measurement of vital signs and observations is a key component of the role of children's nurse that will inform the broader assessment and decision-making process (Royal College of Nursing (RCN), 2017).

This initial assessment – also referred to as triage – is a process in which the children's nurse assesses the risk of deterioration and prioritises the nursing care. Within the standards of proficiency, the NMC has incorporated two Annexe sections, Annexe A (page 27–30) and Annexe B (page 31–37).

Annexe B is titled 'Nursing procedures' and incorporates a set of nursing procedures that newly registered nurses are required to demonstrate to meet proficiency outcomes (NMC, 2018a). These nursing procedures, as with all the NMC proficiency outcomes, should be applied to all four fields of practice. See Box 8.1 for an example from the procedures for assessing people's needs for person-centred care, then complete Activity 8.5.

Box 8.1

Nursing Procedures: Annexe B, Part 1 - Procedures for Assessing People's Needs for Person Centered Care

1. Use evidence-based, best practice approaches to take a history, observe, recognise and accurately assess people of all ages:

   1.2   *physical health and wellbeing*
   1.2.1 *symptoms and signs of physical ill health*
   1.2.2 *symptoms and signs of physical distress*
   1.2.3 *symptoms and signs of deterioration and sepsis.*

2. Use evidence-based, best practice approaches to undertake the following procedures:

   2.1   *take, record and interpret vital signs manually and via technological devices*
   2.7   *undertake a whole-body systems assessment including respiratory, circulatory, neurological, musculoskeletal, cardiovascular and skin status.* (NMC, 2018a: 32)

Activity 8.5

1. Think about the procedures taken from Annexe B in Box 8.1 and determine how these apply to the care of Katie in Scenario 1(a).
2. Consider how you would assess Katie for signs of physical stress or how you may recognise symptoms and signs of deterioration.
3. Now consider the care of a 15-year-old boy with a similar history to Katie. What would be different about the application of these procedures to his care, and how would this differ from your assessment of Katie? It might help at this point to make a note comparing any differences.

The nurse is often the first health care professional to have contact with children and young people in health care and therefore often the professional making initial decisions. The nurse is accountable for ensuring that information gathered during the assessment process is used appropriately to plan and prioritise needs, and to communicate information to the wider interdisciplinary team.

Consider the NMC (2018a) outcomes identified in Box 8.2 and determine how the EBP practice assessment procedures (in Box 8.1: Annexe B: Part 1) are important to gaining these proficiencies outcomes (NMC, 2018a).

Box 8.2

Platform 3: Assessing needs and planning Care

At the point of registration, the registered nurse will be able to:

3.11 undertake routine investigations, interpreting and sharing findings as appropriate
3.12 interpret results from routine investigations, taking prompt action when required by implementing appropriate interventions, requesting additional investigations or escalating to others
3.13 demonstrate an understanding of co-morbidities and the demands of meeting people's complex nursing and social care needs when prioritising care plans
(NMC, 2018a: 15)

Assessment of children and young people with complex needs is often difficult. They may have several underlying health conditions, their anatomy and physiology may differ from what would be expected due to those conditions, and different methods of communication may be required (RCPCH, 2014). To consider these communication needs when planning the care of a child, undertake Activity 8.6 which again focuses on the needs of Katie (Scenario 1(a)).

Activity 8.6

1. Return to Scenario 1(a) and consider the different ways in which Katie may communicate her needs to you.
    Make a note of these as we will be returning to the care of Katie in Scenario 1(b), which continues to provide us with information concerning her situation.
2. It may be helpful to check through your thoughts by visiting NHS Scotland's Children with Exceptional Healthcare Needs (CEN) website and read 'Communication with children with complex and exceptional healthcare needs', which provides a useful guide and further resources for professionals working with these children (see the Web resources section at the end of this chapter for the link).

We will now continue to consider Katie's ongoing care needs, as well as how her mother is involved in communication with her (see Scenario 1(b)).

Scenario 1(b): Katie and her Ongoing Care

During your assessment of Katie, her mother notes that Katie appears uncomfortable. She informs you that Katie has been unsettled for most of the night and this is unusual for her. Your observations of Katie appear to be in the normal ranges and are not scoring abnormal on the paediatric early warning system. Katie's mother, however, is concerned about her and highlights that she is needing more tracheostomy suction and is difficult to settle. She communicates to you that she feels Katie may need some chest physiotherapy.

Working in partnership with Katie's mother, as well as sharing decisions about Katie's care, is an essential outcome to learn to achieve proficiency in platform 4: Providing and evaluating care (NMC, 2018a:16). This is identified as:

4.2 work in partnership with people to encourage shared decision-making to support individuals, their families and carers to manage their care when appropriate. (2018a: 17)

Parents and carers of children with complex health needs are experts in their child's medical needs (RCPCH, 2014), and including them in the assessment and decision-making processes is an important aspect of the nursing role. The nurse must recognise additional needs and implement measures to ensure that the child is assessed appropriately, and that they and their family are included in the decision-making practices.

The Together for Short Lives' Charter (2012) identifies the importance of recognising the rights of children and young people with a life-limiting condition. The Charter places emphasis on the need to ensure that, 'Children and families should always be listened to, and be encouraged to talk through their wishes and care choices.' Using the child's preferred method of communication and understanding behavioural cues will ensure that the child is involved in decisions made about their care (RCPCH, 2014).

The prevalence of children living with disabilities and complex health needs is rising. Although ascertaining prevalence on an international level is problematic, it is a widely held view that, within the UK, there is an increasing number of children living with life-limiting or life-threatening illness or who are technology dependent (Whiting, 2019). Therefore, it is vital that children and families living with such long-term conditions are engaged in the management of their care and supported to make decisions relating to their condition (Garnett, Smith and Ormandy, 2016).

In Scenario 1(b), Katie's mother actively voices her concern regarding her child's condition to the nursing staff. It is paramount that health care professionals, although they are experts in their areas of practice, remember that carers and families know their children best and have their best interests at heart (Gormley-Fleming and Campbell, 2011).

Parents and guardians are given the responsibility for the welfare of their child and all that entails. Though they do possess superior knowledge of their children, they may not always have the knowledge of health care that is needed. It is therefore paramount that decisions are made alongside health care professionals (Gormley-Fleming and Campbell, 2011). Parents are best placed to convey what is in the best interests of their child when that child is unable to convey this themselves; they know their child best by virtue of being their parents (Highe, 2018). Ensuring that you work alongside children and their families in the decision-making process is a vital skill for children's and young people's nurses and collaborating with them should be applied to all elements of the nursing process. To this end, proficiency outcomes of the NMC's platform 3: Assessing needs and planning care require that nurses at the point of registration will be able to:

3.4 understand and apply a person-centred approach to nursing care, demonstrating shared assessment, planning, decision-making and goal setting when working with people, their families, communities and populations of all ages

3.5 demonstrate the ability to accurately process all information gathered during the assessment process to identify needs for individualised nursing care and develop person-centred evidence-based plans for nursing interventions with agreed goals

3.6 effectively assess a person's capacity to make decisions about their care and to give or withhold consent

3.7 understand and apply the principles and processes for making reasonable adjustments. (2018a: 14)

To continue to understand the ongoing care of Katie, and how we can see the importance of achieving all the proficiency outcomes considered so far when caring for a child with similar needs, undertake Activity 8.7.

Activity 8.7

1. First re-read Scenario 1(a) concerning Katie's admission to the assessment unit as a reminder of some of her health challenges and what has brought her to the unit.
2. Now read Scenario 1(b) again and consider the information that Katie's mother has communicated to you.
3. What action would you take regarding the information Katie's mother has provided?

You may have considered taking the following actions concerning the information provided by Katie's mother (Activity 8.7):

- completing a pain assessment using an appropriate pain tool, as Katie's mother communicated Katie's discomfort to you;
- communicating the assessment to members of the interdisciplinary team;
- requesting a review from the physiotherapy team.

Platform 5 of the NMC's Standards of proficiencies focuses on 'Leading and managing nursing care and working in teams' and it states that nurses 'play an active and equal role in the interdisciplinary team, collaborating and communicating effectively with a range of colleagues' (2018a: 19). One of the outcome statements for platform 5 identifies that the registered nurses must be able to:

> 5.4 demonstrate an understanding of the roles, responsibilities and scope of practice of all members of the nursing and interdisciplinary team and how to make best use of the contributions of others involved in providing care (2018: 20).

We can see from both scenarios of Katie's care that the decision-making process in children's and young people's nursing is multifaceted. Nurses in this field must possess expert knowledge and skills in caring for children across the lifespan from infancy, through childhood, adolescence and the transition into adulthood. Highe (2018) emphasises that nurses are accountable to children and their families for the care they give. It is paramount that children's and young people's nurses apply their specialist expertise and knowledge in their field of practice to the individual needs and preferences of children and young people. In addition to this, Söderbäck, Coyne and Harder (2011) remind us that we must not always assume that adults know what is in the child's best interest and should always consider the child's perspective during the decision-making process. They go on to highlight that children's and young people's nurses should ensure that they are applying a child centred approach which safeguards the rights of the child. Coulter and Collins inform us that 'the most important reason for practicing shared decision-making is that it is the right thing to do' (2011: 11).

Communicating with Children and Young People

The importance of communicating effectively with children, young people and their families to ensure that they can participate and be involved in decision-making is paramount. Ineffective communication is one of the barriers to children's and young people's involvement in the decision-making process. Listening to their needs and preferences will promote their involvement, but it is important to recognise that they may feel overwhelmed and stressed by this process. Children's and young people's nurses should be able to recognise this and tailor their involvement to avoid or resolve such difficulties (Coyne and Gallagher, 2011; Moore and Kirk; 2010).

According to the NMC's (2018a) Annexe A (p27), nurses, using a range of skills and strategies, should be able to communicate effectively with people at all stages of life and who have a range of mental, physical, cognitive and behavioural health challenges. The Nurses should also have the ability to demonstrate the knowledge, communication and relationship management skills required to provide people, families and carers with accurate information that meets their needs before, during and after a range of interventions.

Children and young people want to have their voices heard. To ensure that this happens, the nurse must communicate effectively with them. It is vital to respect their views and rights to be involved in decisions about their care and treatment. Receiving information and having their views respected changes children's understanding and, in turn, their level of involvement in decisions about their care (Coyne and Livesley, 2010).

According to Coyne and Gallagher (2011), lack of involvement in the communication and decision-making process has negative effects – children report feeling disappointed, sad, confused, angry, worried, shocked, betrayed, lonely, ignored and rejected. Children need information if they are to know what to expect about their care. Children who are involved feel happy, valued and less anxious.

It is important to avoid only involving children and young people in a tokenistic way. You should acknowledge children's preferences about their care and listen and let them have their say. The importance of such communication cannot be underestimated. Indeed, it is crucial that nurses adopt the principle 'no decision about me, without me' (Department of Health, 2012). In the consultation document *Liberating the NHS: No decision about me, without me*, the Department of Health (2012) outlined detailed proposals to make this a reality and increase opportunities for children and their families to have more involvement in decisions about their care.

For effective communication with children and their families it is necessary to establish a therapeutic relationship. Children's nurses must recognise the child and young person as a pivotal member in the family unit. Establishing and maintaining dynamic, reciprocal therapeutic relationships not only with the child but also with the family is important (Roberts, Fenton and Barnard, 2015).

Essential interpersonal skills that ensure effective communication skills include questioning, explaining, reassuring and listening (Lambert, 2012). Skills in giving explanations, in particular, are a prerequisite for children, young people and their families' increased participation in health care decisions that affect them directly (Mikkelson and Frederickson, 2011). The nurse is required to build trust, empower children and their families and demonstrate respect so they can have an active role in their care. The nurse should always attempt to engage children and young people fully in decision-making and care planning and give them time to express their views.

Decision-making in the context of communication and interpersonal skills involves considering the significance and consequences of decisions – the perceived risks and levels of uncertainty. It is about weighing up what can and cannot be achieved and then deciding the best plan of action and how to achieve a successful outcome (Bach and Grant, 2010). Therefore, for children and young people to be involved in this complex process, there needs to be effective communication of all the risks and benefits of the treatment and it is important to explore the best plan of action with them and their families.

Now consider from your own learning experiences in practice how you carried out communicating effectively with children, young people and their families by undertaking the reflection in Activity 8.8.

Activity 8.8

1. Reflect on a situation in practice when you communicated with a child or young person.
2. Write down what you considered in relation to the following:

    *   What went well
    *   What you found difficult
    *   What you enjoyed or did not enjoy about the experience
    *   What feelings it provoked for you
    *   What interpersonal skills of questioning, listening, explaining and reassuring you used.

    You could use a reflective framework to support this activity (see Chapter 4 for examples).
3. In addition, refer to the NMC's *Standards of proficiency*: Annexe A: Section 3: Communication and relationship management skills (2018a: 27-30), and determine how many of these skills, in relation to a child or young person, that you achieved during the placement. Here are some examples:

    1.1 actively listen, recognise and respond to verbal and non-verbal cues
    1.2 use prompts and positive verbal and non-verbal reinforcement
    1.3 use appropriate non-verbal communication including touch, eye contact and personal space
    1.4 make appropriate use of open and closed questioning
    1.5 use caring conversation techniques
    1.6 check understanding and use clarification techniques. (2018a: 28)

In order to explore various possible scenarios encountered in practice consider the one with a young person in a different age group in Scenario 2.

Scenario 2: Communicating with Young People with Mental Health Challenges

You have been asked to admit a 13-year-old boy, named Charlie, to an acute children's ward following an incident of self-harm. He tells you that he feels unhappy, anxious at school and explains that home life is complicated. Also mentioned during this initial discussion are concerns about the pressures of social media.

In Box 8.3 are key aspects from the NMC's Standards of proficiencies and procedures that can be considered in your decision-making activities in relation to the care of the young person in Scenario 2.

Once you have considered the initial issues raised with Charlie, and the expectations of a nurse at the point of registration, complete Activity 8.9.

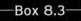

Box 8.3

NMC's *Standards of proficiency* 2018a: proficiencies, outcomes and procedures

Platform 2: Promoting health and preventing ill health

Outcome: 2.6 understand the importance of early years and childhood experiences and the possible impact on life choices, mental, physical and behavioural health and wellbeing. (2018a: 12)

Platform 4: Providing and evaluating care

Outcome: 4.4 demonstrate the knowledge and skills required to support people with commonly encountered mental health, behavioural, cognitive and learning challenges, and act as a role model for others in providing high-quality nursing interventions to meet people's needs. (2018a: 17)

Annexe B: Nursing procedures

Part 1: Procedures for assessing people's needs for person-centred care

1. use evidence-based, best practice approaches to take a history, observe, recognise and accurately assess people of all ages:

1.1 mental health and wellbeing status

1.1.1 signs of mental and emotional distress or vulnerability

1.1.4 behavioural distress-based needs

1.1.5 signs of mental and emotional distress including agitation, aggression and challenging behaviour

1.1.6 signs of self-harm and/or suicidal ideation. (2018a: 32)

Activity 8.9

1. Consider how you might develop a therapeutic relationship with the young person <Charlie> in Scenario 2 and ensure that you make a commitment to encourage participation in the ensuing decision-making process.
2. To do this, it may be helpful to use Shier's (2001) model for enhancing children's participation in decision-making in: H. Shier (2001). Pathways to participation: Openings, opportunities and obligations. *Children and Society*, 15(2), 107–117 and the article by J. Roberts, G. Fenton and M. Barnard (2015) (see the Web resources section for the direct links). Access both these articles and read them to help you to understand what is involved in this engagement between nurse and young person.

From your actions and reading for Activity 8.9, we can see that developing a therapeutic relationship includes the key elements of empathy, trust, respect, developing a rapport, being open and honest, whilst also ensuring that professional boundaries are maintained (Roberts, Fenton and Barnard, 2015). From Shier's (2001) article you may have identified that it would be important to listen, to enable and support the young person to express views and opinions on relevant matters and take those views into account. You may also have discerned that it is important to ensure that the young person is involved in the decision-making process and shares the power and responsibility for the decision made.

According to NICE (2004), regarding self-harm, all children and young people who have self-harmed should be assessed by health care practitioners experienced in the assessment of children and adolescents who self-harm. These assessments should include a full assessment of the family, their social situation and any child safeguarding issues. The child and adolescent mental health team should also undertake an assessment and provide where appropriate, ongoing information and support for the young person, their family, the paediatric team and social services and education staff.

Despite the policy recommendations highlighting the benefits of participation and involvement (Coulter and Collins, 2011), children and young people who self-harm are rarely actively involved in decisions about their care and treatment with mental health services (Gondek et al., 2017). Factors affecting their involvement include:

- information sharing in an appropriate amount and at the right time;
- their ability to listen;
- respecting and validating their decisions;
- assessing their capacity to be involved in their care;
- developing effective therapeutic relationships.

These issues now become neutral ones and apply to any involvement with mental health services in general.

The Legal, Ethical and Professional Issues of Involvement of Children and Young People in Decision-Making

The ethical principle of autonomy and respect for persons is at the heart of all decision-making. 'Autonomy' refers to the respect that should be shown for individuals' ability for self-determination and his or her own personal goals (Gillon, 1994). Children and young people have this right to self-determination and choice with regard to their care, support and treatment. Bou-Habib and Olsaretti (2015) maintain that most children possess some meaningful degree of autonomy, even in early childhood. A relatively young child would have sufficient maturity and intelligence to be capable of being involved in some decisions about their health care. Therefore, there is a responsibility to respect the autonomous free choices of all who are competent to make them. Fairness, justice and respect for persons would lead to the conclusion that children and young people who are competent to make a choice should have their choice honoured (Griffith and Tengnah, 2017).

However, the courts in the UK acknowledge that no child under 18 is a wholly autonomous being but recognise that the right of a child to be involved and consent to treatment develops with maturity and age. Newborn babies and young children lack the abilities required to make autonomous decisions and so can be described as having limits to their autonomy or limited autonomy (Hendrick, 2010). Therefore, it is important to ensure that their ability to *become* involved is facilitated and developed over time. Children's capacity to be involved in decision-making can develop with the cognitive and evaluative skills to make choices that others should respect.

When making decisions, it is important to act in ways that ensure the principles of beneficence and non-maleficence are respected. 'Beneficence' refers to the duty to provide benefit and 'non-maleficence' refers to the duty of not inflicting harm (Wyatt, 2010). (See also Chapter 5 for further explanation.)

The fundamental obligation to act positively for the benefit or best interests of others underpins *The Code* NMC (2018e). In upholding *The Code*, nurses have an ethical duty and are expected to promote children and young people's well-being and best interests. Balancing benefits and harm means making sure that benefits outweigh harm (Hendrick, 2010). *The Code* adds that it is important to encourage and empower people to share in decisions about their treatment and care, and nurses should respect the level to which people receiving care want to be involved in decisions about their own health, well-being and care.

It is vital to remember that parents have a central role in participating in all treatment decisions, and health care professionals must develop an open, respectful and collaborative relationship with parents from the beginning in order for the best decisions to be reached (Wyatt, 2010). In these situations, it is important that parents fully understand the decisions they are making, and they have the right to refuse consent.

Gormley-Fleming and Campbell (2011) state that if parents are not fully informed of the treatment for which they are consenting, they will find it difficult to reach an informed decision. The decisions revolve around the parents or person with parental responsibility to act in their child's best interests whilst protecting them from harm and recognising the child's varying ability to participate in decisions about their health care (Gormley-Fleming and Campbell, 2011). Some parents and, indeed, health care professionals may have difficulty supporting children's participation because they feel that children should be protected. Such views need to be respected and explored sensitively.

Children are dependent on adults to advocate for them until they have the verbal and cognitive abilities to give voice to their needs (Coyne, 2011). Coyne (2011) highlights that children are at risk of being unable to evaluate options and make informed decisions if they are not given opportunities to participate.

Conclusion

This chapter has explored the concept of decision-making in the field of children's and young people's nursing practice. It is paramount for children's nurses to ensure that the child's voice is considered. However, parents and families have a central role to play and should be able to participate in all treatment decisions. Health care professionals must develop therapeutic relationships with children and their families and find ways to work with them so that the best decision can be reached. A children's nurse must be committed to ensuring that they involve children and young people in decisions about their care. This complex process requires effective communication skills.

It is each child's and young person's right to participate in decision-making – a right underpinned by legal, ethical and professional standards. The best interests of the child must be a priority in all decisions and actions that affect children. From critical reflection on your practice as a student nurse and working alongside your practice supervisors and others in the health care teams, you will have seen for yourself the complexity of decision-making in action. As you become more exposed to various experiences with children, young people and their families, you will be able to achieve the proficiencies expected of a future qualified children's and young people's nurse.

References

Alderson, P. (2017). Children's consent and the zone of parental discretion. *Clinical Ethics*, 12(2): 55–62.

Alderson, P., Sutcliffe, K. and Curtis, K. (2006). Children as partners with adults in their medical care. *Archives of Disease in Childhood*, 91: 300–303.

Bou-Habib, P. and Olsaretti, S. (2015). Autonomy and children's wellbeing. In A. Bagattini and C. Macleod (eds), *The Nature of Children's Well-being: Theory and practice*. New York: Springer.

Brierley, J. and Larcher, V. (2016). Adolescent autonomy revisited: Clinicians need clearer guidance. *Journal of Medical Ethics*, 42(8): 482–485.

Corlett, J. and Twycross, A. (2006). Negotiation of parental roles within family-centred care: A review of the research. *Journal of Clinical Nursing*, 15(10): 1308–1316.

Coulter, A. and Collins, A. (2011). *Making Shared Decision-making a Reality: No decision about me, without me*. London: King's Fund.

Coyne, I. (2006). Children's experiences of hospitalization. *Journal of Child Health Care*, 10(4): 326–336.

Coyne, I. (2011). Children's experience of hospitalisation and their participation in health care decision making. I. In G. Brykczynska & J. Simons, Ethical and Philosophical Aspects of Nursing Children and Young People (1st ed., pp. 127–143). Wiley.

Coyne, I. and Harder, M. (2011). Children's participation in decision-making: Balancing protection with shared decision-making using a situational perspective. *Journal of Child Health Care*, 15(4): 312–319.

Coyne, I. and Livesley, J. (2010). Introduction to the core principles in children's nursing. In I. Coyne, F. Neill and F. Timmins (eds.), *Clinical Skills in Children's Nursing*. Oxford: Oxford University Press.

Coyne, I., Amory, A., Kiernan, G. and Gibson, F. (2014). Children's participation in shared decision-making: children, adolescents, parents and healthcare professionals' perspectives and experiences. *European Journal of Oncology Nursing*, 18: 273–280.

Department of Health (2012). *Liberating the NHS: No decision about me, without me*. London: The Stationery Office.

Ehrich, J., Pettoello-Mantovani, M., Lenton, S., Damm, L. and Goldhagen, J. (2015). Participation of children and young people in their healthcare: Understanding the potential and the limitations. *Journal of Pediatrics*, 167(3): 783–784.

Garnett, V., Smith, J. and Ormandy, P. (2016). Child–parent shared decision-making about asthma management. *Nursing Children and Young People*, 28(4): 16–22.

Gillon, R. (1994). Medical ethics: Four principles plus attention to scope. *British Medical Journal*, 309: 184–188.

Gormley-Fleming, L. and Campbell, A. (2011). Factors involved in young people's decisions about their health care. *Nursing Children and Young People*, 23(9): 19–22.

Gondek, D., Edbrooke-Childs, J., Velikonja, T., Chapman, L., Saunders, F., Hayes, D. and Wolpert, M. (2017). Facilitators and barriers to person-centred care in child and young people mental health services: A systematic review. *Clinical Psychology and Psychotherapy*, 24(4): 870–886.

Griffith, R. and Tenghan, C. (2017). *Law and Professional Issues in Nursing*, 4th edn. London: Sage.

Hendrick, J. (2010). *Law and Ethics for Children's Nurses*. Cheltenham: Nelson Thornes.

Highe, L. (2018). Decision-making and accountability in children and young people's nursing. In J. Price and O. McAlinden (eds). *Essentials of Nursing Children and Young People*. Thousand Oaks, CA: Sage.

Lambert, V. (2012). Theoretical foundations of communication. In V. Lambert, T. Long and D. Kelleher (2012), *Communication Skills for Children's Nurses*. Buckingham/New York: Open University Press/McGraw-Hill.

Mårtenson, E. K. and Fägerskiöld, A. M. (2008). A review of children's decision-making competence in health care. *Journal of Clinical Nursing*, 17(23): 3131–3141.

Mikkelson, G. and Frederickson, K. (2011). Family-centred care of children in hospital: a concept analysis, *Journal of Advanced Nursing*, 67(5): 1152–1162.

Moore, L. and Kirk, S. (2010). A literature review of children's and young people's participation in decisions relating to health care. *Journal of Clinical Nursing*, 19(15–16): 2215–2225.

National Institute for Health and Care Excellence (NICE) (2004). *Self-harm in over 8s: short-term management and prevention of recurrence* (CG16). London and Manchester: NICE.

Nursing and Midwifery Council (NMC) (2018a). *Future Nurse: Standards of proficiency for registered nurses*. London: NMC.

Nursing and Midwifery Council (NMC) (2018e). *The Code: Professional standards of practice and behaviour for nurses, midwives and nursing associates*. London: NMC.

Popejoy, E. (2015). Parents' experiences of care decisions of care decisions about children with life-limiting illnesses. *Nursing Children and Young People*, 27(8): 20–24. London: RCN.

Roberts, J., Fenton, G. and Barnard, M. (2015). Developing effective therapeutic relationships with children, young people and their families. *Nursing Children and Young People*, 27(4): 30–35.

Royal College of Nursing (RCN) (2017). *Standards for Assessing, Measuring and Monitoring Vital Signs in Infants, Children and Young People*. RCN: London.

Royal College of Paediatrics and Child Health (RCPCH) (2014). *Children and Young People with Complex Medical Needs*. London: RCPCH.

Royal College of Paediatrics and Child Health (RCPCH) (2017a). *State of Child Health Report*. London: RCPCH.

Royal College of Paediatrics and Child Health (RCPCH) (2017b). *Standards for Short-stay Paediatric Assessment Units (SSPAU)*. London: RCPCH.

Rycroft-Malone, J. (2004). Research implementation: Evidence, context and facilitation – the PARIHS framework. In B. McCormack, K. Manley and R. Garbett (eds), *Practice Development in Nursing*. Oxford: Blackwell. pp. 118–147.

Shapcott, J. (2018). Effective communication with children and young people. In J. Price and O. McAlinden (eds), *Essentials of Nursing Children and Young People*. Thousand Oaks, CA: Sage.

Shier, H. (2001). Pathways to participation: Openings, opportunities and obligations. *Children and Society*, 15(2): 107–117.

Söderbäck, M., Coyne, I. and Harder, M. (2011). The importance of including both a child perspective and the child's perspective within health care settings to provide truly child-centred care. *Journal of Child Health Care*, 15(2): 99–106.

Together for Short Lives (2012). *Together for Short Lives Charter*. Bristol: Together for Short Lives (available online at: www.togetherforshortlives.org.uk/get-support/supporting-you/family-resources/together-short-lives-charter, accessed 28 January 2022).

Törnqvist, E., Månsson, Å. and Hallström, I. (2015). Children having magnetic resonance imaging: A preparatory storybook and audio/visual media are preferable to anaesthesia or deep sedation. *Journal of Child Health Care*, 19(3): 359–369.

Whiting, M. (2019). Caring for children – '24-7': The experience of WellChild Nurses and the families for whom they are providing care and support. *Journal of Child Health Care*, 23(1): 35–44.

Wyatt, J. (2010). Neonatal ethics. In M. Meeks, M. Hallsworth and H. Yeo (eds), *Nursing the Neonate*, 2nd edn. Chichester, West Sussex: Wiley-Blackwell. pp. 334–344.

Further Reading

Carter, B., Bray, L., Dickinson, A., Edwards, M. and Ford, K. (2014). *Child-Centred Nursing: Promoting critical thinking*. London: Sage.

Children's Commissioner (2017). Children's voices. *The wellbeing of children with mental health needs in England*. London: Children's Commissioner.

Coyne, I., O'Mathúna, D., Gibson, F., Shields, L., Leclercq, E. and Sheaf, G. (2016). Interventions for promoting participation in shared decision-making for children with cancer (Review). *Cochrane Database of Systematic Reviews 2016*, 11: Article No. CD008970.

Martin, K., Morton, L., Reid, J., Feltham, A., William Reid, J., Jeremy, G. and McCulloch, J. (2019) The Me first communication model. *Nursing Children and Young People*, 31(2): 38–47.

Further Reading: Decision-making Experiences during the COVID-19 Pandemic

Agostoni, C., Bertolozzi, G., Cantoni, B., Colombo, C., Montini, G. and Marchisio, P. (2020). Three months of COVID-19 in a paediatric setting in the center of Milan. *Paediatric Research*, 89: 1572–1577.

Conlon, C., McDonnell, T., Barrett, M., Cummins, F., Deasy, C., Hensey, C., McAuliffe, E. and Nicholson, E. (2021). The impact of the COVID-19 pandemic on child health and the provision of care in paediatric emergency departments: A qualitative study of frontline emergency care staff. *BMC Health Services Research*, 21, Article No. 279.

Jalongo, M. R. (2021). The effects of COVID-19 on early childhood education and care: Research and resources for children, families, teachers, and teacher educators. *Early Childhood Education Journal*, 49: 763–774.

Warrillow, S., Austin, D., Cheung, W., Close, E., Holley, A., Horgan, B. et al. (2020). ANZICS guiding principles for complex decision making during the COVID-19 pandemic. *Critical Care and Resuscitation*, 22(2): 98–102.

Web Resources

Mental Health Foundation (2021). *Children and young people*: www.mentalhealth.org.uk/a-to-z/c/children-and-young-people (accessed 22 June 2022).

NHS (2019). *The NHS Long Term Plan*: www.longtermplan.nhs.uk (accessed 22 June 2022).

Scotland's CEN website – see *Communicating with children with complex and exceptional healthcare needs,* in its *National Managed Clinical Network* section. Provides a useful guide and further resources for professionals working with these children: www.cen.scot.nhs.uk/communicating-with-children-with-complex-and-exceptional-healthcare-needs (accessed 22 June 2022).

Office for Health Improvement and Disparities (2022). Chapter 4: Children and young people, *COVID-19 Mental Health and Wellbeing Surveillance Report* (updated 12 April): www.gov.uk/government/publications/covid-19-mental-health-and-wellbeing-surveillance-report/7-children-and-young-people (accessed 22 June 2022).

Roberts, J., Fenton, G., and Barnard, M. (2015). Developing effective therapeutic relationships with children, young people and their families. *Nursing Children and Young People*, 27(4), 30–35 at: https://pubmed.ncbi.nlm.nih.gov/25959488 (accessed 22 June 2022).

Royal College of Paediatrics and Child Health (RCPCH) – has a wide range of up-to-date resources (see *Resources* and *Key topics* tabs), including posters and a child protection portal: www.rcpch.ac.uk (accessed 22 June 2022).

Impact of COVID-19 on child health services tool: www.rcpch.ac.uk/resources/impact-covid-19-child-health-services-tool (accessed 22 June 2022).

Impact of COVID-19 on child health services between December 2020 and February 2021 – report: www.rcpch.ac.uk/resources/impact-covid-19-child-health-services-part-2-report (accessed 22 June 2022).

RCPCH (2020). *State of Child Health Report* – full report and update: https://stateofchildhealth.rcpch.ac.uk/wp-content/uploads/sites/2/2020/03/SOCH-ENGLAND-02.03.20.pdf (accessed 22 June 2022).

Shier, H. (2001). Pathways to participation: Openings, opportunities and obligations. *Children and Society*, 15(2), 107–117 at: http://cmspres-vir-1.it.gu.se/digitalAssets/1429/1429848_shier2001.pdf (accessed 22 June 2022).

World Health Organization (WHO). Improving the mental and brain health of children and adolescents: www.who.int/activities/improving-the-mental-and-brain-health-of-children-and-adolescents (accessed 12 July 2022).

9

DECISION-MAKING IN LEARNING DISABILITY NURSING

Louise Cogher and Dale Nixon

Chapter objectives

The aims of this chapter are to:

- explain the value base underpinning decision-making with people with learning disabilities;
- provide examples from practice of how and why decisions are made, and the thought processes involved, including top tips;

- draw attention to some of the particular challenges that you may encounter when making decisions with and in the best interests of people with learning disabilities;
- consider the evidence and best practice to support achieving Nursing and Midwifery Council (NMC) proficiencies.

Introduction

People with learning disabilities have the same rights to health care as anyone else. However, there are health inequalities for people with learning disabilities and these are now well documented. In particular, there is the Learning Disabilities Mortality Review (LeDeR) Programme (Healthcare Quality Improvement Partnership, 2019; LeDeR, 2021), which reviews the deaths of people with learning disabilities to identify any issues where there may have been concern in relation to the care received prior to these deaths and makes recommendations for service improvements. This is in line with the introduction of the National Guidance on Learning from Deaths framework in England in 2017 (National Quality Board, 2017), which arose from a growing concern regarding unexpected deaths within the NHS.

The importance of good decision-making, therefore, with and in the best interests of people with learning disabilities, is paramount in ensuring that health inequalities are addressed and, hopefully, reversed to achieve optimum health outcomes, avoid premature death and achieve a good life for all people with a learning disability (NIHR, 2020).

For the most part, people with learning disabilities can make their own decisions about their health care, but the assumptions of health and social care professionals, albeit misguided or misinformed about individuals' capacity to do so, are a major factor attributed to people with learning disabilities not receiving the care that someone without a learning disability would or should receive. In 2001, the Department of Health (2001) identified an above average death rate for people with learning disabilities and Mencap (2004) identified that an inquiry into the premature deaths of people with a learning disability was required.

Mencap's (2007) *Death by Indifference* report highlighted the unnecessary deaths of six people with learning disabilities and said that it was a 'national disgrace' of 'institutional discrimination'. In response, the Michael report (2008), published after the Independent Inquiry into Access to Healthcare for People with Learning Disabilities, found an increased likelihood that these deaths could have been avoided and stated that:

> Sometimes, treatment is not offered to people with a learning disability because a judgement, albeit an inaccurate one, is made about its value. Such judgements imply that a life lived with learning disability is a life less valued. (2008: 8)

(See the Web resources section at the end of this chapter for links to both the reports.)

Historical Care of People with Learning Disabilities

The values underpinning any decisions made by learning disability nurses today requires us to reflect on the historical care of people with learning disabilities.

Prior to reflecting on this history, it is pertinent to offer a brief explanation of what a 'learning disability' is, to ensure that anyone reading this chapter and indeed the whole book is able to have a point of reference for understanding the issues being discussed. The National Institute for Health and Care Research (NIHR) (2020) refers to the National Institute for Health and Care Excellence's (NICE) (2018) explanation of what is a learning disability in their themed review - *Better Health and Care for All: Health and care services for people with learning disabilities*:

> NICE refers to the formal diagnostic criteria for learning disability that people
> with learning disabilities (also called intellectual disabilities) have lower intellec-
> tual ability (an IQ of less than 70). The disabilities are 'global, causing significant
> difficulties in managing a wide range of everyday health tasks and self-care, and
> starting in childhood' (1). Most definitions include not only lower intellectual
> ability, but associated limitations in adaptive skills, that together manifest during
> childhood or adolescence (essentially before age 18 years). (NIHR, 2020: 7)

For their report they exclude learning difficulties as used by education services and refer to the *Learning Disabilities Observatory* where you can see further explanation concerning terminology and recording of learning disability. (See the Web resources section at the end of this chapter for the links for both the NIHR 2020 report and the Public Health England *Learning Disabilities Observatory report: People with learning disabilities in England 2015.*)

Prior to the 1980s in the UK, people with learning disabilities were essentially housed in long-stay hospitals, often located in remote and rural geographical locations. While, undoubtedly, the majority of the nursing staff attempted to provide the best care they could, due to the institutional nature of these hospitals it was often impossible to provide genuine choices, shared decisions and individualised care to the very many people who were resident in these settings (Brend, 2008).

The 1960s saw the beginning of a major change in both the philosophy and policy regarding the care of people with learning disabilities. A service dominated since the 1900s by long-stay institutional care was to be replaced by a range of community-based services. This new philosophy of care, and resultant change in practice regarding services for people with learning disabilities, was largely based on the principle of normalisation developed by Nirje (1969) and expanded on by Wolfensberger (1972). Wolfensberger defined this principle of normalisation as 'the utilisation of means which are as culturally normative as possible, in order to establish and/or maintain personal behaviours, and characteristics which are as culturally normative as possible' (1972: 28). In other words, people with learning disabilities should be present and participating in ordinary community settings, including accessing regular health care services, and making choices about their own lives.

Following a number of scandals surrounding the level of care provided within these institutions and the increasing awareness of 'normalisation', or the 'principles of social role valorisation' (Wolfensberger, 1983), a nationwide process began to close down the large hospitals and relocate individuals with a learning disability to smaller community group home settings, accessing ordinary services. A central theme to these newly developed services was to enable choice and decision-making by people with learning disabilities themselves.

So given the move away from institutionalised care, there were more opportunities for people with learning disabilities and they more to be meaningfully engaged in ordinary services and activities, but we continue to see them experience discrimination on an institutional scale and poor health outcomes. While awareness and understanding of people with learning disabilities is improving within the general population, health and social care professionals acknowledge that they have little understanding of learning disability, fail to recognise when someone with a learning disability is unwell, fail to make the correct diagnosis and lack confidence in caring for people with a learning disability (Heslop et al., 2013). There is also a lack of understanding in making reasonable adjustments. The Advisory, Conciliation and Arbitration Service (ACAS) defines a reasonable adjustment on its website as:

> *A reasonable adjustment* is a change that must be made to remove or reduce a disadvantage related to:
> * an employee's disability when doing their job
> * a job applicant's disability when applying for a job
> A reasonable adjustment could involve making changes to the workplace equipment or services provided (both current and new services), for example an appropriate keyboard for someone with arthritis
> * the ways things are done
> * make sure you can provide information in an accessible format (ACAS: Reasonable adjustments at: https://www.acas.org.uk/reasonable-adjustments)

The duties that were brought in under the Equality Act 2010 must be adhered to in terms of reasonable adjustments being made for people with a learning disability, and again it is recognised that there are significant failings in doing so within the NHS. Indeed, the learning disability improvement standards (NHS Improvement, 2018) have been introduced to provide a benchmark by which the NHS can be measured against and focus on respecting and protecting rights, inclusion and engagement and improving the poor health outcomes. This is reflective of the rights-based approach and underpins Section 1 of *The Code* (NMC, 2018e): 'Prioritise People'.

In terms of the practical implications of the legal duty to make reasonable adjustments in the area of health, people with learning disabilities may, for example, require appointments that are longer than standard ones, for literature in relation to a particular treatment to be easy-to-read and support with managing issues regarding consent. To this end, Mencap launched a campaign *Treat Me Well* with the intention of revolutionising the way people with learning disabilities are treated within the NHS, not least by means of making such reasonable adjustments. (For examples of easy-to-read resources and more information about Mencap's campaign and report, see the Web resources section at the end of this chapter.)

Another contributing factor is lack of understanding in relation to the capacity of the individual with a learning disability and, in England and Wales, appropriate application of the Mental Capacity Act (MCA) 2005, in Scotland, the Adults with Incapacity (Scotland) Act 2000 and, in Northern Ireland, the Mental Capacity (Northern Ireland) Act 2016. Indeed, the former Department of Health (2005) identified that health services were failing to comply with the Mental Capacity Act (MCA) for decisions on health care.

Prior to these pieces of legislation, it was wrongly assumed that people with a learning disability lacked capacity to make decisions. While it still presents challenges, the NHS is required to demonstrate that members of staff have training in human rights, mental capacity and best interests (NHS Improvement, 2018). The Mental Capacity Act 2005 has a Code of Practice (Department for Constitutional Affairs, 2007) that should be followed by all health care staff (2007). Its five key statutory principles are summarised in Box 9.1.

── Box 9.1 ──

Mental Capacity Act (2005): Summary of Key Principles

- *Assume capacity:* the expectation should be that patients can make their own health care treatment decisions.
- *Provide all possible support for people to make their own decisions:* take time to make information accessible and explain the treatment options, including potential risks and benefits, using plain English, real objects, photographs and symbols.
- *People can make unwise decisions:* patients who have capacity may go against the advice of doctors and nurses.
- *Decisions must be made in a person's best interests:* nurses and doctors are required to provide treatment in the best interests of patients whom they have assessed as being unable to make specific health care decisions.
- *Consider whether a decision can be made in a way that is less restrictive of a person's freedom.*

(See Web resources at the end of the chapter to access full UK Legislation documents on the Mental Capacity Act.)

The five principles must inform all health care decisions involving people who may or may not be able to make decisions themselves (see the Web resources section at the end of this chapter for links to sources of information about the Act (in the UK, Scotland and Northern Ireland), the five principles, examples of capacity and an overview of learning disabilities).

Given the evidence, within England, Scotland and Wales, the legal requirements to uphold the Equality Act 2010 and make reasonable adjustments, together with the professional requirements of the nurse as stated in *The Code* (NMC, 2018e), there has to be a better understanding and application of the Mental Capacity legislation. These requirements along with the learning disability improvement standards (NHS Improvement, 2018), should see health and social care professionals working within and outside the NHS begin to contribute to improved health care outcomes for all people with a learning disability going forward in the future.

The basis for decisions being made with and on behalf of people with a learning disability in relation to their care and treatment, needs to be fundamentally underpinned by these and applied equally regardless of the setting.

Making Decisions with and on Behalf of People with a Learning Disability

Following a major review of the role of the nurse for the future, and the proficiencies required to fulfil this role, the NMC published the *Standards of proficiency for registered nurses* (2018a), whereby all new programmes leading to registration as a nurse had to be implemented from September 2020 (see Chapter 14 for changes that had to be put in place with regards to student nurses following the impact of the global pandemic).

To enable students to focus on decision-making and attaining their required proficiencies, we have identified specific examples from the seven platforms (NMC, 2018a). These can be referred to in Box 9.2. It is important to note that these are not the only ones that need to be achieved to become a qualified nurse, but they provide an insight into what you can plan to learn from your placement learning experiences. This book has many other examples for you to consider in relation to your achieving the learning outcomes and becoming proficient as a future nurse.

You will need to refer to the proficiencies and outcomes listed in Box 9.2 as you read the case studies that follow. They have been provided to enable you to see members of multidisciplinary teams put decision-making into practice and to focus on activities that will challenge your own decision-making knowledge and skills as a learning disability nurse. In addition, information provided earlier in the chapter, as well as in the Further reading and Web resources sections at the end, can contribute to your understanding of what the challenges might be.

Box 9.2

Platforms, Proficiencies and Outcomes (NMC, 2018a): Examples

Platform 1: Becoming an accountable professional

Outcomes

> 1.8 demonstrate the knowledge, skills and ability to think critically when applying evidence and drawing on experience to make evidence informed decisions in all situations (2018a: 8)

> 1.9 understand the need to base all decisions regarding care and interventions on people's needs and preferences, recognising and addressing any personal and external factors that may unduly influence their decisions (2018a: 8)

Platform 2: Promoting health and preventing ill health

Outcomes

- 2.4 identify and use all appropriate opportunities, making reasonable adjustments when required, to discuss the impact of smoking, substance and alcohol use, sexual behaviours, diet and exercise on mental, physical and behavioural health and wellbeing, in the context of people's individual circumstances (2018a: 11)
- 2.10 provide information in accessible ways to help people understand and make decisions about their health, life choices, illness and care (2018a: 12)

Platform 3: Assessing needs and planning care

Outcomes

- 3.4 understand and apply a person-centred approach to nursing care, demonstrating shared assessment, planning, decision-making and goal setting when working with people, their families, communities and populations of all ages (2018a: 14)
- 3.5 demonstrate the ability to accurately process all information gathered during the assessment process to identify needs for individualised nursing care and develop person-centred evidence-based plans for nursing interventions with agreed goals (2018a: 14)
- 3.6 effectively assess a person's capacity to make decisions about their own care and to give or withhold consent (2018a: 14)
- 3.7 understand and apply the principles and processes for making reasonable adjustments (2018a: 14)
- 3.8 understand and apply the relevant laws about mental capacity for the country in which you are practising when making decisions in relation to people who do not have capacity (2018a: 14)

- 3.15 demonstrate the ability to work in partnership with people, families and carers to continuously monitor, evaluate and reassess the effectiveness of all agreed nursing care plans and care, sharing decision-making and readjusting agreed goals, documenting progress and decisions made (2018a: 15)
- 3.16 demonstrate knowledge of when and how to refer people safely to other professionals or services for clinical intervention or support (2018a: 11)

Platform 4: Providing and evaluating care

Outcomes

- 4.10 demonstrate the knowledge and ability to respond proactively and promptly to signs of deterioration or distress in mental, physical, cognitive and behavioural health and use this knowledge to make sound clinical decisions (2018a: 11)

Decision-Making in Action: Case Studies to Support Learning

The case studies that follow have been written as narratives, offering detailed background and ongoing care and decision-making options for you to consider. They are based on our collective experiences in the field of learning disability nursing. In each case, read the case study and all the integrated sections in the ongoing narrative and then complete the relevant activities. The first one is Case study 9.1 and Activity 9.1.

▬▬▬▬▬ CASE STUDY 9.1: GEORGE'S STORY ▬▬▬▬▬

Background

George is 24 years old and lives with his father, Barry, in a second-floor flat. George has a diagnosis of a severe learning disability and autism. George has no verbal communication, but he will walk to his object of need. Barry is George's main carer and George is reliant on him for all aspects of his care. George's mother, Lisa, left when George was 12 years old and reported that she could not cope with George and his level of disability. It was around this time that George started to punch his parents. Barry has periods of anxiety and will often become upset if George does not want to do what is expected from him. George attends a day service Monday to Friday between the hours of 11 a.m. and 3 p.m. Following an annual review at the day service by the social worker, Barry reported that George has an ingrown toenail on his big toe. The toe was causing George pain and Barry was managing with simple analgesia, but both Barry and day service staff reported that there had been a difference in George's behaviours. This included screaming, crying, biting his own hand

and attempting to punch day centre staff and Barry. Barry also reported that George has been to his GP, who assessed the toe and referred George to the hospital for removal of the toenail under a general anaesthetic. Barry informed the social worker and day centre staff that George did attend the hospital last week for removal of the toenail, but it did not take place as George walked onto the day surgery Unit, then turned around and walked back to Barry's car. At the review, the social worker suggested a referral to the community learning disability team (CLDT). The social worker assessed George's capacity to consent to the referral and deemed that George did not have capacity regarding the referral. The social worker therefore asked Barry and day service staff if they felt that it was in George's best interest for the referral. Barry, the day service staff, and the social worker all agreed that it was in George's best interest for the referral. The social worker completed the referral to the CLDT.

Activity 9.1

1. Read and consider George's story in Case study 9.1, then answer the following questions.
2. What are the issues for George and for the nursing and medical staff at the hospital?
3. The social worker referred George to the CLDT. What roles do members of the CLDT play and can you predict which member of the team George's case will be allocated to?
4. Try to predict what main, key decisions need to be made in this case?
5. Identify which of the outcomes in Box 9.2: Platforms, Proficiencies and Outcomes you could achieve, working with your practice supervisors, to support a person who has the same kinds of overall care and needs as George.

Ongoing Narrative About George: Issues to Consider

The members of the CLDT were unclear as to whether or not the GP had considered any desensitisation with George regarding the ingrown toenail, as an alternative to referring George to the hospital for removal of the toenail under a general anaesthetic.

On further investigation, the CLDT duty worker had spoken to the ward sister on the day surgery ward and stated that pre-admission staff confirmed that George was attending, and reasonable adjustments would be required on admission. The following reasonable adjustments were identified at pre-assessment:

*   side room;
*   first on the theatre list;
*   later admission time.

The ward sister had allocated George and Barry a side room and ensured that George was first on the theatre list. Pre-assessment had informed Barry to bring George to the ward at 9 a.m., not 7 a.m., as Barry reported that George would have difficulty waiting.

The ward sister had spoken with the anaesthesia team and informed them of George's admission, that he would be assessed first and possibly require a pre-operative sedation. The ward sister confirmed that George had walked into the day surgery ward, but immediately returned to the car. The ward sister also reported that Barry was clearly upset and was not willing to attempt to persuade George to return to the ward, even with the support of staff on the ward.

Ongoing Narrative Regarding George: Decisions that were Considered Necessary

1. Appropriate referral

On receiving the referral from the social worker, the members of the CLDT had to determine whether the referral was appropriate.

The criteria for referral to the CLDT was that a person has to have a diagnosed learning disability, with a health need that cannot be met by primary and secondary health care services. The members of the CLDT needed to identify whether it was the role of a community learning disability nurse (CLDN) or an acute liaison nurse for adults with a learning disability (ALN) to work with George.

It was decided to refer George's case to the acute liaison nurse. This decision was based on the fact that if the referral went to the CLDN, the case would need to be handed over to the ALN anyway to work in partnership with George and staff on the day surgery ward. This way, the ALN would be able to establish a rapport with George and Barry and maintain a level of continuity throughout the process of the removal of the ingrown toenail.

The CLDT therefore accepted the referral and George's case was allocated to Raj, an acute liaison nurse.

2. Determining the urgency

The timescale for the removal of the ingrown toenail was unclear from the initial referral.

For example, had the GP considered a less restrictive intervention along with some desensitisation to the process, working in partnership with a podiatrist?

Had members of staff on the day surgery ward relisted George to attend day surgery again?

Raj (the acute liaison nurse) decided that she would make contact with George's GP to discuss the rationale for the referral to day surgery. In addition, Raj felt that it would be appropriate to make contact with George and Barry and complete a home visit to discuss whether any other reasonable adjustment was required and to obtain information from Barry regarding the previous attempted admission.

Raj also felt that it would be beneficial to make contact with members of staff on the day surgery ward, to determine whether or not George had been relisted for admission.

Raj understood that making contact with George and Barry, the GP and the day surgery staff would determine the urgency of the referral and give her a better understanding of George and his presenting condition.

Raj made contact with George's GP, Dr Smith, who reported that the ingrown toenail was a chronic condition and she had been trying to manage it for the last two years. Dr Smith also noted that she had tried to remove the nail, but with little success as George became agitated. Dr Smith had referred George to the podiatrist, who had completed six home visits with George, but without success. The podiatrist reported to Dr Smith that, on his final visit, George had been physically aggressive towards Barry.

Dr Smith also reported that the toenail could get infected and antibiotic treatment has been prescribed as a prophylaxis.

Having obtained the clinical history, Raj decided that addressing the ingrown toenail was urgent and acting without delay was essential.

3. Planning the interventions

Telephone contact was made with Barry, who agreed to a home visit to meet George. Barry suggested visiting when George returned from the day service.

Prior to the home visit, Raj reflected on the conversation she had had with Dr Smith and information obtained from the ward manager at the day surgery unit. Raj considered some questions that she would like to ask Barry in relation to George. Raj decided that the questions would be used as a reminder, to prompt herself, if George did not openly disclose any information in discussion.

Raj considered that the questions, which were written down, were to be open for Barry, to enable information to be shared.

Preparing for a visit is good practice and helps to support it, ensuring that no information is overlooked.

On arrival at George's and Barry's home, the initial observation of George was that he was limping. On discussion with Barry, the leg that George was limping on was the one with the foot that had the ingrown toenail. Raj asked if George had received pain relief, as it suggested that he would likely be in pain. Barry reported that George was not prescribed any pain relief as he felt that at the time George was not in pain.

Raj discussed the interventions Dr Smith and the podiatrist had organised and Barry shared that he felt, that at this time, the toe had become infected, and George was in pain. At this time, Barry reported an increase in George becoming agitated and physically aggressive.

Barry told Raj the same account of the previous attempt of admitting George to the day surgery unit that was included in the referral. However, Barry expanded on this to include that he does not like to see his son in pain and gets very anxious when challenging George as he does not want to be physically assaulted by him or see him upset and distressed.

Barry reported that he was unsure what the options were with regard to re-admission for day surgery. He also said that he wanted George to have his toenail removed.

Raj had summarised the information given by Barry with regard to George and suggested the following interventions:

- speak with Dr Smith (GP) to discuss prescribing pain relief, as it is clear that George is limping as he does not want to put weight on his foot because it is painful, plus this would avoid a possible increase in behaviour associated with the pain;
- speak to staff on the day surgery ward to identify a date for George to be to re-admitted for the procedure;
- consider showing a familiarisation video of the unit to George and Barry, so that they would both know what to expect;
- arrange a multidisciplinary meeting to discuss reasonable adjustments and the possibility of an action plan should George return to the car as he did the previous time.

4. Liaising with the multidisciplinary team (MDT)

Following on from the home visit, Raj contacted Dr Smith to discuss George and pain relief and his current presentation – limping and not putting any weight on the foot. Dr Smith suggested that the toe may be infected again, as this had been how George had presented himself before.

Dr Smith agreed with Raj that George would be in pain and reported that she would make a home visit to assess his toe, discuss pain relief and prescribe some for George.

Raj also contacted the day surgery ward at the hospital and spoke to the ward manager. Raj explained that George had been allocated to her care and she had obtained the history in relation to the ingrown toenail from Dr Smith and George's father.

The ward manager reported that George would come into the day surgery ward under the care of Dr Singh. Dr Singh's usual theatre list would be on a Tuesday. The ward manager and Raj agreed to aim for admission in one month's time. Within this time, Raj would arrange an MDT meeting with Dr Singh, the ward manager and a member from the anaesthetic team to look at a plan for admission to day surgery. The team would also consider whether George would require any sedation prior to coming to the hospital.

The ward manager confirmed that the reasonable adjustments identified for George's previous admission remained in place and that George would be first on the theatre list, have a bed in a side room and be offered the later admission time.

Read the whole scenario from the beginning again as related to George and his care and complete Activity 9.2 in order to determine the way forward for the multidisciplinary team.

Activity 9.2

Consider what the key issues are at this point in George's care. Make a note of these so you can refer to them – refer back to all the information you have been given concerning his care.

1. What do you think the MDT will discuss in relation to George if he does return to the car?
2. Do you think that any other reasonable adjustments could be made for George to enable him to access the day surgery unit?
3. Does a capacity assessment need to be completed again?

Consider your answers and options chosen in relation to decisions to be made by the multi-disciplinary team (MDT) and based on what was already known.

5. Decisions to be made by the Multi-disciplinary Team (MDT)

- There was no record that the GP had assessed George's capacity with regard to removal of the toenail. The Mental Capacity Act requires that all decisions made are decision specific and are carried out by the clinician undertaking the procedure.
- As Dr Smith has referred George to Dr Singh, it was agreed that these clinicians would carry out a joint capacity assessment for removal of the toenail.
- If it was assessed that George does not have capacity to consent to removal of the toenail, then Dr Singh would arrange a 'best interests' meeting.
- In addition to the reasonable adjustments identified, the following decisions were agreed by the MDT. All staff were not to wear uniform, to reduce anxiety for George. If George does return to the car, then assessments would be completed in the car by Dr Singh, nursing staff to complete admission and the anaesthetic team would assess and administer prescribed sedation prior to the procedure.
- It was suggested that a hospital passport be completed by Raj. A hospital passport supports individuals with a learning disability when accessing any health care service. The findings from the hospital passport would be shared with the MDT and will focus on George's likes and dislikes, so that all hospital staff, when working with him, do not do anything to increase his anxiety.

6. Mental capacity assessment by Dr Smith and Dr Singh

Dr Smith and Dr Singh agreed to undertake and complete a home visit for George to assess his mental capacity. This was suggested as a reasonable adjustment, and George and Barry would be less anxious in their own environment.

The mental capacity assessment undertaken involved asking the following questions.

1. Is there an impairment of, or disturbance in, the functioning of the person's mind or brain?

    As George has a severe learning disability, Dr Singh and Dr Smith both answered 'Yes' to the first question.

    Dr Singh and Dr Smith continued with the capacity assessment questions. The question that George was being assessed against was, 'Does George have the capacity to consent to removal of the toenail under general anaesthetic?'

2. Was George able to:

    - understand the information given to him
    - retain the information long enough to be able to make a decision
    - weigh up the information available
    - communicate his decision.

These questions are fundamental to a mental capacity assessment and all assessments are decision specific.

George's responses indicated that he did not have the capacity to consent to treatment. Dr Singh and Dr Smith then agreed that a 'best interests' meeting was required to discuss whether treatment was or was not in George's best interests.

Complete Activity 9.3 to give some thought to the issues that need to be considered in George's overall care at this time. Make a note of your responses and refer to them when you are reading the outcome of the best interests meeting arranged by Dr Singh.

Activity 9.3

1. What would you think if, as a nurse, you started a capacity assessment and the person did not have an impairment of, or disturbance in, the functioning of their mind or brain?
2. What would you do in this case, given that George does not have capacity to consent to the removal of his toenail?
3. Considering all the evidence presented so far in this case study, do you feel that it would or would not be in George's best interests to have the toenail removed?
4. Who do you think needs to be invited to a best interests meeting?
5. Who should chair the meeting?
6. Does a referral need to be completed for an independent mental capacity advocate (IMCA)?

To enable you to assess your responses to the questions in Activity 9.3, it is advised that you undertake further reading regarding the assessment and placement guidelines in your learning environment to support the possible actions you could take. Discuss some of the issues of mental capacity of a person with your practice supervisors and other health and social care professionals in the MDT.

Following all the steps taken so far to determine how to support George and the ongoing health problem of his ingrowing toenail, it had been agreed that a 'best interests' meeting needed to take place to discuss the next steps and decisions to help him.

7. Best interests meeting arranged by Dr Singh

Dr Singh had invited the following individuals to George's best interests meeting. Barry (father), Raj (ALN), a day care service staff member, a social worker and a member of staff from the anaesthetic team. Dr Smith was unable to attend the meeting but had written what he thought was in George's best interest to be shared at the meeting.

Dr Singh reported that an IMCA (Independent Mental Capacity Advocate) was not required as George's next of kin was present and able to contribute to the decision. All present contributed to the meeting, commenting on how the toenail was affecting George from their perspective.

The member of the anaesthetic team shared the risks of having a general anaesthetic. All present were in agreement that it was in George's best interest to have the toenail removed. The GP was in agreement in her written statement, which was shared.

Dr Singh followed the guidelines for decision-making in relation to best interests, which are part of the Mental Capacity Act and include the following statements:

- I have encouraged and assisted the patient to participate in the decision.
- I have considered all factors relevant to the decision.
- I have attempted to find out the views of the patient, including his past and present wishes and feelings, and taken these into account.
- I have not based my assessment solely on the patient's age, appearance, condition or behaviour.
- I have considered whether or not the patient might regain capacity and, if so, whether the decision can be delayed.
- The decision is not motivated in any way by a desire to bring about the patient's death.

Dr Singh added the mental capacity assessment and best interest assessment to George's medical file, then documented that the meeting had taken place, and all were in agreement that it was in George's best interest to have the toenail removed under general anaesthetic.

Dr Singh shared the action plan for George – what to do whether he did or did not get out of the car – with those who were at the meeting. Dr Singh recognised the importance of gaining information about George, to prepare for how he may react to being assessed in the car, so asked all present about this, to obtain their views regarding this approach.

A member of staff from the day care service shared with the meeting that George's current interest was dinosaurs, and if clinicians were to have a book about dinosaurs with them, to redirect him if he became anxious, then that would be a good approach to take with George. Raj had completed the patient passport with Barry and had noticed, too, that dinosaurs had been identified as an item that may redirect George.

All present were in agreement that George needed to have the toenail removed, as he was in pain and there had been an increase in negative aspects of his behaviour.

8. Summary of the Outcomes from George's overall care

The scenario described and discussed in Case study 9.1 has shown how setting up a simple treatment plan for George and following the requirements of the Mental Capacity Act made for a positive outcome for George. It showed how family, health and social care professionals worked together to support a decision made in his best interests. The outcome for George was that he had his toenail removed.

To achieve this, George was assessed in the back of the car, an appropriate prescription of midazolam was prescribed and administered as a sedative prior to the procedure, and he was able to be transferred into a wheelchair and taken to the anaesthetic room. Previously, the day centre staff had gone with George to the library and taken out books on dinosaurs, which the medical and nursing team used to distract George with when waiting to complete any intervention.

George went home after the procedure and his behaviour improved. Subsequently he appeared to be pain-free and no longer walks with a limp.

As noted at the beginning of the Case study section of this chapter it is important to show the various kinds of decision-making that can be taken or seen in the care of a person with a learning disability. The following Case study 9.2 narrates the story of Stacey. As with Case study 9.1 it includes decision-making by a multidisciplinary team including nurses.

━━━━━ CASE STUDY 9.2: STACEY'S STORY ━━━━━

The number one principle of the Mental Capacity Act 2005 is to assume that individuals have the capacity to make decisions regarding their health care. When unwise decisions are made by individuals with a learning disability, this challenges health and social care professionals, as they are likely going against their advice. However, the right to make such decisions is supported in the Mental Capacity Act 2005, in its third principle.

This case study, telling Stacey's story, highlights exactly this kind of ethical dilemma, one faced by health and social care professionals when individuals are making unwise decisions and pressure is being applied by families and other public services on the learning disability nurse involved. Persons making unwise decisions can be particularly challenging for the learning disability nurse and their value base in relation to Section 3 of *The Code* (NMC, 2018e) 'Preserve safety', which requires the nurse to protect the individual. It can be noted that in the initial case study narrative, there will be an opportunity to share and discuss options the learning disability nurse can take in making decisions regarding Stacy's safety in making her own decisions.

Background information for Stacey

Stacey is a 29-year-old woman with a mild learning disability. She has been known to the community learning disability team for the past six months, following a referral from a social worker to support Stacey moving into her own flat.

Stacey's flat is in a complex of five flats with other people with learning disabilities living there. The flat complex is in a city centre and Stacey has easy access to shops, public houses and activity centres, such as the library and a gym.

Stacey receives four hours of help a week from a support worker – two hours each Monday and two hours each Friday. The hours on Mondays are to support Stacey with household tasks and the hours on Fridays are to support her with doing her weekly shopping. Stacey is enjoying her new flat and personal space and is fiercely independent: she does not like to refer to herself as having a learning disability.

Stacey previously lived with her parents, who had concerns about her moving into her own flat. To try and alleviate those concerns, Stacey's parents pay for the weekly support she receives. Stacey really likes not having to ask her parents for permission to do things.

In the past two months, Stacey has been employed on a part-time basis in a public house. Stacey enjoys socialising with the customers and has made some friends, who she has started to see socially when she is not working. Stacey tends to meet her friends in the pub and will have an alcoholic drink. Stacey enjoys a gin and orange juice. Stacey's parents and support workers are concerned about her working in the public house and the increase in her consumption of alcohol.

The community learning disability team received a telephone call from the police as they are increasingly concerned about Stacey. The police have had to deal with Stacey being drunk and committing public order offences. They reported that Stacey was on the high street, swearing at members of the public. The police responded and took Stacey to her parents' house. The police inform the community learning disability team that they have also contacted Stacey's social worker to 'sort it out and stop Stacey drinking'.

Stacey was already known to the community learning disability team and had been allocated to Steve, a community learning disability nurse, as one of a 'caseload' he is responsible for. Steve contacted Stacey and reported that the police had contacted him, and a home visit was arranged with Stacey in two days' time. Stacey said that she had been drunk and spent the night at her parents' house. She also said that the police had not charged her with any offence, and she was heading back to her flat that day and would be working at the pub later that same day.

Steve's Action Plan or Next Steps

Steve read Stacey's case notes. There was no evidence of a history regarding consumption of alcohol from the nursing assessment he had completed when Stacey was first referred to the community learning disability team six months ago. Stacey's response when asked about alcohol consumption was that she enjoyed a social drink and liked the feeling alcohol gave her. She reported that it relaxed her, and she was able to be more social. This would suggest that Stacey did not have a previous dependence on alcohol.

Stacey was known to the community learning disability team and initial nursing assessments had been completed but such information may not be available, and this was a new referral from the police. If it was not available, the community learning disability team would have had to obtain this information from the individual and/or carer at an initial assessment.

Steve also contacted Stacey's social worker, Asha, to determine what action she had taken following the telephone call from the police. Asha reported that she, too, had looked through Stacey's case notes and found no evidence of alcohol consumption or dependence either.

Steve informed Asha of his planned visit to Stacey in two days' time. Asha said that she was able to do a joint visit with Steve.

The following day, Steve received a call from a member of staff at the local hospital, who informed him that Stacey had been admitted overnight, as she had fallen in the high street, had been drunk and disorderly and banged her head. A 'CT' scan of her head detected no abnormalities. Stacey's mum had been contacted by staff at the hospital, against Stacey's wishes, and she was with Stacey.

The caller also reported that there had been a conversation with the police, who informed them about the incident yesterday, and the hospital has referred Stacey to the local safeguarding team.

The hospital caller noted that Stacey's mum was not happy; she was suggesting that Stacey should return home to live and had said that it was Asha's and Steve's fault that Stacey lives in her own flat and had been drunk the last two nights and lives in her own flat.

Given the developing scenario with Stacey and the outcomes of her alcohol consumption consider the questions in Activity 9.4 in relation to her background and behaviour.

Activity 9.4

1. Consider the dilemma of Stacey's continued alcohol consumption and concerns raised by the police, staff at the hospital and Stacey's mum.
2. What would Steve's response be to the police, staff at the hospital and Stacey's mum?

3. Consider the evidence base to inform Steve's response and decision-making to actively work with Stacey. You may wish to refer to earlier Chapters 1, 2 and 3 to support your evidence.
4. Consider the referral to the safeguarding team. Is this an appropriate referral?

Issues to Consider When Making Decisions about Stacy's Care

In Case study 9.2 we can see that Steve and Asha discussed with Stacey if there was any reason for her getting excessively drunk. They asked if there had been a significant life event that she was not happy about or wanted to block from her thoughts and was using alcohol to do this. Stacey reported that she was really happy living in the flat on her own, with her job at the pub and the new friendships she had developed. Steve noted that if she was using alcohol instead of addressing an issue, he could refer Stacey to the psychiatry/psychology team. Stacey also said that she did not have a dependence on alcohol, and she liked the feeling alcohol gave her. This mirrored the response that Stacey had given in the original nursing assessment.

If Stacey had reported that she had become dependent on alcohol, then Steve could have considered a referral to the substance misuse team and worked with them to address the issue.

Ongoing Narrative: Decisions that were Considered Necessary

1. Mental capacity

Steve and Asha discussed whether or not Stacey has the mental capacity to make decisions regarding alcohol consumption and the effects alcohol has on her.

Steve was aware of the five statutory principles of the Mental Capacity Act 2005 and the relevance of the first, second and third principle:

- the first principle being: 'A person must be assumed to have capacity unless it is established that he lacks capacity.'
- the second principle being: 'A person is not to be treated as unable to make a decision unless all practicable steps to help him to do so have been taken without success.'
- the third principle being: 'A person is not to be treated as unable to make a decision merely because he makes an unwise decision.' (Mental Capacity Act 2005)

The Mental Capacity Act was the evidence base required to support Steve's decision-making in his nursing practice.

Stacey agreed to meet with Steve and Asha to discuss alcohol consumption.

2. Alcohol use education: meeting with Stacey

Steve and Asha made a home visit to Stacey and discussed the potential effects of drinking alcohol to excess in detail. Steve had prepared for the visit and obtained accessible information to support education, such as the guidance for making reasonable adjustments for people with a learning disability and other Internet resources (see the Web resources section at the end of this chapter for links).

Steve and Stacey discussed the effects of short- and long-term use of alcohol at length. Stacey showed that she had good knowledge regarding alcohol and was able to retain information when questioned. A detailed communication assessment may be required to establish the level of an individual's communication before considering any education.

3. Mental capacity assessment: Stacey's decision-making and drinking alcohol

Following the alcohol use education that Steve had completed with Stacey, Steve and Asha completed a mental capacity assessment with regards to drinking alcohol.

This assessment involves answering some questions, the first of which was:

1. Is there an impairment of, or disturbance in, the functioning of the person's mind or brain?

As Stacey had a mild learning disability, the answer to this question was 'Yes.' When completing a capacity assessment, it is worth remembering that if the answer to this question is 'No', then the individual does have capacity to consent and so the practitioner would not have to complete the remainder of the assessment. In this case, however, Steve and Asha continued with the capacity assessment questions.

The main question that Stacey was being assessed against here was, 'Does Stacey have the capacity to consent to drink alcohol to excess?' Some further questions help to answer this one. Was Stacey able to:

* understand the information given to her;
* retain the information long enough to be able to make a decision;
* balance out and consider the information available and communicate the decision?

Stacey responded appropriately to all the questions in the capacity assessment, which indicated that Stacey did have capacity to consent to drink alcohol to excess.

4. Next steps: Making the next nursing decision

Consider the dilemma of Stacey's unwise decision to drink alcohol to excess against the requirements of a nurse set out by *The Code* (NMC, 2018e).

What do you think Steve's next nursing decision will be? What are the key issues that Steve needs to be aware of?

In this case, it is worth noting that Stacey drinking excessively could have further ramifications if it continues. Stacey could become subject to the criminal justice system if she were to be charged with a public order offence committed while she was drunk. Stacey could injure herself significantly while drunk, which may have a life-changing effect. When intoxicated, Stacey is vulnerable, compromising her personal safety, and she may become a victim of crime, such as being assaulted.

Stacey was aware of all these possibilities as she had discussed them with Steve as part of her alcohol use education and capacity assessment. Steve wanted to discuss these matters further, to minimise the risk to Stacey and look at strategies that she could use when she is drunk. Stacey agreed to this.

5. Decisions made following shared discussion

a.   Alcohol and previous incidents

Steve and Stacey discussed the incidents that had resulted in her being picked up by the police and the fall that resulted in her going to hospital. Stacey reported that her friends drink quickly and described being fine, then not being able to remember what happened.

Steve and Stacey discussed a strategy that she could try. She could have a soft drink as an alternative or choose a drink that does not have a high percentage of alcohol.

b.   Other social activities

When Steve had completed Stacey's nursing assessment, it was identified that Stacey enjoyed exercise, going to the gym and riding her bike. Steve suggested that Stacey ask her friends if they wanted to exercise instead of going to the pub. Steve also suggested that her friends may have hobbies or activities that Stacey has not done before and she could give those a try. Stacey agreed that she would discuss this with her friends.

c.   Informing Stacey's parents, the police, and hospital of the outcome of the capacity assessment

Stacey also agreed to the content of the capacity assessment being shared with her parents, the police and the hospital. Steve and Asha later met with Stacey's parents, the police and the hospital staff to do this.

Stacey's parents and the police were very unhappy that Steve and Asha could not intervene and physically control and stop Stacey from drinking. Steve explained the principles of the Mental Capacity Act in relation to Stacey, that Stacey appears to be making an unwise choice, but she can fully understand the implications of her actions with regard to drinking alcohol. Steve said that he had discussed strategies with Stacey that may reduce the number of times she gets excessively drunk.

Stacey's parents were quite damning in their response to the outcomes of the assessment and Steve's and Asha's subsequent actions, saying that they had failed Stacey and if anything should happen to her while she was drunk, that they would be responsible.

Case study 9.2 in all its sections highlights that the principles of the Mental Capacity Act must be upheld as Stacey has been assessed as having capacity. Steve in this case may have difficulty knowing that Stacey is making an unwise decision that conflicts with his role as a nurse which is to safeguard a person.

If Stacey had been assessed as not having capacity and there was a conflict of interest from her parents, a referral to an independent mental capacity advocate (IMCA) would be required. IMCAs safeguard individuals who lack capacity when significant decisions need to be made, such as those concerning where to live or medical treatment options.

Our final case study (Case study 9.3) exploring decision-making as a learning disability nurse concerns a gentleman called Harry, who has a mild learning disability and lives in a rural environment.

CASE STUDY 9.3: HARRY'S STORY

Background

Harry is a 44-year-old man with a mild learning disability. He lives independently in a flat in a rural village. He is known in the local community as his job is maintaining people's gardens in the village.

Harry goes to the pub every night and has a couple of alcoholic drinks. He smokes tobacco and will roll his own cigarettes, and will smoke more than ten cigarettes a day. He also has a poor diet and goes to the local cafe daily to have a cooked breakfast. Harry is overweight and does not do any exercise other than his gardening job.

The local authority has allocated Harry just two hours of help a week from a support worker. Those hours are to take Harry shopping, which consists of buying tobacco for the week, plus some fizzy drinks and snack-type food. As Harry lives in a rural area, an hour of that time is taken up travelling to and from the shops. Harry is happy that he spends his money on tobacco, alcohol and food from the local cafe.

Harry first became known to the learning disability team more than 20 years ago. This was due to presenting with symptoms of hearing voices. An assessment at that time by the learning disability psychiatrist suggested a diagnosis of a psychosis and so commenced Harry on antipsychotic medication and referred him to a psychology team. Unfortunately, Harry did not commit to going to his psychology sessions but, for the past two years, he has attended a men's group for individuals with a learning disability (based on a community psychology model) that meets once a month.

Harry reports that he does not always remember to take his antipsychotic medication and does not have any other health needs. He is eligible for an annual health check by his GP, but the support worker has noted that, although Harry receives a letter inviting him to the practice for this, he does not attend.

Initial decisions made by support workers

A referral was made to the community learning disability team by one of the support workers who helped Harry to go shopping.

The support worker made the referral as he had noticed a deterioration in Harry's personal hygiene. Harry had given verbal consent for referral to the learning disability team. The support worker reported that Harry appeared to have been wearing the same clothes for more than six weeks, as it had been six weeks since the last time that support worker had taken him shopping.

As Harry had not been known to the learning disability team for over six months, it was evident that an updated assessment was required. Procedures for assessment may differ in learning disability teams. The process the community learning disability team followed was to meet and to decide how to respond to a referral.

Decisions on new referrals in a community learning disability team

The community learning disability team's new referral meetings were multidisciplinary. All disciplines, psychiatry, psychology nursing, speech and language, occupational therapy, physiotherapy are represented. Some community learning disability teams may also include a representative from the local authority and a social worker may also attend referral meetings.

The referral was discussed against the criteria for referral, and it was agreed that Harry would be invited for an initial assessment. This assessment is a person-centred health assessment, which someone from any of the disciplines can complete, together with recording vital signs and observations. A patient passport is also completed at this initial assessment. Its purpose is to support patients if they need to go to hospital. A basic risk assessment is completed as well as the outcomes of the Health Equalities Framework, which is underpinned by an evidence base. This measures the contribution of the MDT in reducing exposure to known determinants of health inequality, as well as baseline or initial admission to the community learning disability team and any following health intervention. This will show whether the member of the MDT had a positive or negative outcome on the individual with a learning disability.

MDT team meeting discussion

The MDT team meeting discussed whether any reasonable adjustment would be required to support Harry at the initial assessment meeting. Reasonable adjustments may include completing the assessment in the home environment. The assessments can be quite lengthy, due to obtaining a large amount of information. In Harry's situation, it was agreed that the MDT would invite him to the Community Learning Disability home base for the initial assessment.

The members of the team try to predict which discipline will undertake an initial assessment in a referral. In Harry's case, it was agreed that psychiatry and nursing would complete this initial assessment. An appointment was considered, and a letter sent to Harry informing him of the preferred date, and a copy to his support worker requesting their support at this appointment.

The initial assessment

The initial assessment was completed with Harry, who attended the appointment with his support worker. A person-centred health assessment and basic risk assessment document had been developed by the community learning disability team and was used at this referral.

The aim of the assessment was to obtain information in relation to Harry's health and determine what support is required from the Community learning Disability team. This assessment is holistic – looking at all aspects of physical and mental health as well as considerations for referral to social care.

Prior to the health assessment and risk assessment, the following clinical observations were completed: weight, height, blood pressure, temperature, pulse, oxygen saturation levels and respiratory rate. The clinical observations showed that Harry was overweight, his BMI indicating that he was in the obese range. His blood pressure was high, with an initial reading of 155/95 mmHg, and all other clinical observations were within normal limits.

The health assessment indicated a deterioration in Harry's personal hygiene and that he had still not attended an annual health check at his GP surgery. Harry reported, however, that he had not been hearing voices and there had been no deterioration in his mental health. A baseline HEF was completed, in readiness for the decision as to which discipline would take the lead in Harry's care.

Decisions made following team discussion and the initial assessment

A decision was made by the team to act immediately with regard to Harry's high blood pressure. The community nurse contacted Harry's GP and discussed the blood pressure results. It was agreed that Harry would go to see the GP that day and an appointment was made.

Harry reported that he did not like going to the GP's surgery as the members of staff talk in words that are not clear and he does not understand what is being said. It was agreed that the community nurse would support Harry at the appointment.

Community learning disability teams may have daily duty workers who may be able to respond in such situations when required. The process of the initial assessment would have been to take the findings of the assessments back to the multidisciplinary team to discuss before allocating to a discipline. Due to the need to respond quickly to

Harry's high blood pressure and his inability to understand the information given to him, the community nurse took the initial lead.

The community nurse supported Harry at his appointment with the GP practitioner. The GP took his blood pressure and requested that this needed to be taken on a daily basis for two weeks. A discussion was had as to whether the community nurse had the capacity to undertake this daily or whether Harry could attend the GP surgery daily and take his own blood pressure reading in the self-service area. Harry agreed to go to the surgery daily.

The GP also discussed Harry's lifestyle choices and he told the GP that he smoked, drank alcohol and ate fried bacon and eggs daily. The GP suggested that Harry reduce his alcohol and tobacco intake and consider having a more balanced diet.

The community nurse reduced all this information down into a basic communication format which Harry understood. The nurse also told the GP that Harry had only been assessed by the community learning disability team that day, and that the health assessment suggested that some further work was needed with regards to Harry's alcohol, smoking and lifestyle choices, in line with the NHS agenda 'making every contact count' approach to changing behaviour to improve health being used in the NHS, local authorities and other relevant agencies.

After the GP, the community nurse showed Harry the self-service area, which had a blood pressure machine and height and weight scales. The community nurse demonstrated the blood pressure machine on himself and then Harry, and the process required Harry to write the reading down and leave it in the post box for collection. He was happy with this and reported that he would go to the GP surgery daily to do this for two weeks. The community nurse then agreed to take Harry home.

On returning Harry to his home, it was found to be flooded, with no electricity and all furniture either turned upside down or smashed to pieces. Harry reported that his neighbours had destroyed his property and he had been living in this home environment for the past six weeks.

To consider what might now be necessary to help Harry's situation answer the following decision-making questions in Activity 9.5, as if you were the student nurse accompanying the community nurse during placement.

Activity 9.5

Imagine that you have accompanied this community nurse, who is your practice supervisor.

1. What do you think will be the community nurse's response to this situation?
2. What is the immediate concern for Harry and how will the community nurse safeguard him?
3. What do you think will be the community nurse's next decision?

Issues to Consider by the Community Nurse

You may have considered the following issues regarding safeguarding Harry following the evidence seen and his disclosure about the neighbours destroying his home.

Consider the safeguarding process in place, noting that they may be different to other areas with their own individual safeguarding policies and procedures.

1. Is Harry at immediate risk? If the answer is 'Yes', the community nurse would contact the police and they would be required to respond. If it is 'No', the next question to consider would be is Harry at risk of serious harm? If the answer is 'Yes', a referral needs to be made to adult safeguarding.
2. What is the level of help required to safeguard Harry? Is he at immediate risk or risk of significant harm?
3. What will the nursing decision be by the community nurse? Imagine that you, as a student nurse, have been asked by the nurse, as your supervisor, to assess Harry's situation and identify the key areas to consider when making such decisions. The following information and observations will help you with this identification.

The Decisions Considered Necessary to Safeguard Harry

Safeguarding

It was unclear whether Harry was at risk of immediate or significant harm, so the community nurse contacted the local authority's adult safeguarding team. The safeguarding team suggested that there was an immediate risk and reported that they would contact the police and respond within the hour.

The community nurse started to tell Harry that his neighbours' behaviour was not acceptable and what they had been doing was abusive in nature. Harry said that he thought his neighbours were his friends and he did not want to leave his flat. He also did not want to leave his flat because of his work and presence in the community and going to the public house and cafe.

The police and the social worker responded and arrived at Harry's home. They assessed Harry and the situation with his neighbours. They deemed the threat from his neighbours to be an immediate risk and a decision was made to offer him short-term temporary accommodation away from his neighbours while the police investigated.

In line with the lone working policy, the community nurse took the opportunity to contact the community learning disability team's base office or main office to inform them of the situation. He reported that he would contact them again when safe and that he will be returning to base.

Transition to New Accommodation: Decisions Made with Harry

The community nurse advocated on behalf of Harry with the police and social worker, informing them that Harry did not want to move out of the village due to his work and social life. The social worker suggested some short-term, temporary bed and breakfast accommodation in the village and made enquiries to see if any rooms were available.

In this case study we can see that Harry's preferences were respected as the community nurse advocated on his behalf. He did not have any family. If his wishes and preferences were not respected, the community nurse may have chosen to refer an independent advocate to work with Harry.

The community nurse informed Harry that his home was not fit for human habitation at the moment and so he would have to move to somewhere else for the short-term. The community nurse suggested that Harry pack some of his belongings and the things that he could not take with him would be made secure after talking to the police and the community nursing team.

At this point, Harry said that he had not been attending to his personal hygiene or washing his clothes as he had no water or electricity.

The social worker managed to secure a place at the bed and breakfast and, together, the social worker and community nurse supported Harry with the transition to this accommodation. He was happy that he could remain in the village and reported that he would attend the GP surgery to record his blood pressure, as had been agreed earlier that day.

As Harry's high blood pressure had needed to be addressed immediately and then the safeguarding team needed to be contacted, the community nurse had not yet completed any of the required clinical records for these interventions. On returning to base and completing the clinical records, the nurse also completed the referral to the safeguarding team, which made the process a formal referral. Even though emergency action had been taken already to support Harry due to the circumstances, this meant that the referral was completed in line with the safeguarding pathway. In addition, the community nurse recognised the situation had been a clinical incident. An incident form, outlining what had happened at all stages since meeting Harry, was also fully completed by the nurse. ·

Outcome for Harry Following Decision-Making by the Nursing and Multidisciplinary Team

The outcome for Harry was that he remained in the bed and breakfast accommodation until his flat was made habitable. He attended to his personal hygiene needs as he had access to water for a shower and to wash his clothes.

The police investigated the neighbours' actions and were looking to charge the individuals in relation to hate crime offences. As the police were pursuing this action, it was found that the neighbours were in breach of their tenancy agreement and had to move out of their flat.

In due course, Harry would be able to return to his flat. In the meantime, he attended the GP surgery for two weeks, as agreed, and recorded his blood pressure. The community nurse made a follow-up appointment with the GP for Harry, who kept the appointment. The blood pressure readings indicated that it was now within normal limits. The GP suggested that the high blood pressure readings could have been a result of the home environment and the situation with Harry's neighbours.

Conclusion

The case studies in this chapter have demonstrated how learning disability nurses make decisions with and on behalf of people with learning disabilities, their families and carers, and work together with other professionals to achieve optimum health outcomes. While what we have been able to cover here cannot be exhaustive, links can be made to the proficiencies set out in the NMC Standards (NMC, 2018a) and the seven platforms for all registered nurses, regardless of their field. We advise that you read each of these again to determine outcomes that you can set as learning goals for your placements. These will, in the main, be related to your field of practice, but could also be associated with the three other fields. Both adults and children with learning disabilities can be found in a wide range of placements, and as we saw with George, he would have probably been cared for in a surgical nursing type of environment rather than a specialist setting.

In concluding this chapter which focused on the care of three individuals with learning disabilities, we are conscious that the future for the field of learning disability nursing continues to be a topic for debate as to whether it should or should not be one of the fields of nursing practice as defined by the NMC. In this chapter we have offered some important insights into the role of the nurse in decision-making and working within a multi-disciplinary team.

Health and care outcomes, with the learning disability nurse being well positioned to enable these to happen, occur both directly and through working with the other members of the multidisciplinary team. We hope that through considering the lives of these three individuals and the range of decision-making required to enable them to live their lives has helped to expand your knowledge of the field of learning disability nursing.

References

Brend, M. (2008). *First and Last: Closing learning disabilities hospitals*. London: Choice Press, Choice Support.

Department for Constitutional Affairs (2007). *Mental Capacity Act 2005: Code of practice*. London: The Stationery Office.

Department of Health (2001). *Valuing People: A new strategy for learning disability for the 21st century*. London: Department of Health.

Healthcare Quality Improvement Partnership (2019). *The Learning Disabilities Mortality Review (LeDeR) Programme: Annual report 2018*. Bristol: University of Bristol.

Heslop, P., Blair, P., Fleming, P., Hoghton, M., Marriott, A. and Russ, L. (2013). *Confidential Inquiry into Premature Deaths of People with Learning Disabilities (CIPOLD): Final report*. Bristol: University of Bristol Norah Fry Centre for Disability Studies.

Learning Disabilities Mortality Review Programme (LeDeR) Team (2021). *The Learning Disabilities Mortality Review Programme (LeDeR) Programme: Annual report 2020*. Bristol: University of Bristol.

Mencap (2004). *Treat Me Right! Better healthcare for people with a learning disability*. London: Mencap.

Mencap (2007). *Death by Indifference: Following up the Treat Me Right! Report*. London: Mencap.

Michael, J. (2008). *Healthcare for All: Report of the Independent Inquiry into Access to Healthcare for People with Learning Disabilities*. London: Aldridge Press.

National Institute for Health and Care Excellence (NICE) (2018). *Learning Disabilities and Behaviour that Challenges: Service design and delivery*. NICE guideline [NG93]. London: NICE.

National Institute for Health Research (NIHR) (2020). *Better Health and Care for All: Health and care services for people with learning disabilities*. London: NIHR.

National Quality Board (2017). *Learning from Deaths Guidance for NHS Trusts on Working with Bereaved Families and Carers*. London: NHS England.

NHS Improvement (2018). *The Learning Disability Improvement Standards for NHS Trusts*. London: NHS Improvement.

Nirje, B. (1969). The normalization principle and its human management implications. *SRV-VRS: The International Social Role Valorization Journal*, 1(2): 1994.

Nursing and Midwifery Council (NMC) (2018a). *Future Nurse: Standards of proficiency for registered nurses*. London: NMC.

Nursing and Midwifery Council (NMC) (2018e). *The Code: Professional standards of practice and behaviour for nurses, midwives and nursing associates*. London: NMC.

Public Health England (2016). *Learning Disabilities Observatory: People with learning disabilities in England 2015: Main report. Version 1.0/November 2016*. London: Public Health England.

Wolfensberger, W. (1972). *The Principle of Normalization in Human Services*. Toronto: National Institute on Mental Retardation.

Wolfensberger, W. (1983). Social role valorization: A proposed new term for the principle of normalization. *Mental Retardation*, 21(6): 234–239.

Further Reading

Picton, A. (2011). Decision-making support for patients with learning disabilities. *Nursing Times*, 107(32/33): 12–14.

Wagemans, M. A., van Schrojenstein Lantman-de Valk, H. M. J., Proot, I. M., Metsemakers, J., Tuffrey-Wijne, I. and Curfs, L. M. G. (2015). End-of-life decision-making for people with intellectual disability from the perspective of nurses. *Journal of Policy and Practice in Intellectual Disabilities*, 12(4): 294–302.

Williams, R. W., Roberts, G. W., Irvine, F. E. and Hastings, R. P. (2010). Exploring decision making in intellectual disability nursing practice: A qualitative study. *Journal of Intellectual Disabilities*, 14(3): 197–220.

Further Reading: Decision-making Experiences during the COVID-19 Pandemic

Bond, C., Stacey, G., Gordon, E. and Harling, D. (2021). COVID-19: Experiences and contributions of learning disability nurses during the first wave of the pandemic. *Learning Disability Practice*, 24(4): 17–25.

Godbold, R., Whiting, L., Adams, C., Naidu, Y. and Pattison, N. (2021). The experiences of student nurses in a pandemic: A qualitative study. *Nurse Education in Practice*, 56: 103186.

Web Resources

Advisory, Conciliation and Arbitration Service (ACAS) – information about and explanations of reasonable adjustments information with examples: www.acas.org.uk/reasonable-adjustments (accessed 22 June 2022).

Challenging Behaviour Foundation – see 'Support through the pandemic' for resources: www.challengingbehaviour.org.uk/information-and-guidance/covid-19 (accessed 22 June 2022).

Easy Health resources www.easyhealth.org.uk (accessed 22 June 2022).

Making a difference together: A health toolkit: http://aldhc.co.uk/repos/guide.pdf (accessed 22 June 2022).

Learning disabilities – overview from the NHS's health A to Z: www.nhs.uk/conditions/learning-disabilities (accessed 22 June 2022).

Mencap – access its resources for health care professionals for a wide range of reports and publications, as well as linked resources from other organisations and its *Treat Me Well* campaign and report: www.mencap.org.uk/learning-disability-explained/resources-healthcare-professionals (accessed 12 July 2022).

www.mencap.org.uk/learning-disability-explained/research-and-statistics/health/health-inequalities (accessed 29 January 2022); www.mencap.org.uk/get-involved/campaign-mencap/current-campaigns/treat-me-well (accessed 29 January 2022).

Mencap (2007) *Death by Indifference report*: www.mencap.org.uk/sites/default/files/2016-06/DBIreport.pdf (accessed 29 January 2022).

Mental Capacity Act – full explanation in relation to the Act and examples of people who may lack capacity: www.nhs.uk/conditions/social-care-and-support-guide/making-decisions-for-someone-else/mental-capacity-act (accessed 29 January 2022)

Principles – information about and examples regarding the meaning of each of the Act's five principles: all accessed 22 June, 2022, Northern Ireland – the Mental Capacity Act Northern Ireland 2016 draft code of practice was due for implementation in 2020. Phase 1 was implemented in 2019: https://www.legislation.gov.uk/nia/2016/18/contents/enacted.

Scotland – for guidance on the Act for Scotland, see Adults with incapacity: Code of practice for medical practitioners (2010): www.gov.scot/publications/adults-incapacity-scotland-act-2000-code-practice-third-edition-practitioners-authorised-carry-out-medical-treatment-research-under-part-5-act (accessed 29 January 2022).

Michael report (2008) *Healthcare for All: Report of the Independent Inquiry into Access to Healthcare for People with Learning Disabilities*: https://webarchive.nationalarchives.gov.uk/ukgwa/20130105064250/http://www.dh.gov.uk/en/Publicationsandstatistics/Publications/PublicationsPolicyAndGuidance/DH_099255 (accessed 12 July 2022).

National Learning Disability Nursing Forum – the go to place for all the latest information about learning disability nursing. The forum serves as a first-class communication resource and has been developed to support learning disability nurses everywhere, as well as those interested in pursuing a career in this unique and highly rewarding branch of nursing: https://learningdisabilitynurse.co.uk/noticeboard (accessed 19 August 2022).

Public Health England (2016). *Learning Disabilities Observatory: People with learning disabilities in England 2015: Main report*. Version 1.0/November 2016: https://assets.publishing.service.gov.uk/government/uploads/system/uploads/attachment_data/file/613182/PWLDIE_2015_main_report_NB090517.pdf (accessed 22 June 2022).

Royal College of Nursing (2021). *Connecting for Change: The future of learning disability nursing*: www.rcn.org.uk/professional-development/publications/connecting-for-change-uk-pub-009-467 (accessed 22 June 2022).

10

DECISION-MAKING IN THE FIELD OF ADULT NURSING

Deborah Atkinson and Jane McGrath

Chapter objectives

The aims of this chapter are to:

- help you to understand why clinical decision-making is an important element in nursing practice;
- consider the complexities of clinical decision-making in the field of adult nursing;
- consider how to recognise the factors influencing clinical decision-making in practice;
- provide a strategy to improve your clinical decision-making ability;
- consider the importance of including the patient in the decision-making process, wherever possible (shared decision-making).

Introduction

This chapter explores clinical decision-making in the field of adult nursing practice. It draws on the actual experiences of student nurses prior to qualifying, to provide real-world examples of the types of decisions that you will face while out on placement as a student nurse and then once qualified. The case studies include learning activities for you to complete, the aim of which is to explore how you might make decisions. This will help you to develop skills for safer professional practice and to put the patient at the centre of your decision-making.

The Role of the Nurse in Decision-Making

The role of the nurse has grown significantly as a result of changes in health policy, enabling the nurse to take on far greater levels of responsibility, such as non-medical prescribing and advanced levels of nursing practice (Wood, 2021). This has resulted in nurses working in an increasingly complex clinical environment.

On a daily basis, nurses are required to make decisions in relation to the care that they provide and how they manage their individual workloads (Banning, 2005; Evans et al., 2020). Clinical judgement, therefore, is considered an essential skill (Tanner, 2006). Nurses now have far greater independence regarding the decisions they make in clinical practice owing to the influence of the changing policy context (Thompson, 2001; Wood, 2021).

With this level of independence, however, comes increased responsibility for the nurse, who will be judged and held accountable for their actions. Nurses are frequently required to make decisions in practice, often with limited information available to them (Ellis, 1997; Gurbutt, 2006). This requires critical thinking and problem-solving abilities, which are important elements of student nurse education (Garrett, 2005).

Clinical decision-making is a highly complicated process, not yet fully understood, and there is considerable debate relating to its constructs and definitions in the literature (Shabban, 2005). Furthermore, a variety of terms are used interchangeably in the literature referring to clinical decision-making, confirming that there is a lack of consensus, and which may cause confusion. The phrases 'clinical judgement', 'clinical decision-making' and 'clinical reasoning' are used interchangeably to discuss and describe similar activity (Maharmeh, 2011).

Consequently, there is a confusing array of theory, opinion and terminology relating to the decision-making process (Buckingham and Adams, 2000). While the definition of 'clinical decision-making' varies among authors, there is some agreement that the process involves a deliberate choice between a range of options and acting within this choice (Thompson and Dowding, 2004).

Nurses make a clinical decision based upon their initial assessment of a situation, using prediction to gauge the likely impact of that decision in the future (Shabban, 2005), and they are responsible and accountable for those decisions (Thompson, 2001; Watson, 1994). Clinical decisions may be based on various types of knowledge, the sources of which have been the subject of considerable philosophical enquiry. The quest to understand the different types of knowledge within nursing continues, on the basis that there remains much to be discovered about the nature of nursing knowledge (Liaschenko, 1998; Thorne and Hayes, 1997).

The initial nursing assessment relies upon the gathering and interpretation of patient data by the nurse using sophisticated cognitive processes to produce a communicable account of the patient's condition (Chase, 1995). A decision can then be made based on the judgement at the time. An accurate nursing assessment and judgement of the situation are therefore critical to effective decision-making. However, when nurses make decisions in daily practice, they are influenced by many things. For example, we may be pressured to make a decision by the patient, relative or colleague. Many other factors may exert some influence over our decisions. What is important for us to consider is that all our decisions have consequences. We therefore want to be confident that the decision we make will result in a positive outcome.

Effective decision-making in practice is essential to improve clinical outcomes for patients and develop and improve nursing practice. There are many theories that have attempted to discover and explain how and why we make decisions in clinical practice. However, exploring how and why we make certain decisions in practice can help us to learn from experience and develop our decision-making skills for the future.

An important consideration for nurses, at all levels, is that the patient should be at the centre of all we do. Wherever possible, we must involve the patient in the decision-making process and always act to ensure that the patient's best interests are preserved. Involving patients in the decision-making relating to their care has been shown to improve patient outcomes (see the Web resources section at the end of this chapter for links to NHS England for information on this and the statutory guidance on patient outcomes).

We have chosen to consider some of the decision-making situations that occur in practice through a series of case studies, based on lived learning experiences of student nurses in various placements.

Case study 10.1 depicts a commonly occurring event in a busy accident and emergency (A&E) department, but one that requires highly effective decision-making from the clinical team in order to maximise the outcome for the patient. It highlights some major learning themes, including the concept of family-witnessed resuscitation (FWR), the breaking of bad news and the emotional impact on family members, nurses and patients when someone dies. These are all situations that explore the need for decision-making by the student supported by the practice supervisor.

CASE STUDY 10.1 (PART 1): DECISION-MAKING IN AN EMERGENCY SITUATION

Background

A third-year student nurse has commenced a placement in an A&E department. Today is her second day and she is working alongside her practice supervisor learning how the department functions. The student has also set some personal learning goals to achieve during the placement.

A phone call had just been made in the department that her supervisor had answered to inform the department that an ambulance was on its way with a patient who appeared to have had a cardiac arrest.

The practice supervisor had told the student nurse that he wants her to be involved in managing the care of this person alongside him as a learning experience and explains that this would be an example of a situation that could happen a number of times while she was in the department.

The student nurse made a decision to reflect on this experience later as there would not be an opportunity to discuss it with her supervisor as the patient had arrived in the ambulance with the paramedic team.

Next is the description, with some observations, that the student nurse wrote down later of what unfolded from the time that the phone call was received in the A&E department.

The Emergency Scenario: Description of the Event by a Student Nurse

The incident began when a call arrived in A&E announcing the imminent arrival of a patient in cardiac arrest, with an estimated arrival time of 1 minute. Immediately, urgent preparations began for the patient's arrival and the team began to assemble in readiness to respond. It was briefly explained to me what to expect and I was fully encouraged to be involved from the beginning. This was my first experience of a resuscitation situation.

My practice supervisor went with me to meet the ambulance. I held open the doors and helped with transporting the patient by stretcher. As I did so, I observed how all members of the team rushed into action, each with their own roles and responsibilities.

In the resuscitation room, the doctors and nurses worked well together as a team, endeavouring to resuscitate the patient. The patient was subsequently intubated and chest compressions were then carried out continuously. Throughout these events, I ensured that I was not 'in the way' and stood at the side of the room in order to observe. Although I had undertaken basic life support training at university in preparation for such events on several occasions, I realised that the reality of cardiopulmonary resuscitation (CPR) in an emergency 'life or death' situation was very different from the calm, safe surroundings of a clinical skills laboratory, and I began to experience feelings of self-doubt and inadequacy. I didn't offer to help with the chest compressions until the senior nurse asked me to pass her a waters circuit. I was grateful for the opportunity to assist and, a short time later, I offered my help. I then began performing chest compressions under the supervision of the qualified nurse.

The patient's son was very distressed in the waiting room and asked to be present while CPR was taking place. The son was then invited into the room during the resuscitation attempt of his mother. While both doctors and nurses continued with the ventilation and chest compressions on the patient, her devastated son was crying and begging his mum not to die, and to hold on to life. He was clearly very distressed. The son's presence and his obvious desperation intensified what was already a highly emotional situation. Once again, I took the role of observer. I felt as though I should have shown him support or said words of comfort, but I simply observed and said nothing.

Having read Case study 10.1 (Part 1), complete Activity 10.1 to reflect on the issues raised, especially the decisions taken by the student.

Activity 10.1

Imagine yourself as the student nurse in this situation. Consider the following questions and make notes prior to considering possible responses:

1. Why did the student not get involved in the resuscitation attempt at first?
2. What happened to prompt the student to get involved?
3. What are the factors that may have influenced this decision?
4. What could the student have done to improve her decision-making for the future?
5. What helps you to make decisions in practice?
6. Have you identified any learning points from the case study?

Issues to Consider

The student nurse in Case study 10.1 (Part 1) initially observed the resuscitation attempt play out before her, rather than immediately offering to participate. Let us consider the factors that influenced her decision-making throughout this situation, which will help you in your responses. They could also be considered to be the kind of issues that you could write about in your reflective diary, because they include the context and actions, as well as possible rationales, for how the student acted. (See Chapter 4 for further advice about reflection and reflective writing.)

1. Knowledge, skills and prior experience

The case study illustrates what could be called a life-and-death situation in an A&E department. The student nurse involved had only ever practised basic life support in a controlled classroom environment before that day. The real-world situation was a very different experience, with serious consequences for the person who arrived at that A&E department.

When we are faced with a clinical decision-making situation, one of the first considerations that we make as nurses is whether we have the required level of knowledge and skill to perform the nursing intervention.

In this instance, the student nurse felt confident about the underpinning rationale for undertaking CPR and had practiced the skill required on previous occasions, but not in a real-world situation. It was her lack of experience of the situation that prevented her from actively participating in the resuscitation attempt at first. The speed of events meant that, in this case, there was not an opportunity to discuss this with her practice supervisor or mentor before the patient arrived. However, it was only her lack of experience that prevented her from volunteering to join at the outset. She did however decide to go to help open the doors to enable the person to be brought into the department.

2. Confidence

The student nurse was new to the A&E department. She was in awe of the members of the clinical team around her and their level of skill and confidence in managing this critical situation. The student felt that she was less able than they were.

The lack of prior experience in resuscitation caused the student nurse to lack the necessary confidence in her ability to resuscitate the patient. The other team members were clearly all very accomplished in their field of practice, and familiar with the resuscitation scenario. They also clearly worked well as a team and were all clear about their individual roles and responsibilities during the resuscitation attempt. As a newcomer to the department, the student nurse had not yet established her place within the team and was concerned that her actions might hinder the other team members.

3. Fear and apprehension

The student nurse was worried that if she were to participate actively in the resuscitation, she might make a mistake or be in the way of the other clinicians, hindering the resuscitation, and making the outcome less favourable for the patient. The fact that other staff were present who had the necessary skills allowed the student an element of choice. However, if the student had been alone in the presence of a patient in cardiac arrest, she would have probably behaved quite differently. For example, here are optional decision-making choices based on her being alone in a cardiac arrest situation:

- It would have been far quicker for her to make her decision as she would not have had to consider other members of staff, but her options would have been limited. It would also have depended very much on where this had happened.
- Ultimately, in the same situation, should the student have opted not to perform CPR, the patient would probably have died without urgent help from another member of staff.

Case study 10.1 (Part 1) discussed the student's lack of experience and confidence that made her apprehensive and fearful, asking herself, 'what if …?' Yet she also knew that her experience and confidence would not improve unless she grasped the opportunity to learn from the clinical situation in which she was involved. This opportunity was essential for her to gain practical skills experience for the future.

Having to make decisions as a qualified nurse can often mean 'facing the unknown', but we know from Benner's (1984) work that as experience, knowledge and skills are gained, the more 'expert' decision-making becomes (see Chapter 1 for more on how proficiency and competence develop).

One aspect that needs to be considered in decision-making is the context and place where a situation occurs. A student nurse, or even a qualified nurse, who comes across someone in cardiac arrest at a shopping centre has very different issues to consider, and that scenario can happen to a nurse from any field of practice. Making decisions such as CPR are now essential proficiencies to achieve for qualifying and working as a future nurse (NMC, 2018a).

Let us briefly consider how the student nurse felt in this first experience of a person in cardiac arrest.

An example from the student nurse's reflection on the CPR situation

The situation felt surreal, and I was in awe of everyone knowing their role, rushing around in an acute situation … I felt frustrated with myself for not taking the opportunity to offer to participate and to take over performing chest compressions.

As we saw, the student later overcame her fear and reticence, offering to participate in the resuscitation attempt. This was prompted by the senior nurse involving the student in the rescue, which occurred when the student was asked to pass a piece of equipment from the trolley. At that point, the student made a conscious decision to get involved because she:

- felt valued;
- was overcoming her fear and apprehension;
- recognised that this was an important opportunity to gain experience.

The student understood the importance of gaining authentic experience while under the supervision of others. She knew that this would provide the opportunity to learn from others, as well as a chance to practice the skills she had previously learnt in a controlled environment.

The senior nurse's inclusion of the student in the situation felt like an invitation to participate. Being included in the team demonstrated that the student was accepted by the other clinicians as a colleague with a valuable contribution to make.

The student was able to overcome her fears of inadequacy because there was sufficient support and supervision available to her. A supportive environment is essential for inexperienced staff to develop their clinical skills and decision-making abilities. This was clearly demonstrated when the student nurse wrote her reflection on a subsequent resuscitation event in the same environment.

The student nurse's reflection on a later CPR situation

This time, I reacted totally differently. I felt focused and confident, and I felt able to become involved immediately. Because I'd already been on placement in the area for a few weeks, the environment felt familiar and I was also familiar with the other staff, which helped. On this occasion, I felt able to become involved from the beginning, helping to prepare the area before the patient arrived. Once the patient had arrived in resus, I made myself available to help out where I could and performed chest compressions along with another staff member, alternately, for 30 minutes. I then asked if I could be involved with the family and observed breaking bad news and helping to support the relatives. The initial experience gave me the confidence to do that, and I think my self-doubt and feelings of inadequacy were an initial hurdle that the original experience helped me to overcome.

Clinical Decision-Making in Action

The clinical decision-making processes illustrated by Case study 10.1(Part 1) follow the 'hypothetico-deductive' model (see Chapter 1). This model processes information made by the nurse during the initial assessment of the situation and generates tentative hypotheses for the various decision-making options available at the time. The decision-making process is somewhat laboured, with careful consideration being given to all of the known possible outcomes. The main problem with this, of course, is that, as an inexperienced student or newly qualified nurse, it is not possible to know all the possible decisions or the influence of other variables on a decision.

As a nurse becomes more proficient in recognising specific risks, managing certain situations or practicing particular skills, the clinical decision-making process becomes easier and less evident. It also becomes more difficult for the nurse to articulate. At this point, the decision-making process has become a more intuitive process (Benner, 1984) or based on tacit knowledge gained from practical experience (Eraut, 2000). This ability has been largely associated with expertise in nursing practice.

As you progress through your nursing education and eventually qualify as a nurse, it will be necessary for you to practice independently, to analyse situations, to make assumptions and to solve problems through the use of critical thinking, clinical judgement, and decision-making (Gabr and Mohamed, 2011). Problem-based learning, or enquiry-based learning, is a strategy that can be used to help with clinical decision-making in practice. Traditionally used in educational settings, it requires a collaborative approach between the student and teacher or mentor and requires the student to take the initiative for defining their own learning goals, and to become a self-directed learner, rather than to be passive in the learning environment.

Problem-based learning has been shown to have a positive influence on learning outcomes, including the development of logical and critical thinking ability, problem-solving, and decision-making (Yuan et al., 2008). These skills are extremely important for nurses, who ought to aspire to be lifelong learners, responsible for their self-directed learning throughout their nursing careers. Additionally, these skills benefit nurses in the constantly changing clinical environment, helping them to make decisions in atypical clinical situations.

The next two activities (Activity 10.2 and 10.3) invite you to use a problem-based or enquiry-based learning approach relating to Case study 10.1 (Part 1), and its relevant sections, to generate critical thinking and self-directed learning, empowering you by allowing you to decide what you need to learn.

Activity 10.2

Read through Case study 10.1 again then answer these questions, which follow a problem-based learning approach.

1. What knowledge would be essential for you, as a student, to participate in CPR for the patient?
2. Where might you locate this essential information?
3. What other knowledge or information would be useful, but not essential in making the decision to participate in giving CPR to the patient?

Knowledge and information to inform your decision-making

When faced with a clinical decision in practice, consider what knowledge you *already have* relating to the presenting problem or issue. Then, work out what other *essential* information you require to make sure actions you decide to take will be safe. Once you have this information, give some thought to what *additional information* might be beneficial, but not essential. This information can be researched at a later point, during home study or discussed with your practice supervisor or mentor. It is useful to jot down any gaps in your knowledge for future reference.

This strategy adopts a 'problem-based learning' or problem-solving approach to making decisions in your clinical practice. It incorporates the learning that you have acquired as a student nurse and builds upon that. Being 'reflective in action' (Schön, 1983) highlights the areas of your knowledge that require additional learning.

Useful information resources include libraries and the Internet – but be sure that any online resources are appropriate and reliable. Some useful websites that you may wish to visit to locate research evidence for practice can be found in the Web resources section at the end of this chapter and others in the book, which may also be relevant to decision-making in practice.

In your answers for Activity 10.2, you should have noted the need for the following.

- **Essential knowledge:** Practical skills experience in performing chest compressions and rescue breaths in a cardiac arrest situation (learnt in a classroom, clinical skills laboratory-based situation or learning through undertaking these skills with an actual real-life patient) is essential knowledge for the student to make the decision to participate. To operate safely, she needs knowledge relating to anatomy and physiology to enable her to deliver the compressions in the correct place.
- **Important knowledge:** Relating to the various pieces of equipment that may be used in a CPR situation is important, so that the student can assist with passing the equipment to team members and so that the team is safe during the CPR attempt. This is especially important when a defibrillator is being used.
- **Additional knowledge:** Understanding the individual roles and actions undertaken by each of the team members is useful for the student, so that they know to adopt one of these roles at a later stage. This might include being the 'scribe' who records the timings of events as they unfold; it might be 'running through' an intravenous (IV) infusion in readiness for connecting it to the patient's IV access; or it might be knowing how to manage a patient following a successful resuscitation.

Now that we have considered some of the issues concerning what relevant knowledge and skills might be important in decision-making in relation to the Case study scenario 10.1 (Part 1), it is an opportunity to explore what your own are and where you need to gain further knowledge and skills to enhance your experience for the future.

Consider the questions in Activity 10.3 and make notes for future learning needs to discuss with your practice supervisors and your personal tutors when setting future learning goals.

Activity 10.3

1. Write down what knowledge, skills and experience you have relating to CPR, using the following questions as a guide:

   - What essential knowledge do you have?
   - What essential knowledge do you need?
   - What else would be important to learn about?
   - What other information would be useful for the future?

2. Consider how you can gain confidence in undertaking CPR in any situation, using the skills and knowledge already gained to support your decision-making.

3. You may be able to have an opportunity available in your university simulation laboratory outside of your normal learning sessions. Contact your personal teacher or your academic supervisor to determine possibilities and organise additional learning experiences.

Now, in Case study 10.1 (Part 2), let us return to the point where we left the student nurse at the end of Case study 10.1 (Part 1). You will see that the student nurse had stepped back from active involvement and was again in an observation role. She was concerned for the patient's son but was unable to offer any support at that time. Now we will move forwards in this same scenario: See Case study 10.1 (Part 2): Further reflection by the student nurse and in particular the possible actions that could be taken to support the son.

■■■■■ CASE STUDY 10.1 (PART 2): FURTHER ■■■■■ REFLECTION BY THE STUDENT NURSE

(Student reflection notes for the end of the CPR situation which also involved the patient's son (Case study 10.1 (Part 1))

The patient's son was in the waiting room, very distressed, and asked to be present while the CPR was taking place. The son was then invited into the room during the attempt to resuscitate his mother. While the doctors and nurses continued with the ventilation and performing the chest compressions on the patient, her devastated son was crying and begging his mum not to die, to hold on to life. He was clearly very distressed. The son's presence and his obvious desperation intensified what was already a highly emotional situation.

Once again, I took the role of observer. I felt as though I should have shown him support or spoken words of comfort, but I simply observed and said nothing.

Decision-making During and After the Immediate Care: Student Reflection

Eventually, a decision was made by the doctor for the resuscitation team to stop CPR, because it was deemed futile and unsuccessful, and the patient was declared dead. It was at this point that the staff nurse broke the sad news to the patient's son. She turned to him and very sensitively explained that, unfortunately, the resuscitation attempt hadn't worked and how very sorry she was.

The patient's son was offered the opportunity to take time to reflect in a quiet room, was supported at all times by the nursing staff and was given the opportunity to speak to the senior doctor, to help him to come to terms with recent events and to ask any questions that he may have.

The incident was extremely emotional for all involved. Throughout the experience, I was supported by the nurses and was asked several times if I had any questions and how I felt.

I helped one of the nurses to make the patient comfortable and then moved the patient to the prayer room, remaining there with her and her son. It was a very difficult experience to watch the son's very early stage of acceptance, while trying to come to terms with the loss of his mother.

Having read Case study 10.1 (Part 1 and Part 2), complete Activity 10.4 where we would like you to consider the student nurse's experience and her reflections throughout as well as any decision-making that she made.

Activity 10.4

1. The student seems to be disappointed that she did not offer the relative any words of comfort during the witnessed resuscitation. Why do you think that is?
2. Adopting the same approach as that used in Activity 10.3, consider what knowledge and information is needed to make a decision about whether or not to comfort a relative:

   • What knowledge is essential?
   • What knowledge is important?
   • What additional information would be useful?

3. As you become familiar with using problem-based or enquiry-based learning, you might think of these three questions when you need to make a decision:

   • What must I know?
   • Should I know?
   • Could I know?

Being able to comfort a distressed patient or relative is fundamental to nursing care. While death is inevitable for everyone at some stage, health care professionals often find it very difficult to break bad news and to deal with grief. In Case study 10.1 the student felt unable to offer the distressed relative, in this case, the son, any words of comfort during the resuscitation attempt. This may have been the first time the student had been in the presence of a distressed relative, as it was her first CPR event. The student may also have felt ill equipped to answer some of the questions the relative may ask.

It is important to understand that your management of the situation during this type of traumatic event may have a lasting memory for the relative. Showing empathy and giving support is extremely important. However, it is also important to be able to identify cues and understand body language from the relative, in this case, which invites you to show that empathy.

Working towards your future decision-making in similar stressful situations, consider the questions asked in Activity 10.5 to explore this subject further and support your learning in future experiences.

Activity 10.5

1. Have you been involved in comforting a patient or relative, or been present during the breaking of bad news?
2. What did you learn from the experience and what do you think might be helpful to other students?
3. What are your fears, if any, about being in this type of situation and how can you address these?
4. What research evidence is available relating to this area of practice?
5. Use the above questions to guide your reflection on a similar situation that you have been personally involved in (see Chapter 4 for more about reflection). Write about your experience in your reflective diary or as a specific 'significant event', which can help you to achieve some of the NMC's competencies (NMC, 2010) or proficiencies (NMC, 2018a).

Our ability to make decisions in practice is largely reliant on our prior knowledge and experience. It is good practice to have a 'debrief' with your practice supervisor towards the end of each shift. Spend a few minutes discussing what went well for you and identify areas that you feel would benefit from additional learning and experience, to improve your knowledge and decision-making for the future. Your supervisor or mentor can then facilitate an action plan to address those areas of learning with you. You may also wish to undertake some reflection on practice after such an event (see Chapter 4).

The debriefing process is an opportunity for you to reflect on your practice and the decisions that you have made. This will help you to identify those areas of practice about which you are confident, as well as those you may need some additional support for so you can improve on them. This helps you to take responsibility for your own learning and prepare for any practice assessments that you will need to achieve successfully in your journey to becoming a qualified nurse. The practice assessors work closely with your practice supervisors to support your learning in practice (NMC, 2018b).

In order to explore decision-making in an entirely different context read the information in Case study 10.2 and then in Activity 10.6 focus on student nurse decision-making options related to the person involved.

CASE STUDY 10.2: DECISION-MAKING BEFORE A DIAGNOSIS IS KNOWN: IMPLICATIONS FOR THE PATIENT AND THE STUDENT NURSE

An elderly lady had been admitted to A&E with a possible stroke. She was alert and talking and had relatives with her. She was waiting to be transferred to the acute medical unit for a full assessment but had already been in the A&E department for almost three hours. She was now feeling hungry and thirsty, so her relatives asked if I (student nurse) could fetch their mother a cup of tea.

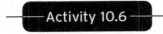

Activity 10.6

1. What should the student nurse do in this situation?
2. Which of the following are appropriate decisions to make?

- Fetch the patient a cup of tea.
- Ask her nurse supervisor or mentor whether the patient is able to have a cup of tea.
- Tell the patient and relatives that it is not yet permissible for the lady to eat or drink anything.
- Explain to the patient and relatives that a swallowing assessment is required before she can have anything to eat or drink, to prevent any risk of aspiration.

Issues to Consider when Making Decisions

What are the risks faced by patients who have been diagnosed with a stroke? The Stroke Association offers a range of information for patients that explains what to expect from an assessment in hospital (see the Web resources section at the end of the chapter for links). Did you consider the following areas of care in your answers to Activity 10.6?

- Pressure area relief and assessment.
- Venous thrombo-embolism prevention.
- Prevention of aspiration and effect of a stroke on the swallowing mechanism.
- Blood glucose management in stroke.
- Maintaining hydration.
- Maintaining nutrition.
- Patient education.
- Personal care.
- Promoting independence.

This list, as well as your other identified risks for a patient who may have experienced a stroke, demonstrates the complexities of clinical decision-making in practice for nurses.

Wherever possible, refer to national guidance or robust research evidence to assist you with clinical decisions. Where practicable, involve your patients in the decision-making process. For this elderly patient and her relatives, however, the most immediate decision needs to be that related to her being able to have a cup of tea.

The possible responses of the student nurse given for question 2 in Activity 10.6 may all be considered appropriate, *except* the first – that is, fetching the patient a cup of tea. To decide to do so may appear logical, as the patient is feeling thirsty, but it would be contraindicated for her care needs at that time because she has not yet had a full assessment, including a full assessment of her ability to swallow, nor possible other issues.

If in your answers you suggested that you would check with your practice supervisor, that shows you are aware that if you are unsure, you are required to check with a qualified nurse.

Either of the other two responses indicate that you may have sought guidance from your supervisor regarding what to say to the relatives, but also that you would offer them an evidence-based rationale for this.

Using the available evidence base to support the decision-making process is essential so we can give a rationale for the decisions that we make (see Chapter 3 for more information about evidence-based practice in decision-making). Research evidence can be published in peer-reviewed journals or reported in other non-peer-reviewed journals and is incorporated into national guidance (available from the Stroke Association, for example). The difficulty for health professionals is keeping pace with the available literature to inform their practice. Additionally, we require the skills to critically appraise the quality of published work in order to evaluate its strengths and weaknesses (Holland and Rees, 2010).

It is necessary to ensure that practices are current, as indicated in the NMC's (2018e) *The Code: Professional standards of practice and behaviour for nurses, midwives and nursing associates*, which sets out the standards of practice and behaviour that need to be upheld. See Box 10.1 for an example of one of these standards: Practice Effectively, that is related to evidence-based decision-making.

Box 10.1

Extract from *The Code* (NMC 2018e: 9)

Practise Effectively
You assess need and deliver or advise on treatment or give help (including preventative or rehabilitative care) without too much delay, to the best of your abilities, on the basis of

best available evidence. You communicate effectively, keeping clear and accurate records and sharing skills, knowledge and experience where appropriate. You reflect and act on any feedback you receive to improve your practice.

6. Always practice in line with the best available evidence.

To achieve this, you must:

6.1 make sure that any information or advice given is evidence-based including information relating to using any health and care products or services

6.2 maintain the knowledge and skills you need for safe and effective practice (NMC, 2018e: 9)

The NMC's professional standards are intended to safeguard the public in our care. We therefore have a professional responsibility to keep up to date with new evidence and to incorporate this into our practice and decision-making. Complete Activity 10.7 to familiarise yourself further with the contents of *The Code*.

Activity 10.7

1. Access *The Code* (NMC, 2018e) and read it in its entirety.
2. Then consider the following questions as they relate to preparation for any new learning placement experience and ensuring that your practice in that placement is underpinned by evidence.

   - How do you keep up to date with new evidence?
   - How do you know whether or not the evidence is reliable?
   - How do you include new research evidence in your practice?

Issues to Consider in your Answers

A useful way to incorporate new research evidence into your clinical practice is to set up a 'journal club'. This is a forum that brings peers together at a dedicated time to consider newly published literature relating to practice issues in a specific placement. The journal club members review relevant publications together, appraising the methodology, results and implications for practice of various studies. The group is usually facilitated by a senior team member in the practice environment, by a tutor at the university, or by a link lecturer from the university. As a student nurse, this format of group learning is maybe something with which you are already familiar. This is also a very good way for students to set a goal for their learning with their practice supervisor, focusing on a patient they are caring for. This could be in a hospital or community environment.

See the Further reading section at the end of this chapter for some examples of developing evidence and see Box 10.2 for some ideas on how to make a journal club successful.

Box 10.2

Ideas for making a journal club successful

1. Focus on the current real patient problems that are of most interest to members of the group.
2. Bring questions, a sense of humour and some snacks and drinks to meetings.
3. Distribute (and redistribute) the time, place and topics for the meeting, and the roles of the group members, in advance.
4. If it is possible bring enough copies of the papers for review for everyone, including both the 'article of the week (or month)' and a back-up article. This may need to be discussed with the leader of the journal club group as there are copyright rules concerning copying multiple copies of an article.
5. Keep handy multiple copies of quick (one-page) quality appraisal tools.
6. Keep a log of the questions asked and answered by the group.
7. Finish with the group's agreed conclusions and develop an action plan for disseminating the knowledge acquired.

Conclusion

This chapter has focused on the clinical decision-making process in the field of adult nursing practice. It has provided some real-life clinical case studies for you to consider, using a problem-solving, enquiry-based learning approach to help you develop your clinical decision-making skills. These case studies can assist students across all the four fields of practice, and the questions asked can be applied to a variety of experiences as you progress along your chosen pathway to becoming a registered nurse. They clearly demonstrate how the evidence base to decision-making (see Chapter 3) and reflection on learning (see Chapter 4) are important as generic learning outcomes that can then be applied in a field-specific context.

Decision-making of any kind is fundamental to the practice of nursing in any context and field of practice (see Chapters 7, and 9 for other fields). It is a skill that we would encourage you to develop from the outset of your programme, and one which you should continue to build once you have qualified as a nurse and take on the responsibility of being an accountable practitioner.

References

Banning, M. (2005). A review of clinical decision-making: Models and current research. *Journal of Clinical Nursing*, 17(2): 187–195.

Benner, P. (1984). *From Novice to Expert: Excellence and power in clinical nursing practice.* Menlo Park, CA: Addison-Wesley.

Buckingham, C. D. and Adams, A. (2000). Classifying clinical decision-making: A unifying approach, *Journal of Advanced Nursing*, 32(4): 981–989.

Chase, S. (1995). The social context of critical care judgement, *Heart and Lung*, 24(2): 154–162.

Ellis, P. A. (1997). Processes used by nurses to make decisions in the clinical practice setting. *Nurse Education Today*, 17(4): 325–332.

Eraut, M. (2000). Non-formal learning and tacit knowledge in professional work. *British Journal of Educational Psychology*, 70: 113–136.

Evans, C., Pearce, R., Greaves, S. and Blake, H. (2020). Advanced clinical practitioners in primary care in the UK: A qualitative study of workforce transformation. *International Journal of Environmental Research and Public Health*, 17(12): 4500.

Garrett, B. (2005). Student nurses' perceptions of clinical decision-making in the final year of adult nursing studies. *Nurse Education in Practice*, 5(1): 30–39.

Gurbutt, R. (2006). *Nurses' Clinical Decision-Making*. Abingdon: Routledge.

Holland, K. and Rees, C. (2010). *Nursing: Evidence-based practice skills*. Oxford: Oxford University Press.

Liaschenko, J. (1998). The shift from the closed to the open body: Ramifications for nursing testimony. In S. Edwards (ed.), *Philosophical Issues in Nursing*. London: Macmillan. pp. 11–30.

Maharmeh, M. (2011). *Coronary care nurses: Developing an understanding of the decision-making process in acute situations*. Unpublished PhD thesis, University of Salford.

Nursing and Midwifery Council (NMC) (2010). *Standards for Pre-registration Nursing Education*. London: NMC.

Nursing and Midwifery Council (NMC) (2011). *Guidance on Professional Conduct: For nursing and midwifery students*. London: NMC.

Nursing and Midwifery Council (NMC) (2018a). *Future Nurse: Standards of proficiency for registered nurses*. London: NMC.

Nursing and Midwifery Council (NMC) (2018b). *Realising Professionalism: Standards for education and training Part 1: Standards framework for nursing and midwifery education*. London: NMC.

Nursing and Midwifery Council (NMC) (2018e). *The Code: Professional standards of practice and behaviour for nurses, midwives and nursing associates*. London: NMC.

Nursing and Midwifery Council (NMC) (2018f). *Realising Professionalism: Standards for education and training Part 3: Standards for prescribing programmes*. London: NMC.

Schön, D. (1983). *The Reflective Practitioner: How professionals think in action*. London: Temple Smith.

Shabban, R. Z. (2005). Theories of clinical judgement and decision-making: A review of the theoretical literature. *Journal of Emergency Primary Health Care*, 3(1–2).

Tanner, C. A. (2006). Thinking like a nurse: A research-based model of clinical judgement in nursing. *Journal of Nursing Education*, 45(6): 204–211.

Thompson, C. (2001). Clinical decision-making in nursing: Theoretical perspectives and their relevance to practice – a response to Jean Harbison. *Journal of Advanced Nursing*, 35(1): 134–137.

Thompson, C. and Dowding, D. (2004). Awareness and prevention of error in clinical decision-making. *Nursing Times*, 100(23): 40–42.

Thorne, S. and Hayes, S. E. (eds) (1997). *Nursing Practice: Knowledge and action*. London: Sage.

Watson, S. (1994). An exploratory study into a methodology for the examination of decision-making by nurses in the clinical area. *Journal of Advanced Nursing*, 20(2): 351–360.

Wood, C. (2021). Leadership and management for nurses working at an advanced level. *British Journal of Nursing*, 30(5): 282–286.

Yuan, H., Kunaviktikul, W., Klunklin, A. and Williams, B. A. (2008). Improvement of nursing students' critical thinking skills through problem-based learning in the People's Republic of China: A quasi-experimental study. *Nursing and Health Sciences*, 10(1): 70–76.

Further reading

Clement, V. J. and Raleigh, M. (2021). The validity and reliability of clinical judgement and decision-making skills assessment in nursing: A systematic literature review. *Nurse Education Today*, 102: 104885.

Garrett, B. (2004). Student nurses' perceptions of clinical decision making in the final year of adult nursing studies. *Nurse Education in Practice*, 5(1): 30–39.

Holland, K. and Roxburgh, M. (2012). *Placement Learning in Surgical Nursing: A guide for students in practice*. Edinburgh: Baillière Tindall Elsevier.

Holland, K. and Rees, C. (2010). *Nursing: Evidence-based practice skills*. Oxford: Oxford University Press.

Nibbelink, C. W. and Brewer, B. B. (2018). Decision-making in nursing practice: An integrative literature review. *Journal of Clinical Nursing*, 27(5–6): 917–928.

Standing, M. (2020). *Clinical Judgement and Decision Making in Nursing*. London: Sage.

Phillips, B., Morin, K. and Valiga, T. M. (2021). Clinical decision making in undergraduate nursing students: A mixed methods multisite study. *Nurse Education Today*, 97:104676.

Joshua, B. (2017). *Nursing students' approaches to learning and clinical decision-making: An intervention study*. Unpublished DEd study, London South Bank University (available at: https://openresearch.lsbu.ac.uk/download/b300aca399db5a7e02de1b5df050e90b9 da109c64f2a1ec7f818f7226a79b101/4043193/2017%20EdD%20Joshua%20.pdf, accessed 30 January 2022).

Joshua, B. and Ingram, A. (2020) An investigation into the impact of approaches to learning on final-year student nurses' clinical decision making. *Nurse Education in Practice*, 49: 102918.

Further Reading: Decision-making Experiences during the COVID-19 Pandemic

Anton, N., Hornbeck, T., Modlin, S., Haque, M. M., Crites, M. and Yu, D. (2021). *Identifying factors that nurses consider in the decision-making process related to patient care during the COVID-19 pandemic. PLoS ONE*, 16(7): e0254077.

Galvin, J., Richards, G. and Smith, A. P. (2020). A longitudinal cohort study investigating inadequate preparation and death and dying in nursing students: Implications for the aftermath of the COVID-19 pandemic. *Frontiers in Psychology*, 11: 2206.

Godbold, R., Whiting, L., Adams, C., Naidu, Y. and Pattison, N. (2021). The experiences of student nurses in a pandemic: A qualitative study. *Nurse Education in Practice*, 56: 103186.

McSherry, R., Eost-Telling, C., Stevens, D., Bailey, J., Crompton, R. et al. (2021). Student nurses undertaking acute hospital paid placements during COVID-19: Rationale for opting-in?: A qualitative inquiry. *Healthcare (Basel)*, 9(8): 1001.

Web Resources

Cochrane Library – source of high-quality information to enhance health care knowledge and decision-making: www.cochrane.org (accessed 22 June 2022).

Joanna Briggs Institute (JBI) – major collection of evidence-based resources, including a special collection concerning COVID-19:
https://jbi.global/ebp (accessed 22 June 2022).
https://jbi.global/covid-19 (accessed 22 June 2022).

NHS Education for Scotland (n.d.). *Clinical Decision-Making*: www.effectivepractitioner. nes.scot.nhs.uk/media/254840/clinical%20decision%20making.pdf (accessed 22 June 2022).

NHS England – Shared decision making and its impact on health: www.england.nhs.uk/ shared-decision-making (accessed 22 June 2022).

NHS England – Shared decision-making statutory guidance: www.england.nhs.uk/ wp-content/uploads/2017/04/ppp-involving-people-health-care-guidance.pdf (accessed 22 June 2022).

National Institute for Health and Care Excellence (NICE): www.evidence.nhs.uk (accessed 22 June 2022).

The Stroke Association (<http://www.stroke.org.uk>)

PART 3

DECISION-MAKING FOR HEALTH CARE

This part will focus on specific areas of healthcare where nurses have an increasing responsibility in ensuring patient safety and managing risk, as well as promoting health. In addition, the role nurses play in health education generally and in relation to their own health and well-being are explored. The chapter on decision-making by nurses in complex situations, offers an insight into the wide range of knowledge and skills that students need to achieve in their proficiencies, all underpinned by an evidence-base.

Given the global health impact of the COVID-19 pandemic, especially on the learning experiences of students in the UK, as well as in other countries, a new chapter has been added which focuses on the direct impact of the COVID-19 virus on nurse education.

11

DECISION-MAKING FOR RISK ASSESSMENT AND PATIENT SAFETY IN PRACTICE

Angela Williams

Chapter objectives

The aims of this chapter are to:

- explore the key features of risk assessment and the decision-making process;
- acknowledge the diverse and different skills needed for patient safety and how to optimise those skills in the clinical environment;
- consider possible models of decision-making that can support student nurse learning and practice to ensure that risks are assessed and managed;
- consider examples of the role of the student nurse in decision-making for risk and patient safety in practice.

Introduction

In 2018, the Nursing and Midwifery Council (NMC) published its new *Future Nurse: Standards of proficiency for registered nurses* (2018a) after an extensive review and consultation exercise to consider the skills and knowledge expectations of future nurses. One of the aspects of the change was the additional focus on their need to gain proficiencies in undertaking risk assessment and ensuring patient safety in decision-making.

This chapter will explore the concept of risk assessment and patient safety within the practice learning environment and provide some examples to aid student nurses, practice supervisors and practice assessors address this proficiency. This applies to all students regardless of which curriculum outcomes are being assessed (NMC, 2010 and 2018a).

Risk Assessment and Patient Safety

The principles of risk assessment are centred on measurable occurrences of hazards and based on factual data (O'Keeffe et al., 2015). While this chapter explores risk assessment in clinical practice, it is important to acknowledge the many complexities of different health care environments in the NHS and this chapter will not be able to cover all areas of risk that may be encountered. The main focus will relate to platform 6: proficiencies and outcomes, which are solely devoted to the improvement of safety and quality of care (see Box 11.1) (NMC, 2018a: 21). That this is included in the standards as a requirement is a major recognition of the importance of assuring the safety of patients when making decisions about their care.

— Box 11.1 —

Nursing and Midwifery Council (NMC): Platform 6: Improving safety and quality of care

Registered nurses make a key contribution to the continuous monitoring and quality improvement of care and treatment in order to enhance health outcomes and people's experience of nursing and related care. They assess risks to safety or experience and take appropriate action to manage those, putting the best interests, needs and preferences of people first. (2018a: 21)

Education providers, in collaboration with practice learning partners, need to ensure that the level of students' proficiency in all aspects of care delivered is safe and person-centred, with the NMC stressing the importance of decisions about student assessments being *'evidence-based, robust and objective'* (NMC, 2018b: 8). It is also important that students learn in a safe and effective way from the professionals around them, to be able to become proficient in the outcomes required for platform 6 and all the other platforms (NMC, 2018a).

All student nurses should be supported in the practice learning environment and provided with safe, effective and inclusive learning experiences (NMC, 2018a: 5). Considering that both student nurses and those in their care are to be 'kept safe', though for different reasons, it is worthwhile exploring what 'risk assessment' means to you in relation to making decisions. Complete Activity 11.1 to begin to give this some thought.

— Activity 11.1 —

1. Firstly, consider the definition of risk assessment and consider what this topic means to you?
2. Think of where you work or are undertaking a learning placement. What risk assessment tools or guidance do you use on a daily basis?
3. What are the main themes that evolve from your initial thoughts? Make a note of these to return to as you read this chapter.

We can consider some of the issues you may have thoughts of in response to Activity 11.1 by focusing on the specific outcome statements that relate to improving safety and quality of care (platform 6), where at the point of registration you will be expected to be able to:

6.5 demonstrate the ability to accurately undertake risk assessments in a range of care settings, using a range of contemporary assessment and improvement tools. (NMC, 2018a: 22)

To be able to achieve this outcome, you will need to learn about the various tools that can be used in various care settings and ensure that your use of them in decision-making is underpinned by effective evidence-based practice (EBP).

An example of an assessment tool used in the health care environment is that published by the Department of Health in 2009, *Best Practice in Managing Risk,* which was issued for the National Mental Health Risk Management Programme. It was developed to provide risk assessment and management advice in a practical way to support services in mental health (see the Web resources section at the end of this chapter for the link to this document).

Another tool utilised in clinical areas nationwide is the Malnutrition Universal Screening Tool (MUST), which was developed by the British Association for Parenteral and Enteral Nutrition (BAPEN) and is used as a nutritional screening tool. The MUST tool is used as a way of assessing if adults are at nutritional risk or are potentially at risk. (See the Web resources section at the end of this chapter for more on this and other types of tools that can be used in different fields of practice.)

Decision-Making and Risk Assessment

Nurses have an integral decision-making role in the delivery of person-centred care within the health care environment (Thompson et al., 2013). It is not only the nurse's sole responsibility to make decisions about patient care but rather a team approach is utilised to work in their best interest. In relation to the delivery of patient care, every aspect involves a certain level of risk dependent on the needs of the person and in some situations the nurse has to manage this risk on their behalf. We can see this clearly in some situations experienced by nurses caring for those patients admitted to hospital with outcomes of COVID-19 illness. Complete Activity 11.2 to consider some of the issues that arose for nurses in relation to patient and personal safety issues during the COVID-19 pandemic.

Activity 11.2

Access and read the following articles:

a. L. Bergman, A.-C. Falk, A. Wolf and I.-M. Larsson (2021). Registered nurses' experiences of working in the intensive care unit during the COVID-19 pandemic, *Nursing in Critical Care*, 26(6): 467–475;

b. N. Anton, T. Hornbeck, S. Modlin, M. M. Haque, M. Crites and D. Yu (2021). Identifying
    factors that nurses consider in the decision-making process related to patient care
    during the COVID-19 pandemic, *PLoS ONE*, 16(7): e0254077.
    Consider how nurses managed risk and ensured patient safety in the two papers and
    how decisions were impacted by the actual context of the clinical area.

One major theme in Anton et al.'s (2021) paper was the importance of identifying
patient care needs within the assessment of the patient using a holistic approach as
critical in decision-making, along with identifying potential risks. As seen in Chapter
6, 'establishing a relationship with patients and their families' was very important, as
they knew the patient and could tell them more information regarding their relative
especially for example as related to their normal health.

Bergman et al., however, in their paper reported that many nurses perceived that,
because of the uncertainties at the time (it was at the beginning of the first wave of the
pandemic in 2020), there were many challenges, stating:

> Participants described how patient safety and care quality were compromised,
> and that nursing care was severely deprioritised during the pandemic. The situ-
> ation of not being able to provide nursing care resulted in ethical stress. Fur-
> thermore, an increased workload and worsened work environment affected
> nurses' health and well-being. (2021: 467)

We do not know whether or not this remained the case but hope that their views of
their current working situation, if they are in the same intensive care unit, hopefully,
have moved forwards. The authors use a phrase from one of their themes which could
also be indicative of how many nurses globally have felt when making decisions during this pandemic – and that was 'tumbling into chaos' where the suddenness of the
situation placed huge stress on them. This is an example of when an issue is not only
one of managing risk for patients but also for the nurses involved.

Platform 6: Proficiency outcome 6.2, illustrates what student nurses need to achieve
to be able to evaluate such situations in their future role, and which can also be seen
in Bergman et al.'s (2021) study:

> 6.2 understand the relationship between safe staffing levels, appropriate skills
> mix, safety and quality of care, recognising risks to public protection and qual-
> ity of care, escalating concerns appropriately. (NMC, 2018a: 22)

Within health care, 'risk' normally refers to potential dangers, threats or perils to
patients and the environment, and risk management aims to reduce their probability.
Risk assessment and management relates to the patient safety agenda. The identification of risk or a hazard is the main aspect of risk management.

There are numerous definitions and terms available that are associated with patient safety and risk. The terms 'risk' and 'hazard' are often used interchangeably and previously the National Patient Safety Agency (NPSA) developed a list of 'Never Events' and applicable tools. This focused on 'learning from what goes wrong in healthcare and preventing future harm' (NHS Improvement, 2018: 2).

However, since 2016 the patient safety aspect has been transferred to NHS Improvement and NPSA no longer exists. However, policies and other information can be found on NHS England's website (see the Web resources section at the end of this chapter for the link to the revised Never Events policy and framework and Never Events list).

As well as reducing risk in the health care environment, the process of risk assessment should be linked to ensuring a level of quality care delivery.

In Mathew Syed's book *Black Box Thinking: The surprising truth about success* (2015), he begins by recounting Elaine Bromiley's story and the list of errors that happened in the course of what should have been a routine operation but ended in her death. Syed shares the story of how Elaine's husband Martin, an airline pilot, continued to ask questions about his wife's death and he came to realise that the answers followed a pattern of events.

As a result, Martin Bromiley set up the charity the Clinical Human Factors Group in 2007 (see the Web resources section at the end of this chapter for the link). The group was established, with the help of the Health Foundation, as a campaign group, which intends to encourage discussion and understanding about human factors and the role these factors have in promoting patient safety.

Decision-Making and Anticipating Possible Risks

The key aspect seen in the papers you have already read, as well as those offered in the Further reading section at the end of the chapter, is that experienced or expert nurses are able to anticipate risk and put mechanisms in place to mitigate this. The clinical judgement model proposed by Tanner (2006) describes four important phases, not just for experienced nurses but also to guide students to gain learning experiences for their future role. There are four aspects to this proposed model (see Tanner, 2006: 208) which are:

- noticing
- interpreting
- responding
- reflecting.

To support an exploration of what these terms mean in relation to decision-making, it is helpful if you return to Chapters 1, 2 and 4, where some of them are also discussed. Let's start by thinking about the first part of the model: *noticing*.

Benner's (1984) influential research, which describes how nurses move from being a novice to expert, demonstrates that experts have a different way of *noticing* to that of their non-expert counterparts. Being able *to notice* as an expert means that you are more likely to grasp the importance of the situation and intervene quickly and appropriately.

In Chapter 1, Benner's notion of proficiency was briefly considered, and it was noted that experienced nurses see situations as 'wholes', so they are able to zero in on the problem and orchestrate what needs to be done in complex situations. Seeing a situation as a whole is an important skill to develop so that you are able to notice cues in either an individual or the environment (or both); cues are collected as data to enable an appropriate course of action.

'Learner nurses', however, have yet to be exposed to a myriad of situations so have not built up what could be termed a 'bank of cues' to then use holistically. It can be simplified to say that an experienced nurse will practice using 'wholes', but a student nurse will be learning in 'parts' (see Chapter 1 for further information).

Complete Activity 11.3 to help clarify what this process involves.

Activity 11.3

a. Try standing in front of a painting or photograph and think about really seeing what it is about. You may find yourself looking in a systematic way – that is, often people doing this will start by looking at the top left-hand corner and then work their way across and down the image, back and forth in horizontal lines, until they reach the bottom right-hand corner. This happens because we use our knowledge of how to read a book and transfer this to 'reading' the painting.

b. Now think about trying to 'read' a patient or a bay of patients or a ward. You might employ a similar systematic technique to enable you to read the cues. Expert nurses are able to rapidly recognise a familiar pattern of cues and compare these to other similar situations that they have encountered. Benner (1984: 102) describes this as being equipped with reality-based expectations and concerns, which means that the nurse can often anticipate future problems.

DeBourgh and Prion point out that beginner nursing students have not had multiple opportunities to develop an awareness of patient risk or safety concerns and so may not act on their responsibilities to manage patient safety. They state that:

> Predicting patient risk for harm and proactively initiating actions to mitigate this risk are actions derived from clinical experience and well-developed thinking skills (predictive reasoning and clinical judgement). (2011: 48)

These thinking skills (which are often hidden to students) can be learned and supported over time.

Tanner points out, however, that:

> Good clinical judgements in nursing require an understanding of not only the pathophysiological and diagnostic aspects of a patient's clinical presentation and disease, but also the illness experience for both the patient and family and their physical, social, and emotional strengths and coping resources. (2006: 205)

This idea reinforces the importance of knowing the patient, knowing them as individuals and the significance they place on their symptoms and or illness, their typical patterns of responses to these and their engagement with health care professionals.

To build on your knowledge and skills in these areas, complete Activity 11.4, which focuses especially on understanding cues.

Activity 11.4

1. When you are working alongside an experienced nurse (perhaps your practice supervisor), ask them to try and articulate their thinking when they approach a patient or clinical situation.
2. Ask them to try and explain the cues that they are noticing, and their thoughts associated with these cues.
3. Ask them what subtle changes in behaviour or appearance they notice.

Benner (1984) asserts that it is often nurses who will initiate emergency procedures, such as resuscitation, because they are present and continually monitoring patients (both formally and informally). You might want to think about how you informally monitor patients next time you are in clinical practice. What is it that you are noticing?

In reality, very little is known about the number and types of cues recognised by student nurses. In an integrative review of literature published between 1964 and 2013 by Burbach and Thompson (2014), only 27 studies were identified in this area. What is known is that students recognise different cues in different situations, but the ability to see, recognise and act on cues can be taught (Burbach and Thompson, 2014).

Having considered the concept of noticing in a broad context, let us start to think about applying a patient safety approach to assessment in specific clinical practice situations.

Silverston (2014) presents a model of safe information gathering and processing for use during clinical assessment. Although the model is shown in use with trainee emergency nurse practitioners, the concepts are important for all nurses. Silverston argues that the clinical assessment is integral to the consultation process and nurses should understand the normal pattern of disease or illness progression. Silverston cites an example:

> In order to learn about a pattern of illness, one has to know how the illness develops and in order to give appropriate safety-netting advice, one needs to know how an illness progresses. A classic example of how this is used in clinical practice is the content of a minor head injury advice sheet, where the patient, or their relative, is asked to look out for the early signs and symptoms of a worsening head injury. The natural history of a progressive head injury is taken into account in the advice that is given. The same applies to the advice that would be given to the mother of a feverish child, in terms of looking for the signs and symptoms of meningococcal disease. One cannot give advice on what to look out for unless one knows what the natural history of the illness is, which is based upon the change in symptoms over time. (2014: 215)

You might want to access the paper by Silverston (see the References section at the end of this chapter for details) and think about his suggestions for a safe approach to patient assessment. He argues that nurses should eliminate the 'worst case' scenarios first and then work towards a diagnosis of the problem. This appears to be very similar to Benner's notion of seeing the whole picture that was discussed earlier.

Some other areas in the NMC's *Standards of proficiency for registered nurses* (NMC, 2018a) whereby knowledge of risk and vulnerability is essential can be found in platform 3: outcome 3.9, and platform 4: outcome 4:10. Let us look at each of these in turn (see Box 11.2 and Box 11.3).

Box 11.2

Platform 3: Assessing needs and planning care

3.9 recognise and assess people at risk of harm and the situations that may put them at risk, ensuring prompt action is taken to safeguard those who are vulnerable. (2018a: 15)

Once again, the theme of noticing can be applied here, as the standard requires you to be able to recognise and, subsequently, assess if people are at risk of harm and also notice and recognise the situations that, effectively, may mean that someone could be vulnerable and at risk. An interesting editorial from Richards, Aronson and Heneghan (2020) describes the consequences of preventable harm going unnoticed, resulting in death. The editorial refers to subsequent papers in the series describing actions to safe-guard vulnerable individuals, including children, elderly people and high-risk patients with substance abuse or histories of self-harm. The authors point out that coroners' reports hold valuable information about cause of death and highlight where health-care outcomes could be improved with better understanding of the causes of prevent-able deaths. There is a legal requirement for coroners to report and communicate a death when it is believed that action should have been taken to prevent the death.

We can see that outcome 3.9 for platform 3: Assessing needs and planning care, highlights the expectation that practitioners will give priority to protecting vulnerable adults so that, within the assessment process, practitioners assess (physical and mental health), protect and safeguard the welfare of vulnerable adults, older people, people with learning disabilities and children. (See the Web resources section at the end of this chapter for the link to the UK Office of the Public Guardian's safeguarding policy, where there are links for Scotland and Northern Ireland.)

Box 11.3

Platform 4: Providing and evaluating care

4.10 demonstrate the knowledge and ability to respond proactively and promptly to signs of deterioration or distress in mental, physical, cognitive and behavioural health and use this knowledge to make sound clinical decisions. (NMC, 2018a: 18)

Detecting changes that indicate rapid deterioration of health status is a commonly required clinical decision. Furthermore, when a patient's condition deteriorates, it is crucial that the decisions are both accurate and timely (Bucknall et al., 2016). *Interpreting cues* that have been noticed, as in Tanner's model (2006), now becomes a critical part of caring for the patient, where ensuring their safety is paramount in the decision-making.

Bucknall et al. (2016) undertook a study of 97 final-year nursing students in Australia while they were taking part in team-based simulations with an actor. The study highlighted three broad categories of influences on the student nurses' decision-making (see Box 11.3: Outcome):

- patient characteristics
- individual students and the team
- context.

Specifically, Bucknall et al. noted that the students recalled 11 types of decision, including:

information seeking; patient assessment; diagnostic; intervention/treatment; evaluation; escalation; prediction; planning; collaboration; communication and reflective. (2016: 2482)

The students appeared to begin collecting information based on visual cues as the patient entered the room, then quickly progressed to recording vital signs, but these were sometimes incomplete as they focused on what they perceived to be the area of concern. Furthermore, for the students in this study, leadership and team communication was absent or lacking. While the students clearly focused on patient safety, decision-making was influenced by patient distress, uncertainty, lack of knowledge and the absence of experienced support staff (Bucknall et al., 2016).

It seems that the students in Bucknall et al.'s (2016) study felt compelled to act rather than spending time to 'take notice' and obtain the 'whole picture'. Benner (1984) describes this as being indicative of the increasing expertise seen in more experienced, qualified nurses. They are potentially *responding to* the cues they recognise or have in fact reasoned out what the cues could be indicative of. This is the third phase in Tanner's study (Tanner, 2006).

When examining the two explanations of how novices become experts at decision-making in practice offered by Benner (1984) and later by Tanner (2006), the outcome found in the more recent study by Bucknall et al. (2016) is not necessarily unexpected. Tower et al. (2019) offer an exploration of what they call situation awareness as a precursor to main decision-making by final-year student nurses. They decided that the students in their study were not yet fully prepared to undertake clinical decision-making once qualified as they did not exhibit certain actions in their learning to make decisions. It is noted that, as in all research with a small group of participants, the results need to be considered in relation to the context in which their learning was taking place, as well as the whole curriculum and learning experiences that they were being exposed to. However, both Benner's (1984) and Tanner's (2006) narratives highlight these differences in learning to become proficient as qualified nurses.

The impact of COVID-19 brought the importance of *reflecting* both 'in action' and 'after action' (see Chapter 4), in relation to safety and risk assessment for patients in practice, to the fore. This kind of learning from reflection can be applied in other situations and can be used by nurses to manage their own safety and make decisions based on assessments relating to their personal risk. These next paragraphs explore this in more detail.

Most working nurses have had to consider the same situation for their families and friends too. In some countries, this assessment of risk to self and others, in local epidemics and pandemics, for example, and decision-making for patient care without causing harm to themselves and others, has been a longstanding challenge that they have needed to manage. The World Health Organization's (WHO) (2018) report *Managing Epidemics* offers a major insight into all aspects of what this involves.

Decision-Making in Assessment of Risk and Safety of Nurses and Students

Nursing, as work, takes place in and across different fields of practice, where it is assumed and expected that the risk to those nurses is at least minimised when caring for individuals. It is recognised that some fields of practice today may be considered more unsafe places to work in, but again actions are put into place to mitigate harm to the self and ensure safety to practice. For example, King's College London has a useful *Lone Working Policy* for pre-registration students that outlines some useful definitions of lone working and advice regarding personal safety (see the Web resources section at the end of this chapter to access the link to the *Lone Working Policy*).

The King's policy cites the NHS (2009a) Security Management Service definition of lone working:

> 2. Definitions
> 2.1 **NHS Security Management Service (2009a, p8) defines lone working as:** 'Any situation or location in which someone works without a colleague nearby; or when someone is working out of sight or earshot of another colleague.'
> 2.2 **Dynamic risk assessment is defined as:** 'A ... continuous process of identifying hazards and the risk of them causing harm and taking steps to eliminate or reduce them in the rapidly changing circumstances of an incident.' (NHS Security Management Service, 2009b p21). (2021: 1)

Student supervision should be flexible and in line with the progression of the student in their pre-registration journey: 'The decision on the level of supervision provided for students should be based on the needs of the individual student. The level of supervision can decrease with the student's increasing proficiency and confidence' (NMC, 2018c: 4). Knight (2022) et al. (see Further reading list) provide an example of what they term long arm supervision to support students in placement in private, independent and voluntary organisations (PIVOs).

The whole King's policy, linked to the student Handbook for Practice Learning, offers an excellent example of proactive support of students while they are in learning placements – and not just for them but also for their clinical colleagues and the patients or clients in their care. Managing and accessing risks prior to students going to learning placements, as well as ongoing processes during that time, is an integral part of the guidance.

In response to the need to manage the risks posed to the nursing, midwifery and allied health professions students during the different stages of the COVID-19 pandemic, the NHS in Scotland produced a number of guidance documents focusing on risk assessment. One of those documents was NHS Scotland's (2020) *Nursing, Midwifery and Allied Health Professions Students' Return to Supernumerary Practice Learning Experiences: Applying the COVID-19 Occupational Risk Assessment Guidance* (see the Web resources section at the end of this chapter for the link). It offered not only guidance on the impact of the pandemic on student learning options but also, most importantly, the decision-making as regards to the personal risk to students in relation to their health and well-being.

Completing Activity 11.5 will enable you to give more thought to assessing risk in relation to one of the most challenging situations nurses have had to work in modern times.

Activity 11.5

1. Access and read the documents listed below (see the Web resources section at the end of this chapter for the links):

    - Scottish Government (2021) *Coronavirus (COVID-19): Guidance on individual occupational risk assessment.*
    - UCL (2022) *COVID-19 Health Advice for Managers.*
    - King's College London (2021) *Lone Working Policy.*
    - Royal College of Nursing, *Clinical Guidance for Managing COVID-19.*

2. Consider the ongoing implications of such assessments of risk at the time of reading this chapter and for the future, in relation to student learning in practice and in relation to the context and country. Note that some of the above are specific documents, while others link to a range of resources to support understanding of managing yourself and supporting others by gaining further knowledge and learning.

Within the scope of the nursing profession, student nurses must learn to deliver care safely, for the patients and for themselves. However, combining new technologies with the delivery of safe care creates an ever-changing situation (noted during the COVID-19 pandemic).

Students adapt when in a learning environment, often using skills of observation, communication and reasoning. They adjust their decision-making skills depending on the situation and the cues they pick up from it. O'Keeffe et al. predict that due to the limited experience of student nurses in the learning environment, student nurses 'will be more likely to seek help when judging their own safety to be at risk' (2021: 7).

Conclusion

Nurses are essential members of the health care team, making critical decisions based on the best evidence and best practice in patient care. As seen in this chapter, managing risk and safety as a student applies as much to the support and guidance available from their assessors and supervisors as it does to actual experiences met in their practice learning placements.

Living and working as nurses globally during the COVID-19 pandemic has meant that another common factor has become more prominent: decision-making related to managing risk and safety applied to our own personal situations. This has needed to be considered alongside assessing risk and safety for those nurses have had to care for. The skills and knowledge required, however, remain common factors in such assessments but, of course, as a global incident, there has been a major cultural and societal context difference to manage in each situation. The impact on learning to become proficient and competent in this important aspect of a nurse's role has taken on a new meaning as countries face both their own challenges as well as the unpredictable outcomes of a major pandemic.

References

Anton, N., Hornbeck, T., Modlin, S., Haque, M. M., Crites, M. and Yu, D. (2021). Identifying factors that nurses consider in the decision-making process related to patient care during the COVID-19 pandemic. *PLoS ONE*, 16(7): e0254077.

Benner, P. (1984). *From Novice to Expert: Excellence and power in clinical nursing practice.* Menlo Park, LA: Addison-Wesley.

Bergman, L., Falk, A.-C., Wolf, A. and Larsson, I.-M. (2021). Registered nurses' experiences of working in the intensive care unit during the COVID-19 pandemic. *Nursing in Critical Care*, 26(6): 467–475.

Bucknall, T. K., Forbes, H., Phillips, N. M., Hewitt, N. A., Cooper, S. and Bogossian, F. (2016). An analysis of nursing students' decision-making in teams during simulations of acute patient deterioration. *Journal of Advanced Nursing*, 72(10): 2482–2494.

Burbach, B. E. and Thompson, S.A. (2014). Cue recognition by undergraduate nursing students: An integrative review. *Journal of Nursing Education*, 53: 73–81.

DeBourgh, G. A. and Prion, S. K. (2011). Using simulation to teach prelicensure nursing students to minimize patient risk and harm. *Clinical Simulation in Nursing*, 7: 47–56.

Domoney, J., Howard, L. M., Abas, M., Broadbent, M. and Oram, S. (2015). Mental health service responses to human trafficking: A qualitative study of professionals' experiences of providing care. *BMC Psychiatry*, 15: 289.

Dovydaitis, T. (2010). Human trafficking: The role of the health care provider. *Journal of Midwifery and Women's Health*, 55(5): 462–467.

King's College London (2021). *Lone Working Policy* https://www.kcl.ac.uk/nmpc/assets/practice-learning/lone-working-for-pre-registration-nursing-and-midwifery-students-policy.pdf (accessed 21 August 2022).

Makary, M. A. and Daniel, M. (2016). Medical error: The third leading cause of death in the US. *British Medical Journal*, 353: i2139.

Nabhan, M., Elraiyah, T., Brown, D. R., Dilling, J., LeBlanc, A., Montori, V. M., Morgenthaler, T., Naessens, J., Prokop, L., Roger, V., Swensen, S., Thompson, R. L. and Murad, M. H. (2012). What is preventable harm in healthcare?: A systematic review of definitions. *BMC Health Services Research*, 12: 128.

NHS Improvement (2018). *Never Events Policy and Framework*. London: NHS Improvement.

NHS Improvement (2019). *The NHS Patient Safety Strategy: Safer culture, safer systems, safer patients*. London: NHS Improvement.

NHS Wales (2016). *An Overview of the Healthy Child Wales Programme*. Cardiff: NHS Wales.

Nursing and Midwifery Council (NMC) (2010). *Standards for Pre-registration Nursing Education*. London: NMC.

Nursing and Midwifery Council (NMC) (2018a). *Future Nurse: Standards of proficiency for registered nurses*. London: NMC.

Nursing and Midwifery Council (NMC) (2018b). *Realising Professionalism: Standards for education and training Part 1: Standards framework for nursing and midwifery education*. London: NMC.

O'Keeffe, V., Voyd, C., Philips, C. and Oppert, M. (2021). Creating safety in care: Student nurses' perspectives. *Applied Ergonomics*, 90: 103248: 1–9.

Richards, G. C., Aronson, J. K. and Heneghan, C. (2021). Coroners' concerns to prevent harms: A series of coroners' case reports to serve patient safety and educate the public, clinicians and policymakers. *BMJ Evidence-Based Medicine*, 26: 37–38.

Silverston, P. (2014). The safe clinical assessment: A patient safety focused approach to clinical assessment. *Nurse Education Today*, 34: 214–217.

Syed, M. (2015). *Black Box Thinking: The Surprising Truth About Success*. UK: John Murray Publishers.

Tanner, C. A. (2006). Thinking like a nurse: A research-based model of clinical judgement in nursing. *Journal of Nursing Education*, 45(6): 204–211.

Thompson, C., Aitken, L., Doran, D. and Dowding, D. (2013). An agenda for clinical decision-making and judgement in nursing research and education. *International Journal of Nursing Studies*, 50(12): 1720–1726.

Tower, M., Watson, B., Bourke, A. and Tyers, E. (2019). Situation awareness and the decision-making processes of final-year nursing students. *Journal of Clinical Nursing*. 28(21/22): 3923–3934.

Xavier, G. N., Duarte, A. C. M., Melo-Silva, C. A., dos Santos, C. E. V. G. and Amado, V. M. (2014). Accuracy of pulmonary auscultation to detect abnormal respiratory mechanics: A cross-sectional diagnostic study. *Medical Hypotheses*, 83(6): 733–734.

World Health Organization (WHO) (2018). *Managing Epidemics: Key facts about major deadly diseases*. Geneva: WHO.

Further Reading

Fisher, M. (2017). *An exploration into student nurses' perception of patient safety and experience of raising concerns.* PhD thesis, Northumbria University (available at: https://nrl.northumbria.ac.uk/id/eprint/36280/1/fisher.melanie_prof-doct.pdf, accessed 23 June 2022).

O'Keeffe, V., Tuckey, M. R. and Naweed, A. (2015). Whose safety?: Flexible risk assessment boundaries balance nurse safety with patient care. *Safety Science,* 76: 111–120.

Knight, KH., Whaley, V. Bailey-McHale, B. Simpson, A. & Hay, J. (2022). The long-arm apporach to placement supervision and assessment. *Br J Nurs.* Feb24;*31*(4): 247

Further Reading: Decision-making Experiences during the COVID-19 Pandemic

Fagan, A., Lea, J. and Parker, V. (2021). Student nurses' strategies when speaking up for patient safety: A qualitative study. *Nursing and Health Sciences,* 23: 447–455.

McSherry, R., Eost-Telling, C., Stevens, D., Bailey, J., Crompton, R. et al. (2021). Student nurses undertaking acute hospital paid placements during COVID-19: Rationale for opting-in?: A qualitative inquiry. *Healthcare,* 9: 1001.

World Health Organization (WHO) (2018). *Managing Epidemics: Key facts about major deadly diseases.* Geneva: WHO.

Web Resources

British Association for Parenteral and Enteral Nutrition: https://www.bapen.org.uk/

Clinical Human Factors Group – charity working to make health care safer: https://chfg. org (accessed 23 June 2022).

Department of Health (DoH) (2009). *Best Practice in Managing Risk*: https://assets. publishing.service.gov.uk/government/uploads/system/uploads/attachment_data/ file/478595/best-practice-managing-risk-cover-webtagged.pdf (accessed 23 June 2022).

Healthy Child Wales Programme Surveillance Schedule (2016) – other types of tools may be used within other fields of nursing, such as children's nursing, and in Wales the Surveillance Schedule is offered as part of this programme. It is a universal health programme for all families with 0–7-year-old children. It includes a range of evidence-based preventative and early intervention measures, and offers advice and guidance to support parenting and healthy lifestyle choices: https://gov.wales/sites/ default/files/publications/2019-05/an-overview-of-the-healthy-child-wales-programme.pdf (updated regularly at: https://gov.wales/healthy-child-wales-programme, accessed 23 June 2022).

King's College London (2021). *Lone Working policy*: https://www.kcl.ac.uk/nmpc/assets/ practice-learning/lone-working-for-pre-registration-nursing-and-midwifery-students-policy.pdf (accessed 21 August 2022).

www.kcl.ac.uk/nmpc/clinical-education/mentorzone/codh-returning-to-clinical-placements-guide-for-heis.pdf (accessed 29 January 2022).

Malnutrition Universal Screening Tool (MUST): www.bapen.org.uk/pdfs/must/must-full.pdf (accessed 23 June 2022).

NHS Improvement – the website has several tools and resources. Patient safety and improvement tools – there are various tools available to help practitioners explore the relevant application of resources to clinical situations and there are several helpful tools, theories and techniques on the NHS Improvement's website: https://improvement.nhs.uk/resources/quality-service-improvement-and-redesign-qsir-tools (accessed 23 June 2022).

Other resources and tools available to practitioners related to patient safety: https://improvement.nhs.uk/improvement-hub/patient-safety (accessed 23 June 2022).

Revised Never Events policy and framework, plus Never Events list: www.england.nhs.uk/patient-safety/revised-never-events-policy-and-framework (accessed 23 June 2022).

NHS Scotland (2020). *Nursing, Midwifery and Allied Health Professions Students' Return to Supernumerary Practice Learning Experiences: Applying the COVID-19 Occupational Risk Assessment Guidance*: www.nes.scot.nhs.uk/media/hrsjgigz/nmahp-student-placement-risk-assessment-final-version-11-09-20-2.pdf (accessed 23 June 2022).

RCN – Clinical Guidance for Managing COVID-19: www.rcn.org.uk/clinical-topics/infection-prevention-and-control/novel-coronavirus (accessed 23 June 2022).

Scottish Government (2021) *Coronavirus (COVID-19): Guidance on individual occupational risk assessment*: www.gov.scot/publications/coronavirus-covid-19-guidance-on-individual-risk-assessment-for-the-workplace (accessed 23 June 2022).

UCL (2022). *COVID-19 Health Advice for Managers*: www.ucl.ac.uk/human-resources/health-wellbeing/workplace-health/what-we-do/covid-19-individual-health-assessment-tool-managers (accessed 23 June 2022).

UK Office of the Public Guardian's safeguarding policy – there are links for Scotland and Northern Ireland: www.gov.uk/government/publications/safeguarding-policy-protecting-vulnerable-adults (accessed 23 June 2022).

12

DECISION-MAKING IN COMPLEX SITUATIONS IN PRACTICE

Melissa Corbally and Karen Holland

The aims of this chapter are to:

- explain how nursing uses clinical judgement and decision-making in practice;
- demonstrate through examples the variety of complex situations in which nurses have to make decisions;

- illustrate the layers of complexity inherent in the practice of nursing;
- describe how simulation can aid nurses in understanding the challenges of decision-making in complex situations;
- describe how nursing assessment aids decision-making;
- illustrate some tips to help decision-making in complex situations.

Introduction

Nursing is complex and often difficult to define. Florence Nightingale (1859) famously stated that 'the very elements of nursing are all but unknown'. Even all these years later, the challenge in making what nurses do within complex environments visible still remains a challenge. Professor Dame June Clark addressed Florence Nightingale's words in her inaugural professorial lecture (the title of which was 'The elements of nursing are all but unknown' – see Web resources for full digital access) focusing on the nature and development of nursing knowledge itself, and determined that:

> The core of nursing practice is not the ability to measure vital signs, administer medication, dress wounds, or manage complicated machines. It does not lie in our technical skills, many of which will be as obsolete in five years' time as some of the skills I learnt as a student nurse thirty years ago. It does not lie solely in our empathy or caring approach to people, for there are many others who can equal that claim. It lies in our ability to diagnose and deal with human responses to illness, frailty, disability, life transitions, and other actual or potential threats to health, and to do so within a relationship of trust and care that promotes health and healing.
>
> Nursing is now, and will be more than ever in the future, not just a matter of a collection of tasks which anyone with a little training can perform at an acceptable level of competence. (1997: 18)

Of course, Professor Clark makes this statement supported by a background of evidence-based discussion, but it is in her final challenge to nursing itself that we can see her vision that:

> Nursing must now take on the responsibility ... to develop its knowledge base (its science), and take its place as a scientific, as well as a practice, discipline. (1997: 19)

Nursing work, in its broadest context, occurs in a multiplicity of different environments and different fields of practice (as we have seen in Chapters 7–10). It can involve taking care of many patients with multiple health problems (multimorbidities) and requires interaction with multidisciplinary care teams in addition to relatives, management, administrators and other allied health professionals. Invariably, many of the individuals' you interact with are from different cultural backgrounds and this will require you to have a degree of cultural sensitivity when you are managing and delivering their care (Holland, 2018).

This all sounds incredibly complex (and it is), however, during your whole education and training learning experience, you are being prepared to practice as a registered nurse by your practice supervisors, practice and academic assessors, university lecturers and teaching staff who are more than familiar with these contexts. 'Realising professionalism' is a key aspiration of the Nursing and Midwifery Council (NMC) in its *Standards for education and training Part 1* (NMC, 2018b) alongside those in its *Future Nurse: Standards of proficiency for registered nurses* (NMC, 2018a).

Clinical environments, as well as the Higher Education institution you are studying at, are equally responsible for ensuring that you achieve your full potential as a nurse, to make a real difference to patient care. The introduction of *Realising Professionalism: Standards for education and training Part 2: Standards for student supervision and assessment* (NMC, 2018c) explains this collaborative responsibility for ensuring student proficiency at the point of registration.

There is no doubt that you will feel daunted at times when facing competing demands as you progress through your programme (see Chapters 2 and 14). Although all the individuals involved in your education endeavour to foster competence and proficiency, which enables you to reach your potential in effectively managing these competing demands, often students will still struggle with making good decisions. See Box 12.1 for questions that students commonly ask us related to decision-making in practice, and then work through them as indicated in the Activity 12.1.

Activity 12.1

1. Read the examples of questions (listed in Box 12.1) that students have asked us about decision-making in practice.
2. Identify those that you have asked someone either at the university or in practice.
3. Consider what you needed to do and find out to prepare to answer them yourself.
4. Make the subject of one of the questions a goal that you will focus on during your next placement, with the support of your practice supervisor.

---Box 12.1---

Questions commonly asked by final-year students related to decision-making

- How can I develop better time management skills?
- Can you help me with tips for prioritising care of medical patients?
- What do you do when you feel things are getting on top of you and there isn't a lot of support on the ward?
- How do I plan my day's work effectively? That is, how do I go about prioritising care?
- How can I manage a caseload of six patients effectively?
- How do I respond in an emergency?
- Could you please advise us on how to cope when we are given an extra-large caseload in final-year? E.g., patients, paperwork, obs.
- How should I manage the great deal of responsibility that is associated with being a final-year student?
- How do I make sure that I don't panic when I first arrive on a ward, and I don't remember everything? I feel we should know it all.
- How do I go about managing things we have never been trained to deal with?

When you set about considering the kinds of questions students ask given in Box 12.1, you will soon realise that answering them involves more than a single-sentence response. In each of them it can also be determined that the student would need to make an informed judgement as to what decisions will be required.

The questions, in the main, are focused on how the students need to make a decision that impacts on themselves and their actions, for example', How do I respond in an emergency?' This could relate to a patient they are caring for, in which case, it would be necessary for the nurse to ensure that they have the necessary knowledge and skills, and that any decisions they may make in response to an emergency ensure patient safety and demonstrate professional competence and proficiency.

The decision-making required by the nurse in their response to emergency situations involving a patient has also to be considered in relation to what judgements both a student nurse and a qualified nurse need to make regarding their own safety as well as that of a patient's in keeping with the NMC's (2018e) *The Code: Professional standards of practice and behaviour for nurses, midwives and nursing associates. The Code* focuses on four major standards, and related statements that nurses, midwives and nursing associates must uphold within the limits of their competence (NMC, 2018e: 4), which are:

- prioritise people
- practice effectively

- preserve safety
- promote professionalism and trust.

Keeping to all these standards while practicing effectively and using clinical judgement when providing care can, at times, feel overwhelming for a student nurse. This chapter should help you to focus on learning to manage and make decisions through focusing on the initial foundation for decision-making and then leading to those more complex decision-making situations.

We will start by looking at some of the essential components of decision-making in nursing before moving on to complex situations later in the chapter. Often, these situations may appear to novice nurses to be managed by qualified, more experienced nurses in a seamless way, but learning to unpack everything that goes into any clinical decision-making is the first step to achieving future proficiency in practice.

Some of the issues that you will read about in other chapters in this book establish a theoretical and practical foundation necessary for then making decisions in more complex situations. For this reason, it is recommended that, prior to reading this chapter in full, you re-read Chapters 1 to 6 in particular.

Nursing, Judgement and Decision-Making

Nursing has been defined as:

> The use of clinical judgement in the provision of care to enable people to improve, maintain, or recover health, to cope with health problems, and to achieve the best possible quality of life, whatever their disease or disability, until death. (Waters, 2003)

From this definition, it is clear to see that 'judgement' is considered a key feature of nursing. Within the 'provision of care', it is implied that making decisions forms part of the overall practice of nursing. It is important at this point to revisit the meaning of the terms 'judgement' and 'decision-making' briefly (see also Chapter 1 for an extended discussion).

'Clinical judgement' is dependent on collecting information, assessing and interpreting it and considering alternative interpretations of it (Downie and McNaughton, 1993), whereas 'decision-making' is the act of making a choice between alternatives (Thompson and Dowding, 2002). In essence, three elements are required to make decisions:

1. information – that is, facts;
2. judgement – some kind of interpretation of the information or facts;
3. decision – choosing based on the outcomes of our interpretations.

As you progress through your studies, you will realise that dealing with uncertainty is an inevitable part of nursing work. This means that what you can 'know' or 'learn about' becomes even more crucial.

Let's now consider these elements of decision-making in more detail.

Information

'Clinical information' is defined as "those characteristics associated with patients and which have a bearing on the diagnosis or management of health and illness" (Thompson and Dowding, 2002: 14). It can also take the form of laboratory findings, physical symptoms or verbal information. Gathering these could be likened to collecting 'facts' as, like facts, they are (mostly) verifiable.

This is an area in which nurses excel. They are expert collectors of information as they note all kinds of details about patients either explicitly (such as taking a pulse) or implicitly (looking at a person's skin integrity while showering a patient, for example). Also, the first stage of the nursing process is an assessment, which is focused on the importance of collecting detailed information (Holland and Jenkins, 2019).

The importance of that first stage cannot be underestimated, and the collecting of good and accurate information is an essential and critical nursing skill. Arising from the work one of us (MC) has undertaken with nursing students, a framework (Corbally and Timmins, 2016) was devised to help students illustrate the breadth of clinical *information* that needs to be collected when routinely assessing patients. This framework – the 4S model – was created as a result of the fact that, within the word 'assessment', there are four 's's, and it is important to appreciate these four things beginning with 's' when assessing a patient:

- situation
- story
- symptoms
- signs.

In my experience (MC) (and also anecdotally, from feedback from students, practice supervisors and practice assessors), students appear more confident in responding to the complexities of clinical situations when they use these four words as prompts for what information to gather and consider in advance of making decisions. Activity 12.2 will give you some practice in using the 4S model.

Activity 12.2

1. Access and read the paper by M. Corbally and F. Timmins (2016), The 4S approach: A potential framework for supporting critical care nurses' patient assessment and

interprofessional communication, *Nursing in Critical Care*, 21(2): 64-67. (See the Web resources section at the end of the chapter for a link related to the NICC article.)

2. Consider the four 's's of assessment, in order:

    - **Situation** In brief, what is going on around the person being assessed.
    - **Story** This has three elements: the patient history/story being presented, the patient's understanding of their story and, importantly, the nurse's own story, with regard to experience, knowledge and skills, for example, and how it has an impact or influence on the nurse's assessment of the person.
    - **Symptoms** How does the person express what is wrong, what are they feeling or saying, and most importantly, how does the nurse then interpret these in order to intervene for the benefit of the person.
    - **Signs** These vary in significance but rely heavily on nursing skills to understand the clues being presented by the person, in a visual way (such as pallor) and sensory clues (do they exhibit visual signs of pain when a part of their body is touched for example). Clues can also be identified when vital signs are monitored and assessed by technology and mechanical means.

3. Use the content of the paper and the more detailed explanation of these stages of the 4S model and put the model into action by completing the final steps of this activity:

    a. Think about a patient you cared for in a recent placement and reflect on the care provided.
    b. Consider the points discussed by Corbally and Timmins (2016) and write down the kinds of information you would normally collect as part of your routine assessment of a patient in your care.
    c. What information did you have to gather about the patient you cared for and how did you use this to assess their needs?

In completing Activity 12.2, which involved focusing on just one person you have cared for, you will realise that a lot of information is collected in the process of clinical nursing assessment.

As you might have experienced the healthcare setting is an incredibly complex place. Uncertainty seems to be the norm. Although there is much we do know about our patients (date of birth, temperature, pulse, respiration and blood results), there is so much that we do not know and are unaware of.

The quality of our judgements and decisions is inextricably linked to the quality of the knowledge you have, the quality of your assessment skills, the quality of other information you receive (e.g., blood results), and also your ability to interpret the significance of all of the information you receive. Your knowledge, skills and attitudes (which are continually shaped by both placement and university learning) need to enable you to achieve the proficiencies required by the NMC in the UK and other similar professional bodies in other countries.

While at times situations can seem very daunting, always remember that the stages known as the ABCDE approach when assessing (and treating) a patient, and its principles set by the Resuscitation Council (UK), is a valuable place to start to consider complex situations that you may come across. It is essential reading for all student nurses prior to a placement in any field of practice (see the Web resources section for the link). As a student nurse, however, there will be some aspects of obtaining information and deciding on actions to be followed that will only be possible to complete under the supervision of a registered nurse.

Now that we have considered what information may need to be gathered from a number of sources, we can focus on how decisions are to be made using the clinical judgement skills that you have. To consider a focus to exploring your decision-making skills we have adopted a case study approach.

Case Studies: Decision-making in Action

The following series of case studies offer you this focus, and an opportunity to consider decision-making in action. Through the activities linked to each one, you can also evaluate your current practice in making clinical judgements as well as identifying areas where you need to develop and set goals in order to achieve, with practice and academic supervisors, the NMC proficiencies (NMC, 2018a).

Read the first Case study 12.1 and consider the complexity of the patient's health and well-being, then complete Activity 12.3.

**■■■■■■■■ CASE STUDY 12.1: CONSIDERING ■■■■■■■■
COMPLEXITY**

Shauna Butterly a is 65-year-old female retired teacher. She has a previous history of acute coronary syndrome, hypertension and had an angioplasty in 2003. She cut her right foot on holiday two days ago and has just been admitted with cellulitis of her right foot. She is scheduled to commence IV antibiotics and is awaiting her first dose of these. Her IV cannula has not yet been sited. You are a student nurse on the ward.

You walk over to her to say hello, you notice she is grimacing and rubbing her chest, she also seems to look quite clammy, although her skin looks healthy, and she has a suntan. You ask her how she is, and she says that her foot is sore, she has a headache and also the lunch she has recently finished seems to be causing her a lot of indigestion. She explains that her flight and journey to the hospital was very stressful, and she didn't get much time to rest. You perform a set of vital signs on her. Her heart rate is 100, respiratory rate 14, blood pressure 180/115, temperature 38.6 degrees Celsius.

---Activity 12.3---

1. Imagine that you are the student nurse in Case study 12.1 as you answer the following questions.

   - What do you know about Shauna?
   - What do you not know about her situation?
   - What kinds of questions might you ask her?
   - What are the significant observations in relation to this case?
   - Are there any other assessments that you might undertake to give you more information to help make a decision?
   - What do you suspect is going on?
   - What would you do if you had to deal with this situation on a ward?

2. Now write down what you can assume to know from the information given to you. How did you decide that this was important information in relation to what was happening with this patient?

3. What did you need to understand to be able to both read and understand the case study in relation to the clinical information regarding her illnesses?
   (Please note this is not a real person that we are discussing here and ensure that you understand why names and information of real people cannot be referred to: read the NMC *Code* (2018e).)

You have completed Activity 12.3 and read the Case study in order to consider the issues you have understood as a student nurse.

Now we need you to consider the actual case study related to Shauna Butterly (Case study 12.1) and determine what you will need to know in assessing her needs.

Undertake Activity 12.4. Refer back to the 4S framework (Corbally and Timmins) to do this: recall these as Situation; Story; Symptoms; and Signs.

---Activity 12.4---

1. Continue to consider Case study 12.1. (Shauna Butterly). Now, write down how much knowledge you needed to have in order to make your decisions. In other words, write down all the things you needed to 'know' in order to have decided what to do.

2. The first exercise in Activity 12.3 focused on what you considered you knew from the initial information supplied in the case study; now you have to decide what more you will need to know to be able to make decisions concerning this patient. Ensure that you also identify what evidence you are going to gather to ensure that you are following best practice.

3. The NMC proficiencies and Annexe B: Part 1 and Part 2: Nursing Procedures (2018a) make it clear that evidence-based decisions of any kind are essential requirements to attaining future nurse proficiencies. (See Box 12.2 for examples of these evidence-based procedures.)

Box 12.2

NMC (2018a: 32) Annexe B: Nursing Procedures

Part 1: Procedures for assessing people's needs for person-centred care

Use evidence-based, best practice approaches to take a history, observe, recognise and accurately assess people of all ages:

1.1 mental health and well-being status
   1.1.1   signs of mental and emotional distress or vulnerability
   1.1.2   cognitive health status and well-being
   1.1.3   signs of cognitive distress and impairment
   1.1.4   behavioural distress-based needs
   1.1.5   signs of mental and emotional distress including agitation, aggression and challenging behaviour
   1.1.6   signs of self-harm and/or suicidal ideation
1.2 physical health and well-being
   1.2.1   symptoms and signs of physical ill health
   1.2.2   symptoms and signs of physical distress
   1.2.3   symptoms and signs of deterioration and sepsis.

Consider that complex situations can involve assessment of mental health and well-being as well as that of physical health and well-being at the same time. People are themselves complex in their overall health care needs and you will need to learn to respond to and prioritise any decisions to be made.

If we look at Patricia Benner's definitions discussed in Chapter 1, we can see that becoming competent and proficient do not happen overnight and neither would becoming an expert nurse. Benner stated that:

> Capturing the descriptions of expert performance is difficult, because the expert operates from a deep understanding of the total situation ...

An expert nurse, with an enormous background of experience, now has the intuitive grasp of each situation and zeroes in on the accurate region of the problem without wasteful consideration of a large range of unfruitful, alternative diagnoses and solutions. (1984: 32)

Complete Activity 12.5 and consider your views of Benner's categories of nursing achievement.

Activity 12.5

1. Consider Benner's (1984) view on 'expert performance', from her now well-established work, *From Novice to Expert*, and think about where you are in relation to her definitions in each of these categories – competent and proficient. (See Chapter 1 for definitions.)
2. Two of Benner's categories that we have not discussed are 'novice' and 'advanced beginner'. Access Benner's work (see the References section at the end of this chapter) and make a note of her definitions for these two categories as well.
3. During your next placement, consider where you are in relation to these definitions in terms of decision-making and making clinical judgements, in both general and complex care situations.
4. Discuss with your practice supervisors where you think you need to enhance current decision-making skills and develop confidence in others.

Complex Situations in Nursing: The Value of Simulation

Holland (2020) points out that nursing students have to navigate 'two worlds' – the health care setting and the university environment. These two worlds are extremely different such as the difference between a large lecture theatre and that of a hospital ward. However, in some instances, the university intentionally recreates hospital and community-type environments as simulated practice learning settings in order to provide students with an opportunity to enhance both practical and decision-making skills in a safe situation.

These have become known as clinical simulation laboratories where the students can engage in many scenarios and develop skills prior to engaging in practice placements. In the UK, this has also enabled Schools of Nursing to consider some of this carefully planned and organised simulation learning experience as contributing to the number of placement hours nurses are expected to achieve to qualify. (NMC, 2018b) (see Chapter 14 for further information).

There is a large body of literature now available from different countries on this development and the use of innovative technology has become successful in creating real-life scenarios alongside the physical set up of a simulated clinical environment (see the Further reading section at the end of this chapter). So, what is simulation in the context of nursing and health care?

Simulation, according to Lopreiato et al., is:

> A technique that creates a situation or environment to allow persons to experience a representation of a real event for the purpose of practise, learning, evaluation, testing, or to gain understanding of systems or human actions. (2016: 33)

Simulation as a practice was made popular by the aviation industry. Today, it is a well-known term which is used by many practitioners worldwide. It is used a lot in health care and has particular relevance for nursing. Let us consider simulation as it relates to aviation to assist you to understand its relevance in nursing.

Many people have heard of 'flight simulators', which are usually a recreated aircraft cockpit with all of the equipment they would expect to see in a real-life aircraft. Student pilots are then tested on whether they can perform particular skills (such as fly a plane safely) as well as respond to challenging situations (such as changing weather patterns). It is in everyone's interest, especially those of us travelling by air, for pilots to be able to practice in this safe environment.

The poet Alexander Pope coined the phrase 'to err is human' as far back as 1711. Since then, it has been much used to acknowledge the fallibility of human judgement and decision-making and how closely it relates to being human. In reality, everyone makes mistakes, regardless of their level but it is hoped that these do not cause harm to human life. It is essential that this fallibility to 'be human' is factored into learning, as it is clearly impossible for anyone to learn without making mistakes.

In health care settings, patients are vulnerable and unwell. The risk to them is high if someone makes a mistake. Equally however, students need to learn particular skills. That is why simulated settings are useful, because they mimic the real environment but provide a safe place to practice. Students can make mistakes and learn from them without harming anyone. When the consequences of mistakes are serious (such as those where the pilot is no longer able to fly a plane, or where the nurse is not able to recognise a deteriorating patient), these simulated environments are extremely useful as they enable a safe environment from which to practice and learn (see the Further reading and Web resources sections at the end of this chapter for related links).

To help you consider the value of using a simulated learning environment in which to practice the skills needed in any field of practice, consider Activity 12.6.

Activity 12.6

1. Think about the most unwell patient you have looked after recently, in any field of nursing. Write a brief synopsis of their situation and refer to the patient as the person only. You can do this as part of your learning off campus (remember to anonymise it – in both name and any context).
2. List all the tasks and procedures that were undertaken for that patient (such as pulse, blood tests, inserting a nasogastric tube, assessment of physical and/or mental health needs and so on).
3. List the tasks and procedures that you (yourself) carried out for the patient.
4. Reflect and consider the tasks or procedures that you have listed. Carefully consider what the consequences of someone making a mistake might have been by anyone involved in their care, and those that you undertook yourself. Make a list of them.
5. Consider how many of these listed tasks or procedures you could have practiced in a clinical skills laboratory and make a note of all those you have yet to achieve.

While considering your lists, you should now be getting a sense of why simulation is used in nursing. It is good when, for example, a patient may need to be given many different medications at one time or even for how to transfer a patient from a bed to a trolley. Patient safety (as noted in Chapter 11) is one of the seven platforms of NMC standards and their proficiencies that need to be attained to qualify and register as a nurse. So being aware of the consequences of your actions, not just for patients but also other colleagues, has become an ongoing aspect of decision-making in any situation.

The glossary of the NMC's *Realising Professionalism: Standards for education and training Part 3: Standards for pre-registration nursing programmes* defines simulation as follows:

> Simulation: an artificial representation of a real-world practice scenario that supports student development through experiential learning with the opportunity for repetition, feedback, evaluation and reflection. Effective simulation facilitates safety by enhancing knowledge, behaviours and skills. (2018d: 18)

We can see again that facilitating safety is an important aspect of simulated learning and practice. Each of you will have different and varied access to simulation environments, with some of you sharing these with other health professionals. Some may also experience multidisciplinary simulation experiences to help them to learn to become a part of a multidisciplinary team situation in clinical environments. Others may have a very different experience as these learning scenarios may take place in a computer-based learning environment.

However you find yourself able to access safe learning environments, they are now an integral part of learning to become a nurse. Next, consider Case study 12.2, an example of a fictitious safe learning experience, for how you might prioritise care in a clinical placement.

■■■ CASE STUDY 12.2: COMPLEX DECISION-MAKING: ■■■ PRIORITIES AT NURSING HANDOVER

Imagine that you have just arrived on a ward for a two-week placement and are receiving the handover for the following six patients in this busy (fictitious) medical-surgical ward. You will be working with a health care assistant and your practice assessor (a qualified nurse with five years' experience) to care for this group of patients. (See Box 12.3 for the brief information concerning the patients you have been allocated to care for during the nursing handover.)

You will need to note that the patient histories are written in an abbreviated way and include an expectation of you understanding the terminology and language used to describe or explain their content. These histories may also omit certain information that you would normally have access to and may describe situations in an abbreviated format not normally used in a ward setting nor in a full nursing handover. This is an activity to enable you to think about managing the care for a small group of patients and different types of decisions a nurse might have to make in the course of a working shift. You will be working with one health care assistant (HCA) and a qualified nurse who is also your practice assessor.

Please ensure that you read all the brief histories before completing Activity 12.7.

▬▬Box 12.3▬▬

Information on group of patients you will be caring for given to your team at the morning handover (in brief)

In bed one is Michael Kelly, an 89-year-old gentleman who was admitted two weeks ago with an extensive right-sided cerebrovascular accident (CVA). He has not regained consciousness since the event. All nursing care has been continued and he has IV fluids in situ. His family spend a lot of time with him and are very concerned about his condition. The doctor has talked to them, and they are aware of his prognosis. We will continue to keep him comfortable. He has been documented not for resuscitation in the event of cardiac or respiratory arrest. Neurological observations and artificial feeding have been discontinued at the request of the family.

In bed two is Hans De Longhe, a 43-year-old gentleman on holiday with his wife from Amsterdam. He fell yesterday and fractured his right tibia and fibula. He was admitted from A&E overnight and is for elevation, ice and analgesia pending theatre. He can mobilise to go to the toilet with crutches but otherwise is to keep his leg elevated. He is scheduled for theatre at 11 a.m. this morning for open reduction and internal fixation. He has not had a chest X-ray, ECG or consented to the surgery. Hans is partially deaf. His hearing aids have gone missing en route from A&E, so communication with him is difficult. Please contact A&E again about his hearing aids, as he will need them post-op.

In bed three is William Bonner, a 55-year-old gentleman who is one day post a right lower lobectomy. His chest drain is oscillating and draining small amounts of haemo-serous fluid. He has a PCA in situ, giving satisfactory pain relief. He is tolerating light diet and fluids. He had a comfortable night; his respirations are slightly raised from this morning, but his other observations are normal. He is sitting in bed at the moment but is beginning to get a bit agitated. Continue to monitor the underwater seal drainage for fluid. He is for removal of his urinary catheter, PCA and IV fluids today. Oral analgesia has been prescribed.

In bed four is Ahmed Hussain, a 23-year-old male. He fell at a party last night and arrived at A&E at about 1 a.m., unaccompanied, in an ambulance. He was unable to confirm whether or not he lost consciousness. There was a smell of alcohol on his breath. He has been unco-operative, agitated and aggressive since admission. According to notes from his last admission, also for a fall in similar circumstances, he has no medical or surgical history, is not on any medications and has no drug allergies. He was admitted to the ward at 4 a.m. for hourly neurological observations for 24 hours. His neuro-obs have been stable since admission. His GCS is 14, pupils equal and reacting to light, size 3, no limb deficits. He was agitated this morning but is now sleeping. His parents are committed to Islam and the Muslim faith and are keen to know the reason for Ahmed's fall, but he does not want them to receive any information. They were quite angry with us earlier because we explained that we couldn't give them any information.

In bed five is Mark Murphy, a 73-year-old gentleman who was an elective admission for total colectomy and end-ileostomy formation for colonic Ca. He has a history of rheumatoid arthritis and is allergic to penicillin. He has just gone to theatre and his bed needs to be made up and prepared for his return.

In bed six, a single side ward, due to an emergency bed situation across the hospital, which meant moving patients to wards not normally considered for them, is a lady who has had to be admitted to hospital.

Daisy Field, a 68-year-old woman, had a (L) CVA and is being transferred to a nursing home this morning. She now has right-sided paralysis, dysphasia and is doubly incontinent. She needs total nursing care and assistance with nutrition. Her ambulance is booked for 11 a.m. today and the nurses' transfer letter has been started. The doctor's transfer letter and prescription still have to be completed and she also has £100 in the finance department, which has to be returned to her before she is discharged.

To enable you to engage in learning to make decisions and to prioritise care for both individuals and a small group of patients, complete the following Activity 12.7.

Activity 12.7

1. From the information provided in the handover notes (see Box 12.3) first, consider the situation in relation to the usual initial assessment priorities for each patient:

   1. airway
   2. breathing
   3. circulation
   4. disability
   5. exposure.

2. Now answer the following questions in relation to their planned care, which you have to determine.

   - What are your team's decisions initially after the handover from the night staff? What would you do if you were team leader for the day?
   - Considering your assessment priorities, who do you think you need to attend to first? Why?
   - What tasks do you think could be delegated to the health care assistant?

   Use the top tips in Box 12.4 to help you decide whose care to prioritise.

Use this activity to help you to learn about complex decision-making before you are assessed formally by your practice assessor as part of achieving proficiencies. You can ask for feedback from the practice assessor and the HCA on how you carried out decision-making during a shift such as the one involving this small group of patients. On occasion patients may offer comments or testimonials to you as well on the care that they had from you and the team. These are also very important as part of the overall feedback in your assessment of practice learning.

Box 12.4

Top Tips for Decision-making in Complex Situations

- Always use the ABCDE approach to make a quick initial assessment – go to the sickest patient first.
- Understand that the most seemingly demanding person may not be the sickest patient.
- Realise that you will always be working with an element of uncertainty. All health care settings are complex.
- Ascertain who you have to help you. Work and **constantly communicate** with one another to ensure that you all know what work needs to be done and by whom.

- Take charge of your environment. Check all your equipment, remove any unnecessary furniture and so on.
- Don't be afraid to escalate challenging decisions to the manager in charge.

Remember – you are only human! Be honest when you feel overwhelmed and always double check if you are unsure of making decisions, especially when the outcome could impact on the patient or your own safety and well-being.

Conclusion

Decision-making in any situation depends on many things, of course, not least of which is where you are in terms of learning to become a nurse – that is, if you are just starting on a first placement, or one in your final-year. Integral to this of course is what prior experience you have had before starting a course at university, as some of you may already have a lot of experience working in various health care environments. Familiarity is very important, too, because all the issues we have been talking about in this chapter take place in a number of different environments, where you not only have to consider the people you are looking after, and their health problems, but also the impact that their physical situation can have on how you manage their care. You can see this in some of the case studies already discussed – the difference between how you manage complex situations in a medical ward, an acute mental health unit or an intensive care unit, as the context of care also has to be taken into account. Learning to become confident, safe and knowledgeable decision makers, and achieving professional proficiencies that demonstrate this, will, of necessity, be your main goal to becoming a qualified nurse.

References

Benner, P. (1984). *From Novice to Expert: Excellence and power in clinical nursing practice*. Menlo Park, CA: Addison-Wesley.

Clark, Dame J. (1997). 'The elements of nursing are all but unknown', Florence Nightingale. *Inaugural professorial lecture*. Swansea: University of Wales.

Corbally, M. and Timmins, F. (2016). The 4S approach: A potential framework for supporting critical care nurses' patient assessment and interprofessional communication. *Nursing in Critical Care*, 21(2): 64–67.

Downie, R. S. and McNaughton, D. (1993). *Clinical Judgement: Evidence in practice*. Oxford: Oxford University Press.

Holland, K. (2018). Cultural Awareness in Nursing and Health Care: an introductory text. Abingdon: Routledge.

Holland, K. (2020). *Anthropology of Nursing: Exploring cultural concepts in practice*. Abingdon: Routledge.

Jeffries, P. R., Rodgers, B. and Adamson, K. (2015). NLN Jeffries simulation theory: brief narrative description. *Nursing Education Perspectives*, 36(5): 292–293.

Lopreiato, J. O. (ed.), Downing, D., Gammon, W., Lioce, L., Sittner, B., Slot, V. and Spain, A. E. (associate eds.), and the Terminology and Concepts Working Group. (2016). *The Healthcare Simulation Dictionary*. Minneapolis, MN: Society for Simulation in Healthcare.

Nightingale, F. (1859). *Notes on Nursing: What it is and what is not.* London: Harrison.

Nursing and Midwifery Council (NMC) (2018a). *Future Nurse: Standards of proficiency for registered nurses.* London: NMC.

Nursing and Midwifery Council (NMC) (2018b). *Realising Professionalism: Standards for education and training Part 1: Standards framework for nursing and midwifery education.* London: NMC.

Nursing and Midwifery Council (NMC) (2018c). *Realising Professionalism: Standards for education and training Part 2: Standards for student supervision and assessment.* London: NMC.

Nursing and Midwifery Council (NMC) (2018d). *Realising Professionalism: Standards for education and training Part 3: Standards for pre-registration nursing programmes.* London: NMC.

Nursing and Midwifery Council (NMC) (2018e). *The Code: Professional standards of practice and behaviour for nurses, midwives and nursing associates.* London: NMC.

Thompson, C. and Dowding, D. (2002). *Clinical Decision-Making and Judgement in Nursing.* London: Churchill Livingstone.

Further Reading

Canadian Association of Schools of Nursing (2021). *Virtual Simulation in Nursing Education Report.* Ottawa: Canadian Association of Schools of Nursing.

Corbally, M., Kirwan, A., O'Neill, C. and. Kelly, M. (2018).) Simulating troublesome contexts: how multiple roles within ward-based simulations promote professional nursing competence. *International Journal of Practice-based Based Learning in Health and Social Care*, 6(1): 18–23. DOI: https://doi.org/10.18552/ijpblhsc.v6i1.422

Cusatis Phillips, B., Morin, K. and Valiga, T. M. (2021). Clinical decision making in undergraduate nursing students: A mixed methods multisite study. *Nurse Education Today*, 97: 104676.

Higgs, J., Jones, M. A., Loftus, S. and Christensen, N. (2008). *Clinical Reasoning in the Health Professions*, 3rd edn. Oxford: Butterworth-Heinemann.

Holland, K. and Jenkins, J. (eds) (2019). Applying the Roper Logan and Tierney *Model in Practice*. Oxford: Elsevier.

Rushton, M. A., Drumm, I. A., Campion, S. P. and O'Hare, J. J. (2020). The use of immersive and virtual reality technologies to enable nursing students to experience scenario-based, basic life support training: Exploring the impact on confidence and skills. *Computers, Informatics, Nursing*, 38(6): 281–293.

Thompson, C. and Dowding, D. (2009). *Essential Decision Making and Clinical Judgement for Nurses*. London: Churchill Livingstone.

Further Reading: Decision-making During the COVID-19 Pandemic

Anton, N., Hornbeck, T., Modlin, S., Haque, M. M., Crites, M. and Yu, D. (2021). Identifying factors that nurses consider in the decision-making process related to patient care during the COVID-19 pandemic. *PLoS ONE*, 16(7): e0254077.

Godbold, R., Whiting, L., Adams, C., Naidu, Y. and Pattison, N. (2021). The experiences of student nurses in a pandemic: A qualitative study. *Nurse Education in Practice*, 56: 103186.

Pan, D. and Rajwani, K. (2021). Implementation of simulation training during the COVID-19 pandemic: A New York hospital experience. *Simulation in Healthcare: Journal of the Society for Simulation in Healthcare*, 16(1): 46–51.

Web Resources

Male nurse's first day on the ward: Student nurses E1: Our stories (2021). *YouTube* – a series of student nurses' stories of learning to become a nurse, offering an amazing insight into a wide range of decision-making experiences for students at all levels of their learning experiences when on placement. This is the first story, which leads to all the others available: www.youtube.com/watch?v=mhJllmUI1Z4&list=PLGkph1Nt iNFVjNzvq07Uni-IT9LlmqxsW (accessed 23 June 2022).

Oxford Medical Simulation (2021). 'This will translate to the real world': Nursing students learn skills through virtual reality: https://oxfordmedicalsimulation.com/category/vr-nursing-simulation (accessed 23 June 2022).

Resuscitation Council (UK) ABCDE approach – it is essential for all student nurses to have read about this approach prior to a placement in any field of practice: www.resus.org.uk/resuscitation-guidelines/abcde-approach (accessed 23 June 2022).

Resuscitation Council (UK) Lifesaver learning – the interactive training tool Lifesaver, a cutting-edge way to learn lifesaving skills anytime, anywhere: www.resus.org.uk/apps/lifesaver (accessed 23 June 2022).

Student nursing during the pandemic (2021). YouTube: www.youtube.com/watch?v=7YMLfssL1JQ (accessed 23 June 2022).

University of Salford, Simulation suites: Health and social care simulation suites and their use during the COVID-19 pandemic: https://www.salford.ac.uk/our-facilities/simulation-suites (accessed 23 June 2022).

Professor Dame June Clark, Inaugural lecture: 1997 Swansea University – Digital archives: https://rescoll.swan.ac.uk/omeka-s/s/swansea-2020/media/2556 (accessed 10 August 2022).

13

DECISION-MAKING FOR PROMOTING HEALTH AND PREVENTING ILL HEALTH IN PRACTICE

Stephen Prydderch and Daniel Lucy

Chapter objectives

The aims of this chapter are to:

- explore concepts and influences on health and well-being;
- consider theories, models and approaches to health promotion to facilitate decision-making;
- demonstrate, using case studies, how different approaches and strategies can support nurses as they promote health and prevent ill health;
- explore the decision-making role of student nurses in promoting health in practice.

Introduction

Promoting health, protecting health and preventing ill health by empowering people to care for themselves better is firmly embedded in the Nursing and Midwifery Council's (NMC) (2018a) *Future Nurse: Standards of proficiency for registered nurses*. These proficiencies are grouped under platforms, with platform 2: promoting health and preventing ill health, focused on all the proficiency outcomes student nurses are required to achieve on completion of their course to become a qualified nurse.

The NMC's recognition that nurses need to have knowledge and skills related to these specific proficiencies is an important recognition of the health needs of their communities and that the nurse has a role to play in both promoting ill health and preventing ill health.

While it is beyond the scope of this chapter to provide examples and discussion for each of the outcome statements, some are provided here to help you begin to plan your learning journey, if you are a student nurse, or, if you are a practice supervisor, to think about how you could support the learning of students to achieve proficiency in these areas.

The practice of promoting health and preventing ill health applies to all four fields of nursing in the UK, and across the entire lifespan.

Together, the proficiency outcomes ensure that nurses support individuals to make informed choices about managing their own health, with wider reference to public health in the context of protection against disease and ill health at community and global levels. The NMC overarching statement for platform 2 underlines the importance of the role of the nurse in promoting health and preventing ill health:

> Registered nurses play a key role in improving and maintaining the mental, physical and behavioural health and well-being of people, families, communities and populations. They support and enable people at all stages of life and in all care settings to make informed choices about how to manage health challenges in order to maximise their quality of life and improve health outcomes. They are actively involved in the prevention of and protection against disease

and ill health and engage in public health, community development and global health agendas, and in the reduction of health inequalities. (NMC platform 2: Promoting health and preventing ill health, 2018a: 10)

Before we begin to look at how student nurses can achieve the proficiencies related to this statement, we shall take the opportunity to first consider what is meant by 'health' and, indeed, 'ill health.'

What Is Health?

The concept of 'health' is difficult to define and determined by a spectrum of complex physical, mental, social, spiritual, emotional, cultural, societal and environmental dimensions (see Figure 13.1). When you consider these in relation to an individual or

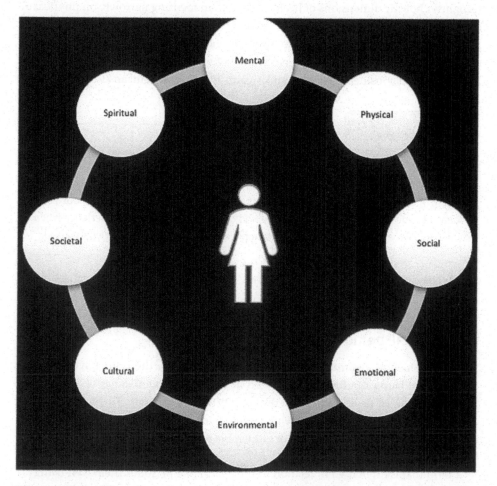

Figure 13.1 Dimensions to consider in relation to health.

a community, it is important to recognise that an individual's perception of 'healthiness' or 'being healthy' is likely to differ from your own. For example, 'lay' perceptions of health will have a direct influence on whether or not a person considers themselves to be 'healthy', with some people thinking of this as merely the absence of a diagnosed medical condition. Others may consider themselves to be healthy if they are able to go walking every day.

Health has been described by the World Health Organization (WHO) as 'a state of complete physical, mental and social well-being, and not merely the absence of disease or infirmity' (1946: 1).

While this definition is sometimes criticised – due to the word 'complete' – it does promote the concept of 'positive health', suggesting that health and well-being can only be achieved by stabilising physical, emotional and social influences that have a negative impact on a person's ability to maintain their health. Achieving such a state of health, therefore, can only be brought about by adopting a social approach that recognises holistic dimensions of health, rather than focusing narrowly on physical or biological components. At this point, you may wish to explore the WHO's resources further (see the Web resources section at the end of this chapter for links), where you will find information and data on a range of world health topics. Also, complete Activity 13.1 to consider what you think health is and what it means to you.

Activity 13.1

1. What does 'being healthy' mean to you?
2. Using the two columns (with their headings) shown, consider what 'health' and 'ill health' mean to you and write down your thoughts. You may wish to think about what it means to you to be 'healthy' and what conditions or events you may experience when you consider yourself 'unhealthy'. An example has been provided to get you started.

Health	Ill health
Attending my yoga class keeps me healthy.	My asthma makes me feel unhealthy.

Health, well-being and wellness

We have seen how definitions of what health is, such as the one above from the WHO, or not being healthy, have emerged in the media and all areas of health care, in particular public health, as a result of the COVID-19 pandemic. This has resulted in a wide range of different policies being adopted according to which group of people have been considered to be healthy or vulnerable to a new illness or anything increasing their current ill health status.

A term that is often used in relation to the health of a person is their 'well-being' as seen in the WHO definition, and Simons and Baldwin (2021) have explored this term in relation to differentiating between the two during the COVID-19 era in relation to doctors and their patients. Their focus was to try and develop a new definition of what this means to people, and they arrived at the following conclusion:

> While overlapping with health, wellness, welfare and quality of life, well-being is separate to these nouns. Well-being is a holistic positive noun, and measurement adopting a salutogenic approach allows further differentiation of the concept from others. The operational definition proposed is not, therefore, limited to doctors, or the workplace, as a definition must allow for all determinants of well-being, whether generic, or specific to a particular group. Society is now global and is described in that way in this proposed definition: 'Well-being is a state of positive feelings and meeting full potential in the world. It can be measured subjectively and objectively using a salutogenic approach.' (2021: 990)

Complete Activity 13.2 and consider these definitions and meanings to help you understand what they might mean to patients in your care.

Activity 13.2

1. Access the paper by G. Simons and D. S. Baldwin (2021), A critical review of the definition of 'well-being' for doctors and their patients in a post COVID-19 era, *International Journal of Social Psychiatry*, 67(8): 984–991.
2. Consider Simons and Baldwin's explanation of the impact of health and related issues on people's lives during the COVID-19 pandemic. Make notes for yourself in relation to this review.
3. Access the Local Government Association's website, where there is an explanation of the term 'salutogenesis' as well as a wide range of examples that illustrate the meaning in more day-to-day examples (see the Web resources section at the end of this chapter for the link). In the most basic meaning this approach refers to a focus on wellness, focusing on health and not ill health or disease.
4. Read about how the meaning of this term can help you to understand how patients you care for, or people that you meet, manage situations that can impact on their health. Some of you may have been on a learning placement caring for patients with a COVID-19 diagnosis where an understanding of the meaning of both health and well-being will have been very relevant to the care given that you will have been part of.
5. Share both the above resources with your practice supervisors and discuss with them how to support patients with their health and well-being to support achieving the proficiency outcomes of platform 2 during the learning placement.

The 'well-being framework,' developed by the Organisation for Economic Co-operation and Development (OECD) as part of its 'Better Life Initiative,' outlined in *How's Life?* (OECD, 2020), uses a range of distinct domains that measure people's well-being against circumstances, such as material conditions, quality of life and the sustainability of well-being over time. This framework depicts health and well-being as being beyond the absence of illness, recognising much wider determinants of health that allow people to be viewed holistically and as 'functioning well' despite any physical restrictions. For example, while we are all different, having close relationships with family and friends may reduce the impact loneliness can have on physical and mental health (see the Web resources section at the end of this chapter to read more about this and other OECD health initiatives).

Research has linked exposure to loneliness with heart disease, depression and low self-esteem, which may lead to hospital admissions or affect a person's ability to work or gain employment. In response to such findings, in 2018 the government announced a strategy to tackle loneliness in England in *A Connected Society: A strategy for tackling loneliness* (HM Government, 2018). This strategy highlighted the importance of social relationships to the health and well-being of individuals and set out proposals to ensure that community nurses, for example, are able to connect people who are experiencing loneliness to community groups and services by means of social prescribing. Consider the issues raised on the various models/frameworks of health in the following activity.

Activity 13.3

There are various implications of using a social model of health and well-being to aid and facilitate holistic practice. Considering this, and the example of how loneliness can have a negative impact on the health and well-being of individuals, answer the following questions. It would help if you had already accessed and read about some of the issues raised in the previous section.

1. What dimensions of health could be affected by a person experiencing loneliness and how might those dimensions relate to one another?
2. Considering the affected dimensions, what are the wider possible physical, mental and social consequences for the health and well-being of an individual?
3. What evidence is there to support your observations?
4. What steps could you take, as a nurse, to promote or improve the health and well-being of people experiencing loneliness?
5. While completing this activity, read *A Connected Society: A strategy for tackling loneliness* (HM Government, 2018) to help you think about this subject.

Before we continue to explore how health and other concepts can help you in your practice experiences, it is important to take a step back for a moment and consider how health relates to you as a professional.

Your Health as a Nurse

Student nurses and their practice supervisors also have an accountability to their own health. This implies that nurses should be healthy in order to promote healthy behaviours in others (ICN, 2010: 37). In addition, the Nursing and Midwifery Council's (NMC) *The Code: Professional standards of practice and behaviour for nurses, midwives and nursing associates* contains a section on the concept of nurses promoting professionalism and trust by means of their own level of health (2018e: 19) – see Box 13.1 for examples.

Box 13.1

Promote professionalism and trust (NMC *Code*, 2018e: 19)

20. Uphold the reputation of your profession at all times...

   To achieve this, you must:

20.8 act as a role model of professional behaviour for students and newly qualified nurses, midwives and nursing associates to aspire to

20.9 maintain the level of health you need to carry out your professional role

---

Kelly, Wills, Jester and Speller (2017) investigated the expectation that nurses should model healthy behaviours using a Delphi study. The findings revealed that participants in the study agreed that being seen as 'human' was of greater importance, together with having an understanding of the challenges of changing health behaviour. The study challenges the expectation and assumption that nurses should be role models for health.

As part of the NMC *Standards of proficiency for registered nurses* (2018a) the platform 1: Being an accountable professional outcomes also ensure that student nurses in their learning experience are expected to care for their own health, adopt a healthy lifestyle and most importantly recognise when others are vulnerable through the 'demands of professional practice' (see examples in Box 13.2).

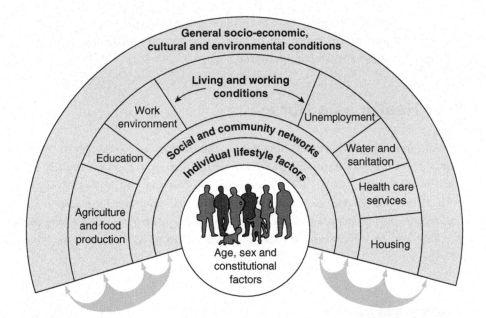

Figure 13.2 The Dahlgren and Whitehead model (Fineout-Overholt, 2019, reproduced with permission).

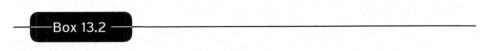

Box 13.2

NMC *Standards of proficiency* (2018a), Platform 1: Being an accountable professional

1. **Outcomes**

   At the point of registration, the registered nurse will be able to:

   1.5 understand the demands of professional practice and demonstrate how to recognise signs of vulnerability in themselves or their colleagues and the action required to minimise risks to health

   1.6 understand the professional responsibility to adopt a healthy lifestyle to maintain the level of personal fitness and well-being required to meet people's needs for mental and physical care

Determinants of Health

'Determinants of health' refers to a broad range of social, economic and environmental factors which impact on the health status of populations or individuals. For example, social and economic resources, such as adequate access to food, clean water and basic human rights, are considered fundamental to achieving health, a view sustained by the Jakarta Declaration, which links social and economic maturity to health (WHO, 1997). However, poverty, education and the social environment in which a person or communities live, equally impact on health and well-being, with people in lower socio-economic groups, for example, experiencing greater levels of ill health. The Dahlgren and Whitehead model of health determinants (1991; see Figure 13.2) shows the interrelationship between the individual, the environment and health and highlights the various influences on health.

It is important that students are able to understand these important relationships so that they can achieve the standards of proficiency required by the NMC (2018a) to qualify and become registered nurses (see examples in Box 13.3).

Box 13.3

NMC Standards (2018a: 11) Platform 2: Promoting health and preventing ill health

2. Outcomes

At the point of registration, the registered nurse will be able to ...

2.2 demonstrate knowledge of epidemiology, demography, genomics and the wider determinants of health, illness and well-being and apply this to an understanding of global patterns of health and well-being outcomes

2.3 understand the factors that may lead to inequalities in health outcomes

---

In 1998, the government published the findings of an independent enquiry into health inequality (Acheson, 1998). It found that, while there is evidence that the overall UK population is 'healthier' than in the past, gender, geographical location and level of income will have direct impacts on the health of an individual or community, suggesting a stark level of health inequality across all societies. Evidence supporting this can be found by exploring statistics, such as those collected and published by the Office for National Statistics (ONS), which suggest that Hull in England and Blaenau Gwent in Wales, had the highest mortality rates in England and Wales, while London and Ceredigion had the lowest mortality rates (ONS, 2017). Such differences are directly attributed to income, socio-economic status and health behaviour. For example, the local authority with the highest proportion of Lower Layer Super Output Areas (LSOAs) in the most deprived 10 per cent of the population in Wales was Blaenau Gwent (Welsh Index of Multiple Deprivation, 2014) (see Web resources for full information on LSOA's).

Explore and familiarise yourself with health statistics by completing Activity 13.4 and using a range of online UK Government data sources such as the Office for National Statistics and the Scottish Public Health Observatory.

Activity 13.4

Using the Scottish Public Health Observatory's (ScotPHO) and the Office for National Statistics' (ONS) websites (see the Web resources section at the end of the chapter for the links), answer the following questions:

1. What is the current average life expectancy of males in Scotland?
2. How does the life expectancy of males living in Scotland compare to that for males in the rest of the UK?
3. What is the average life expectancy at birth for males in Glasgow?
4. How does the life expectancy of males living in Glasgow compare to that for those living in Aberdeenshire?
5. Which of Scotland's local authorities has the highest and lowest proportions of deprivation?
6. How does the prevalence of smoking in males aged 16+ in Glasgow compare to that for males living in Aberdeenshire?
7. Which council areas in Scotland have the highest rates for children living in low-income families?
8. How does child dental health in Orkney compare to that for children living in Fife?
9. How do deaths from suicide in young people living in Aberdeen compare to those for young people living in Orkney?

Understanding some of your answers to the questions in Activity 13.4 will help you to understand the requirements set by the NMC's *Future Nurse: Standards of proficiency for registered nurses* (2018a) in relation to health choices, especially the ones found in platform 2 (see examples in Box 13.4 and 13.5).

Box 13.4

NMC Standards (2018a: 12): Platform 2: Promoting health and preventing ill health

2. Proficiency Outcomes:

    At the point of registration, the registered nurse will be able to:

    2.6 understand the importance of early years and childhood experiences and the possible impact on life choices, mental, physical and behavioural health and well-being

2.7 understand and explain the contribution of social influences, health literacy, individual circumstances, behaviours and lifestyle choices to mental, physical and behavioural health outcomes

Promoting Health

At the point of registration, nurses are required to demonstrate proficiency and skills in the delivery of nursing care that promote health and prevent illness. It is important, therefore, to consider the role of the nurse today as 'promoter of health' (see NMC, 2018a, and the overarching statement for the platform 2 Standard in Box 13.5).

Box 13.5

NMC Standards (2018a: 10): Platform 2: Promoting health and preventing ill health

Registered nurses play a key role in improving and maintaining the mental, physical and behavioural health and well-being of people, families, communities and populations. They support and enable people at all stages of life and in all care settings to make informed choices about how to manage health challenges in order to maximise their quality of life and improve health outcomes. They are actively involved in the prevention of and protection against disease and ill health and engage in public health, community development and global health agendas, and in the reduction of health inequalities.

Public health and health promotion are the responsibility of every registered nurse. These aspects of a nurse's work have provided an integral foundation to nursing practice since the era of Florence Nightingale. In 1869 Ms. Nightingale suggested that recovery from ill health or illness could only occur in clean environments with clean air and good nutrition, stating, according to Monteiro, that, 'The work we are speaking of has nothing to do with nursing disease, but with maintaining health by removing the things which disturb it … dirt, drink, diet, damp, draughts, and drains' (1985: 185).

Since then, nurses have continued to play a key role in managing disease and reducing the risk factors that can have an impact on health. The modern-day public health agenda continues to challenge nurses to consider the role of preventative health care, with emphasis on prevention, early intervention and self-management. Contemporary approaches to public health and health promotion have resulted in the focus moving away from 'treating' and clinician-led interventions to 'preventing' and self-help interventions. This approach to public health and health promotion requires nurses to develop a deeper understanding of the skills and knowledge required to deliver nursing care that is founded upon the premise of public health, promoting prevention, early intervention and resilience across the life course.

In order to consider how these approaches to public health and health promotion have changed over a period of time, consider the outcome of the Ottawa Charter as seen in Activity 13.5.

Activity 13.5

1. Find out more about the changing nature of health promotion by accessing and reading a paper by S. R. Thompson, M. C. Watson and S. Tilford (2018), The Ottawa Charter 30 years on: Still an important standard for health promotion, *International Journal of Health Promotion and Education*, 56: 2, 73-84.
2. Now access the original version, unveiled at the first International Conference for Health Promotion in 1986 - Ottawa Charter for Health Promotion, *Health Promotion International*, 1(4): 405 (see the Web resources section at the end of the chapter for the link) Consider the differences over the 30 years discussed and decide whether you agree that the standard remains an important one for health promotion internationally.

Since the eradication of smallpox by the introduction of a global vaccination pro-gramme in the 1970s, public health continues to present complex and uncertain challenges requiring a skilled nursing workforce to meet contemporary public health challenges. Despite efforts to reduce cigarette use since the 1970's tobacco use remains the leading cause of death, illness and impoverishment worldwide, with one in five people in the UK still addicted to tobacco. Cardiovascular disease remains a significant cause of death within the UK and the USA, too, with more than one in every four deaths being attributed to cardiovascular disease (Public Health England, 2019). New epidemics are also emerging, with obesity affecting 650 million adults worldwide and 41 million children under the age of five. Statistics from NHS Digital (for 2019; see the Web resources section at the end of this chapter for the link) suggest that 10,660 hospi-tal admissions between 2017 and 2018 were directly attributable to obesity, compared to 9,325 between 2013 and 2014. The global obesity epidemic is closely associated with the global increase in the number of individuals living with Type II diabetes, with estimates by WHO suggesting that 366 million will be living with the disease by 2030 – double the figure of 171 million in 2022 (see the Web resources section at the end of this chapter). The microvascular and macrovascular complications of Type II diabetes are associated with increased morbidity and mortality, as they result in diabetic retinopathy, diabetic nephropathy, diabetic foot disease, diabetic neuropa-thy and cardiovascular disease. Mental health conditions and suicide are also on the increase, with suicide attributed to the second leading cause of death among 15- to 29-year-olds globally (WHO – see the Web resources section at the end of the chapter).

It should also be remembered that mortality rates for individuals with a learning disability are significantly higher when compared to those without diagnosed learning needs. According to ONS data for 2013, for people with a learning disability, a substantially higher proportion of deaths were classifiable as avoidable: 50.9 per cent of deaths of men, 36.9 per cent of women and 44.7 per cent of all persons (ONS, 2015). Indeed, due to barriers encountered in accessing and receiving health care, health inequalities continue to be experienced by people with a learning disability.

These figures emphasise the importance of nurses tackling preventable diseases and promoting public health across the life course.

Communicable Diseases

Communicable diseases can be defined as infectious diseases that are transmissible by direct person-to-person contact or indirect contact with contaminated bodily fluids. Socio-economic, environmental and behavioural factors can influence the transmission of a communicable disease, such as travel and crowding.

The transmissible nature of communicable diseases poses a significant threat to international health security, as was experienced in the 2014 Ebola outbreak, which required a global response to contain the virus and protect international health security. Such a global response to communicable diseases is embedded in the International Health Regulations 2005; the 194 member states of the WHO have all agreed to these regulations in preventing and controlling the international spread of communicable diseases and epidemics. The regulations include clear obligations for member states to detect, investigate, respond and report any public health event that may be of international concern.

Disaster and conflict can increase the transmission of communicable diseases by displacing populations, breaking down treatment programmes (such as for HIV, AIDS, TB), damaging infrastructure (such as waste disposal, sewage, water purification), reducing access to health care services, limiting supplies (of food and clean water) and increasing the prevalence of common illness and disease.

To maintain the status quo in communicable disease and reduce the likelihood of an epidemic, are prevention and immunisation programmes and access is provided as well as to fundamental resources, such as food, clean water and sanitation. We have seen of course the unprecedented impact of a global pandemic since the beginning of 2020, with the advent of the COVID-19 virus in its different forms, and as yet the term epidemic, normally reserved for a communicable disease affecting individual countries and not all world countries, has not yet been widely applied. (See the Further reading section at the end of this chapter for sources of information on the impact of the pandemic on the health of nations and global communities.)

Immunisation programmes have been central to the prevention of a number of communicable diseases that threaten both individual and international health security. Yellow fever, measles, mumps and rubella are all examples of communicable diseases that are preventable by means of vaccinations that are available through immunisation programmes globally. The child and adult vaccination programmes in the UK have identified milestones when individuals will be offered vaccinations, starting with babies at eight weeks of age, up to adults aged over 65 for influenza and adults aged 70 for herpes zoster (shingles).

The RCN information on immunisation (see the Web resources section at the end of the chapter for the link and other Department of Health information resources on immunisation) states that: 'Nurses have a major role in advising and promoting immunisation. This includes administering vaccinations included in the childhood immunisation programme and those recommended for adults, including travel vaccines and the annual influenza vaccination.'

There have been concerns raised within areas of the UK regarding the number of individuals who have not received the required two doses of the MMR (measles, mumps and rubella) vaccine. This has meant that there has been an increase in the number of cases of measles, with outbreaks seen in Swansea in 2012–2013 that saw more than 1,219 cases reported within the local area and 88 individuals hospitalised. The aftermath of the Wakefield (1998) MMR scandal, which wrongly suggested a link between the MMR vaccine and autism in an article in the *Lancet* (this was retracted by the journal in 2010) was associated with the lowering of rates of immunisation that resulted in the outbreak in Swansea. The outbreak of measles there was a reminder of the impact communicable diseases can have on health security and the impact the media can have in influencing parents' decisions to vaccinate their children.

Case study 13.1 enables an exploration of some of the aspects of decision-making that can arise for nurses working in the community with regards to vaccinating children.

CASE STUDY 13.1: DECISION-MAKING DILEMMAS FOR THE NURSE

During a general practice nurse's clinic, a 12-month-old child was brought in for immunisation by their parents. The nurse started the process of obtaining informed consent and explained that the child would be receiving the following vaccinations: booster doses of meningitis B (third dose) and pneumococcal (second dose) vaccines plus the first dose of haemophilus influenzae type B with meningitis C, and the separate vaccine for measles, mumps and rubella (MMR). (See the Web resources section at the end of the chapter for a link to the NHS vaccination schedule.)

On learning that the child was to receive four immunisations, the parents became agitated. The nurse invited them to ask questions, allowing them to express that they were not happy for their child to receive four vaccines as they were concerned that it was too many to receive at the same time.

The nurse advised the parents that there is no evidence to suggest that receiving multiple vaccines at the same time is harmful and it enables individuals to be protected against multiple diseases at the same time.

The parents also expressed that they were concerned about an article they had read online about the links between autism and the MMR vaccine.

The nurse advised the parents that there is no proven evidence to suggest a link between the MMR vaccination and autistic spectrum disorders, and that the research attempting to prove that link was proven to be incorrect by international experts.

On discussing their concerns, both parents appeared a lot more satisfied regarding the information they had concerning vaccinations but there was still some uncertainty.

Additional Notes to Consider

This is a common dilemma in clinical practice for nurses involved in giving vaccinations. Obtaining informed consent is the most important part of the vaccination process as it ensures that the individual, parents or guardians are fully aware of and understand the reasons for vaccination, method of vaccination and the disease they will be protected against.

In the situation described here, it would be reasonable to advise postponing the vaccination and providing the parents with written information from the local public health department on the safety of providing multiple vaccinations at the same time and on the MMR vaccine so they can have more time to read these and then organise another appointment to return for the vaccinations as soon as they are happy to do this. By adopting this sharing supportive approach, the appropriate health promotion and health education has been adopted to support informed decision-making.

Case study 13.1 is a very topical one, in the current global COVID -19 virus situation, in terms of questions raised about vaccination status in the UK, Europe and worldwide, of adults of various ages, young people and children. This has been impacted by social media, 'fake news' and fake information about the virus overall with an increase in groups of people in different countries who do not believe in vaccinations of this type. The impact, both during and post the pandemic, has been very much felt in health and social care services worldwide (ONS, 2022). (Please see the Web resources section for a link to this resource.)

There are ongoing debates regarding how many countries have vaccinated their populations against what has clearly become a highly infectious virus, albeit appearing in various guises since the original variant in early 2020. Various names have been given to these changes in the virus, from the Delta to the current Omicron virus.

The initial outbreak was identified as beginning in Wuhan, China, and subsequently spread globally via different means, such as travel between countries, within countries and local communities, to become the pandemic it still is today. The vaccines were developed and approved by medical agencies such as the UK's Medicines and Healthcare products Regulatory Agency (MHRA) in a far shorter time than has ever been achieved before (see the Web resources section for a link to the MHRA's press release in 2020), but despite lockdowns and other precautionary measures instigated by governments worldwide, there have been significant numbers of deaths.

Non-communicable Diseases

Non-communicable diseases are defined as chronic conditions that develop as a result of genetic, environmental and lifestyle factors that an individual may have been exposed to during the course of their life. While non-communicable diseases are not transmitted from human to human, they are a significant burden to public health and are said to be associated with 41 million deaths globally each year, 8.5 million of these being premature (WHO, 2018).

Complete Activity 13.6 to find out some more about this area of health and its importance for the role of the nurse in health promotion and education.

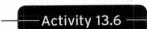

Activity 13.6

1. Access and read a report by the WHO (2018), *Global Action Plan on Physical Activity 2018-2030: More active people for a healthier world* (see the Web resources section at the end of this chapter for the link). It describes the global picture for non-communicable diseases. As it was published in 2018, we have yet to see the possible impact that the pandemic has had on its content and guidance.
2. Consider your own experiences in clinical placements during 2020 and 2021 in particular, and for some of you in 2022, and how the role of a nurse in health promotion and education has had to be adjusted in relation to many chronic health challenges, such as obesity, diabetes, arthritis, cardiovascular disease and chronic respiratory disease. (See Chapter 14 for further information on how the overall programme curriculum and your studies were affected by the pandemic.)
3. Discuss with your practice and academic supervisors how you can meet the NMC 2018a *Standards of proficiency* outcomes for platform 2: promoting health and preventing ill health.

With individuals living longer globally, the prevalence of non-communicable diseases is expected to increase, as they are exposed to the risk factors for developing such diseases for longer. There is, therefore, a growing role for every registered nurse to play in prevention and early intervention to support the growing calls to action in reducing the incidence of non-communicable diseases globally.

Conclusion

This chapter has focused on the concept of decision-making within health education that can enhance the health and well-being of individuals, groups and populations across the life course. It has provided you with an insight into the contemporary public health challenges faced locally and globally and offered useful strategies that can be adopted in clinical practice, as a student or a qualified nurse, to improve public health through health education. The NMC's *Future Nurse: Standards of proficiency* (2018a) articulates the responsibility of every registered nurse in promoting health, health protection and preventing ill health by empowering people and populations to better care for themselves. Health education is central to achieving this responsibility.

References

Acheson, D. (1998). *Independent Inquiry into Inequalities in Health Report*. London: The Stationery Office.

Dahlgren, G. and Whitehead, M. (1991). *Policies and Strategies to Promote Social Equity in Health*. Stockholm: Institute for Futures Studies.

HM Government (2018). *A Connected Society: A strategy for tackling loneliness*. London: Department for Digital, Culture, Media and Sport.

International Conference for Health Promotion (1986). Ottawa Charter for Health Promotion, *Health Promotion International*, 1(4): 405.

International Council of Nurses (ICN) (2010). *Delivering Quality, Serving Communities: Nurses leading chronic care*. Geneva: ICN.

Kelly, M., Wills, J., Jester, R. and Speller, V. (2017). Should nurses be role models for healthy lifestyles? Results from a modified Delphi study. *Journal of Advanced Nursing*, 73(3): 665–678.

Monteiro, L. A. (1985). Florence Nightingale on public health nursing. *American Journal of Public Health*, 75(2): 181–186.

Nightingale, F. (1860). *Notes on Nursing: What it is and what it is not*. New York: Appleton & Company.

Nursing and Midwifery Council (NMC) (2018a). *Future nurse: Standards of proficiency for registered nurses*. London: NMC.

Nursing and Midwifery Council (NMC) (2018e). *The Code: Professional standards of practice and behaviour for nurses, midwives and nursing associates*. London: NMC.

Office for National Statistics (ONS) (2015). *Avoidable Mortality in England and Wales*, 2013, Newport, South Wales. London: ONS.

Office for National Statistics (ONS) (2017). *Death over 100 Years in the United Kingdom*. London: ONS.

ONS (2022). Coronavirus (COVID-19) latest insights: *Vaccines*: www.ons.gov.uk/ peoplepopulationandcommunity/healthandsocialcare/conditionsanddiseases/ articles/coronaviruscovid19latestinsights/vaccines (accessed 23 June 2022).

Organisation for Economic Co-operation and Development (OECD) (2020). *How's Life? Measuring well-being*. Paris: OECD.

Public Health England (now Office for Health Improvement and Disparities (OHID)) (2019). *Cardiovascular Disease Prevention: Applying all our health*. London: Public Health England.

Simons, G. and Baldwin, D. S. (2021). A critical review of the definition of 'well-being' for doctors and their patients in a post COVID-19 era. *International Journal of Social Psychiatry*, 67(8): 984–991.

Thompson, S. R., Watson M. C. and Tilford, S. (2018). The Ottawa Charter 30 years on: Still an important standard for health promotion, *International Journal of Health Promotion and Education*, 56(2): 73–84.

World Health Organization (WHO) (1946). *Constitution of the World Health Organization*. Geneva: WHO.

World Health Organization (WHO) (1997). *The Jakarta Declaration: On leading health promotion into the 21st century*. Geneva: WHO.

World Health Organization (WHO) (2018). *Global Action Plan on Physical Activity 2018– 2030: More active people for a healthier world*. Geneva: WHO.

Further Reading

Bravo, C. A. and Hoffman-Goetz, L. (2015). Social media and men's health: A content analysis of Twitter conversations during the 2013 Movember campaigns in the United States, Canada, and the United Kingdom. *American Journal of Men's Health*, 11(6): 1627–1641.

Cancer Research UK (2019). *Cancer in the UK: 2019*. London: Cancer Research UK.

Charlesworth, L., Hutton, D. and Hussain, H. (2019). Therapeutic radiographers' perceptions of the barriers and enablers to effective smoking cessation support. *Radiography*, 25: 121–128.

Dahlgren, G. and Whitehead, M. (2006a). Concepts and Principles for Tackling Social Inequities in Health: *Levelling Up Part 1*. Geneva: WHO.

Dahlgren, G. and Whitehead, M. (2006b). European Strategies for Tackling Social Inequities in Health: *Levelling Up Part 2*. Geneva: WHO.

Dahlgren, G. and Whitehead, M. (2021). The Dahlgren-Whitehead Model of Health Determinants: 30 years on and still chasing rainbows. *Public Health*, 199: 20–24.

Forum of International Respiratory Societies (2016). *The Global Impact of Respiratory Disease*, 2nd edn. Sheffield: European Respiratory Society.

Gabarron, E. and Wynn, R. (2016). Use of social media for sexual health promotion: A scoping review. *Global Health Action*, 9(1): 32193.

Hurley, S., Edwards, J., Cupp, J. and Phillips, M. (2018). Nurses' perceptions of self as role models of health. *Western Journal of Nursing Research*, 40(8): 1131–1147.

Laverak, G. (2017). The challenge of the 'art and science' of health promotion. *Challenges*, 8: 22.

Office for National Statistics (ONS) (2017). *Death over 100 years in the United Kingdom.*

Hurley, S., Edwards, J., Cupp, J. and Phillips, M. (2018). Nurses' perceptions of self as role models of health. *Western Journal of Nursing Research 2018*, 40(8): 1131–1147.

HM Government (2018). *A Connected Society: A strategy for tackling loneliness.* Available from: https://assets.publishing.service.gov.uk/government/uploads/system/uploads/attachment_data/file/750909/6.4882_DCMS_Loneliness_Strategy_web_Update.pdf (accessed 23 August 2022).

Mackereth, P., Finchett, C. and Holt, M. (2016). Smoke-free hospital site conversations: How nurses can initiate change. *British Journal of Nursing*, 25(21): 1176–1180.

Mikkelsen, B., Williams, J., Rakovac, I. et al. (2019). Life course approach to prevention and control of non-communicable diseases. *British Medical Journal*, 364: 1257.

National Institute for Health and Clinical Excellence (NICE) (2006). *Brief Interventions and Referral for Smoking Cessation in Primary Care and Other Settings*. Public Health Intervention Guidance No. 1. London: NICE.

World Health Organization (WHO) (n.d.). *Cultural Contexts of Health and Well-being: Culture matters: Using a cultural context of health approach to enhance policymaking.* Policy brief No. 1. Geneva: WHO.

Further Reading: Decision-making During the COVID-19 Pandemic

de Campos-Rudinsky, T. C. and Undurraga, E. (2021). Public health decisions in the COVID-19 pandemic require more than 'follow the science'. *Journal of Medical Ethics*, 47: 296–299.

Hargreaves, L., Zickgraf, P., Paniagua, N., Evans, T. L. and Radesi, L. (2021). COVID-19 pandemic impact on nursing student education: Telenursing with virtual clinical experiences. *SAGE Open Nursing*, 7: 1–8.

Medicines and Healthcare products Regulatory Agency (MHRA) (2020). UK medicines regulator gives approval for first UK COVID-19 vaccine, press release. London: MHRA.

Nelson, H., Murdoch, N. H. and Norman, K. (2021). The role of uncertainty in the experiences of nurses during the COVID-19 pandemic: A phenomenological study. *Canadian Journal of Nursing Research*, 5392: 124–133.

Office for National Statistics (ONS) (2022). *Coronavirus (COVID-19) latest insights: Vaccines.* London: ONS.

Swift, A., Banks, L., Baleswaran, A., et al. (2020). COVID-19 and student nurses: A view from England. *Journal of Clinical Nursing*, 29(17–18): 3111–3114.

Web Resources

Dahlgren, G. and Whitehead, M. (2006b), European Strategies for Tackling Social Inequities in Health: *Levelling Up Part 2*: www.euro.who.int/__data/assets/pdf_file/0018/103824/E893 84.pdf (accessed 23 June 2022).

Health in Wales – the objective of the website is 'to provide the people of Wales, including NHS staff, academia, media and partner organisations, with access to links to information from the NHS in Wales and its partner organisations, about the health of the population of Wales, and health and social care services provided by NHS Wales. It is the point of access for information on what we, the NHS in Wales, do, how well we do it, how and who to contact, available jobs and the careers we offer': http://www.wales.nhs.uk/ (accessed 15 July 2022).

Report on the measles epidemic in Swansea in 2013: www.wales.nhs.uk/news/29688 (accessed 23 June 2022).

Local Government Association: Explanation of the term 'salutogenesis': www.local.gov.uk/salutogenesis (accessed 23 June 2022).

Medicines and Healthcare products Regulatory Agency (MHRA) (2020), UK medicines regulator gives approval for first UK COVID-19 vaccine, press release: www.gov.uk/government/news/uk-medicines-regulator-gives-approval-for-first-uk-covid-19-vaccine (accessed 23 June 2022).

NHS Digital – Statistics on obesity, physical activity and diet, England, 2019: https://digital.nhs.uk/data-and-information/publications/statistical/statistics-on-obesity-physical-activity-and-diet/statistics-on-obesity-physical-activity-and-diet-england-2019 (accessed 23 June 2022).

NHS vaccination schedule: https://www.nhs.uk/conditions/vaccinations/nhs-vaccinations-and-when-to-have-them/ (accessed 23 August 2022).

The Organisation for Economic Cooperation (OECD): https://www.oecd.org/sdd/OECD-Better-Life-Initiative.pdf

Office for National Statistics (ONS): www.ons.gov.uk (accessed 23 June 2022).

Ottawa Charter – first unveiled at the International Conference for Health Promotion in 1986: https://academic.oup.com/heapro/article/1/4/405/933881 (accessed 23 June 2022).

Public health, case studies on the transfer of public health from the NHS to local government and Public Health England (PHE): www.local.gov.uk/topics/social-care-health-and-integration/public-health (accessed 23 June 2022).

Public Health Notes – this site has a large number of international Internet resource links in the reference list related to health promotion, including *Ottawa Charter – all you need to know!*: www.publichealthnotes.com/ottawa-charter (accessed 23 June 2022).

Royal College of Nursing (RCN), *Clinical Guidance for Managing COVID-19*: www.rcn.org.uk/clinical-topics/infection-prevention-and-control/novel-coronavirus (accessed 23 June 2022).

Scottish Public Health Observatory's (ScotPHO): www.scotpho.org.uk (accessed 23 June 2022).

World Health Organization (WHO) – information and data on a range of world health topics: www.who.int (accessed 23 June 2022).

The constitution of the WHO: https://apps.who.int/gb/bd/PDF/bd47/EN/constitution-en.pdf?ua=1 (accessed 23 June 2022).

Information about diabetes: http://apps.who.int/iris/bitstream/handle/10665/204871/9789241565257_eng.pdf;jsessionid=7A405AA6C116BCFE5E28E042A23EF38B?sequence=1 (accessed 23 June 2022).

(2018) *Global Action Plan on Physical Activity 2018–2030: More active people for a healthier world*: https://apps.who.int/iris/bitstream/handle/10665/272722/9789241514187-eng.pdf?ua=1 (accessed 23 June 2022).

Information about health-promoting schools: www.who.int/health-topics/health-promoting-schools#tab=tab_1 (accessed 23 June 2022).

Information about obesity and being overweight: www.who.int/news-room/fact-sheets/detail/obesity-and-overweight (accessed 23 June 2022).

Information about suicide: www.who.int/en/news-room/fact-sheets/detail/suicide (accessed 23 June 2022).

Lower Layer Super Output Areas: https://www.data.gov.uk/dataset/c481f2d3-91fc-4767-ae10-2efdf6d58996/lower-layer-super-output-areas-lsoas (accessed 23 August 2022).

14

DECISION-MAKING AND NURSING EDUCATION IN A GLOBAL PANDEMIC

Debbie Roberts and Karen Holland

Chapter objectives

The aims of this chapter are to:

- examine the impact on nurse education in the UK of a global pandemic
- consider various changes in decision-making experiences for student nurses' learning in practice
- consider future learning needs of all nurses in relation to global public health emergencies.

Introduction

The COVID-19 pandemic has without doubt impacted on every aspect of nursing practice globally and in particular on that of nurse education in the UK. The publication of this book was planned for mid-2020 but, as its editors, we soon realised that a textbook designed to support student nurse decision-making would need to consider the impact of the global pandemic on nurse education.

Nearly two years later, as we write, the true impact of the virus and public health response to it is becoming evident. Given the importance of this impact, we decided to include reference to the global pandemic, as appropriate, throughout the book, but also recognised that a new chapter, to examine the impact specifically on student learning in practice, would be a valuable addition to the original text.

During these two years both student nurses and their practice supervisors were suddenly exposed to new decision-making situations on such a large-scale, involving not only patients in their care but also their families. In addition, decisions involving the nursing professional bodies, such as the Nursing and Midwifery Council (NMC) in the UK, in collaboration with all health and social care providers, saw unprecedented emergency actions being implemented to ensure safe practice and continuity of learning to ensure the registration of nurses as well as successful graduate studies. This of course created major tensions for all those involved in supporting learners in practice as qualified nurses in particular were now at the forefront of caring for patients admitted to hospital with the COVID-19 virus.

Managing the Initial Changing Learning Needs of Students

The announcement of the presence of a global pandemic by the World Health Organization (WHO) in March 2020 meant that some universities closed, but some of those where nursing and allied health programmes were taught did initially maintain some semblance of on-site face-to-face learning. For most students however, lessons were delivered and received remotely via online technology, such as Zoom or Teams.

This shift to remote learning happened quickly for both students and those working in Higher Education, now having to deliver learning and teaching at a distance.

It is noted that in many university departments, students were already engaged in online learning, but there was then an urgent imperative to develop such an approach for all.

For some students, the shift to online learning exposed inequalities in levels of information technology infrastructure and access – sometimes referred to as 'digital poverty'. Watts (2020), writing in *The Lancet,* also noted that this digital inequality also impacted the lack of access to health care information by certain groups not only in the UK but globally. This urgency to transfer learning and teaching to online platforms also had a major impact on the need for all those lecturers who had never before used this mode of teaching. Kechi Iheduru-Anderson and Jo Anne Foley (2021: 1) in the USA found the experiences of a nurse faculty to be 'stressful and overwhelming and feeling emotionally and physically exhausted'.

While we recognise that this background information is necessary to have as a context, the focus of this chapter is to explore the context of learning to be a nurse during a pandemic, and while the emphasis is on the experience within the UK, the chapter draws on the global literature to highlight similarities and differences across the world and in so doing brings the extent of the impact of the virus on learning to be a nurse during the pandemic to the fore.

Given the emergency needs of the various services and departments delivering health care, alongside the need for an increase in the workforce to do this both in hospitals and community care, it became evident that the student nurse population as a whole could offer a contribution to this emergency.

This next section of the chapter explains what the professional governing body in the UK for nursing and midwifery did as a direct response to the unfolding global emergency. It soon became clear that as the virus spread, there was an impact on the National Health Service and its ability to deliver planned care because increasing numbers of beds were being used for patients experiencing severe symptoms of COVID-19. Most planned surgery was cancelled, and the designation of wards changed to accommodate patients with the virus. Some nurses were deployed to other services and seven new, large emergency hospitals, known as Nightingale Hospitals, were rapidly built in anticipation of the large numbers of people that might require respiratory support. Staff from the NHS also contracted the virus and as a result were unable to work due to illness and periods of enforced isolation. Appleby (2021) describes the extreme rates of sickness and absence experienced by NHS staff during the early part of the pandemic, where the numbers of nurses and doctors available to deliver care were vastly reduced. In order to boost the numbers of staff available to care for patients there were several initiatives implemented involving nursing and allied health care students.

In the first year of the pandemic, there was no vaccine available to help reduce the impact of the virus but, following rapid and significant investment by scientists in both time and funds, the development of vaccines led to major changes in the pattern of the virus spreading, and in the severity of the symptoms experienced by those contracting the virus, not just in the UK but across the world.

This next section explains what the professional governing body in the UK for nursing and midwifery did as a direct response to the unfolding global emergency.

The Emergency Standards for Nurse Education in the UK

In the UK, the Nursing and Midwifery Council (NMC) published emergency and recovery standards for nurse education (2021) (please see the Web resources section at the end of the chapter for full access to these).

The NMC recognises that wherever possible the delivery of normal nurse education should continue. However, given the ongoing impact on student learning in both university and practice, it was agreed that such emergency and recovery standards were needed and recommended as follows, for the UK government and the full NMC to approve:

> 60. Recommendation: In accordance with its powers set out in the Nursing and Midwifery Order 2001 and subject to any minor drafting changes required by the Privy Council, the Council is recommended to approve the Nursing and Midwifery Council (Emergency Procedures) (Amendment) Rules 2020 Order of Council 2020 (Annexe 3) with a view to making the Rules by correspondence following the passing of the Coronavirus Bill. (NMC, 2020: 12)

One particular Order for the Emergency registration of nurses and other health and care professionals (NMC, 2020 Annexe 1a) would have a major impact on student nurses learning experience. These were the Emergency and Recovery Standards (NMC, 2020) and subsequently the NMC published its initial standards for UK nurse education. These (NMC, 2020) enabled the following to take place:

- First-year nursing and midwifery students were to focus on academic and online learning rather than participating in clinical placements while their normal learning environments were under pressure due to the pandemic. In other words, many student nurses who commenced their programmes of nurse education during 2020 may have spent their first-year studying theoretical modules; rather than gaining experience in practice learning environments. Furthermore, much of that theoretical learning will have taken place through online modules and blended learning approaches. This would, however, have a subsequent impact on the learning experience of these students as they progress through their programmes.

- It should be remembered that the ruling on the use of blended learning will remain in place until the Secretary of State for Health and Social Care declares the pandemic emergency is over. This situation was not unique to student nurses studying in the UK; other countries, such as Canada (Dewart et al., 2020) and the Caribbean (Agu et al., 2021), took the difficult decision to remove students from clinical areas amidst fears over student safety.

- Final-year nursing students could opt in to undertake paid clinical placements while the emergency standards were in place.

- The impact of this rapid acceleration into practice is being investigated in a number of studies, such as King's College London (2020) and Robert Gordon University in Scotland (2020) (see the Web resources section at the end of this chapter for the links.) In Spain, Gómez-Ibáñez et al. (2020) describe the experiences of final-year nursing students called to support Spain's national health care system. The study reports that the students felt a strong sense of altruism in supporting society and the profession of nursing in the fight against the pandemic. The study also reported students feeling it was their duty to help. This was not without personal sacrifice, however, in terms of delaying a consolidation of their studies and being exposed to potentially contracting COVID-19 themselves.

- The decision to respond to national calls for help in the UK (and indeed elsewhere) was a personal decision, taken individually by the students themselves. Students exposed to COVID-19 put themselves and their families at potential risk.

- Furthermore, self-isolation also presented financial hardship to students who would normally also take paid employment to supplement their income (Dewart et al., 2020).

- That decision, therefore, of whether to respond to the call to support the healthcare services was possibly the biggest decision of all facing large numbers of student nurses globally. The dilemma faced (by students) as to whether to opt in or not, is described in detail by Townsend (2020). His insightful reflection describes the emotional, personal and professional journey he experienced as a student nurse during the pandemic (see the References section at the end of the chapter for article access).

- Education institutions and their practice learning partners were given more flexibility to ensure students got appropriate support and supervision. The emergency standards enabled students to receive practice supervision and assessment from the same individual. Some universities also explored innovative practice learning opportunities and models of practice learning.

- It was important to ensure that the next generation of nurses qualify in a timely way with the skills and knowledge they need to deliver safe, effective and proficient care. The International Council of Nursing (ICN), in its policy brief of April 2021 (see the Web resources section at the end of this chapter for the link), suggests that delays in graduation, in many instances, could impact the supply and development of the nursing workforce of the immediate future. In an online survey of 130 associations, 64 responses (a response rate of 49 per cent), from representatives of all the World Health Organization (WHO) regions, reported that 73 per cent of national nurses' associations (NNA) experienced a disruption in undergraduate nursing education, with 46 per cent of countries experiencing delays or cancellations to nursing students' clinical placements. Another 41 per cent of countries reported that placements were restricted to certain areas. A total of 57 per cent of countries reported delays to students graduating, including 7 per cent that reported major delays of 12 months or more (see ICN *Policy Brief: Nursing Education and Emerging Nursing Workforce in COVID-19 Pandemic* (April 2021) in the Web resources section).

- A most important option enabled students to practise and learn through simulated practice learning where conventional clinical practice was not available or not possible. This meant that hours spent in simulation could be treated as clinical hours and contribute towards the requirement within the UK for student nurses to accumulate 2,300 hours in practice learning environments during their pre-registration programmes (NMC, 2018a).

These emergency standards and further reference to some of the issues already raised in this section of the chapter are referred to and explored throughout the next section, especially focused on the context of learning in both practice-based and university settings. It could be said that the nature and impact of decision-making related to patient care entered a new phase in the student journey to become a qualified and registered nurse. Indeed, one where achieving the required proficiencies became a major challenge for all involved in the support of students and the overall management of curriculum delivery to meet the required NMC (2018a) *Standards of proficiency for registered nurses*.

The Context of Learning in Practice: Impact on Student Learning

In the UK, as noted, the NMC issued emergency nursing standards (since updated; NMC, 2022) enabling students to 'opt in' to undertake extended paid clinical placements. During this time, the emphasis for the students was on their becoming paid employees rather than learners, thereby becoming a valuable resource in health care environments. Decisions about whether to opt in or remain on the educational programme involved complex decision-making for many students.

The students in the study by Gómez-Ibáñez et al. (2020) describe a strong sense of altruism in stepping forward to work as health care aides in Spain. These findings are mirrored in a study undertaken by Douglas, Kennedy, Torrance et al. (2021) of students at a Scottish University where there was also a strong sense of moral responsibility among participants. Students in this study however felt pressured into stepping forward to accept a paid clinical post or to enter professional practice early but none the less they did so. The students also acknowledged that there were challenges to achieving the necessary clinical competencies required by the NMC to complete their studies. According to the findings, the authors reported that:

> Hospital-based nursing participants expressed frustration at being directed to work that was consistent with their temporary paid status, but which they felt prevented them engaging in the full range of clinical activities they needed to complete their educational course requirements. Their paid status appears to have acted as a constraint on their educational and professional development. (Douglas, Kennedy and Torrance et al., 2021: 2)

It was also reported that the full range of clinical activities referred to here simply did not exist in hospitals (in their pre-COVID form) at the height of the COVID pandemic, thus creating an overall very different placement learning environment. For example, many children's services were adapted to care for adult patients. This was true of intensive care units in particular. A joint statement from adult and paediatric intensive care societies signalled that paediatric intensive care units in the UK would (if required) care for critically ill adults while simultaneously providing high-quality care for critically ill children (you can read the Paediatric Critical Care Centre's (PCCS's) full statement (2020) – see the Web resources section at the end of this chapter for the link).

Senior-level decision-making would have been evident at this time as 'clinical leads' (people responsible for a particular area of care delivery) would decide who could and should be admitted to a paediatric intensive care bed. Deep, Knight, Kernie et al. (2020) provide some excellent descriptions of how these decisions were made at two paediatric intensive care units in London and New York during the initial pandemic surge of 2019. The role of the clinical leads in decision-making at that time was of paramount importance. The paper highlights how 'just in time education and coaching' was provided to support all staff in this decision-making.

Some staff who had left nursing also chose to return in response to the government's plea to help boost staff numbers at this time. They 'shadowed' other more experienced colleagues as a key mechanism of support.

At the same time as paediatric intensive care units were admitting adult patients, some paediatric nurses (and nurses from other fields of nursing practice) were also redeployed. In response to the pandemic, nurses were sometimes asked to be flexible in terms of where they were asked to work and were moved to work in areas which may have been unfamiliar in response to a surge in the numbers of COVID-positive individuals requiring hospitalisation. Students who were being supervised by those registrants may also have been asked to follow their supervisor, while others may not have been.

Accepting that when you read this chapter that life as a student nurse (following any of the four fields of practice pathways) during the COVID pandemic will have changed, it is important to recognise what part you played in the ongoing support of patients and those helping you to learn to become a nurse. As a future qualified nurse, you will need to understand the context of care that was in place at this time in order to be able to support those individuals that suffer from the long-term effects of the pandemic overall. With this in mind complete Activity 14.1.

Activity 14.1

1. Access and read the extensive guidance offered to nurses by the Royal College of Nursing (RCN) about the decisions associated with redeployment as well as the advice for students during the COVID-19 pandemic (see the Web resources section at the end of this chapter for the links).
2. Access the NHS (2020) document *COVID-19: Deploying our people safely* (see the Web resources section at the end of this chapter for the link), which outlines the key considerations for the safe redeployment of staff and deployment of those joining the NHS in temporary support of the existing workforce – that is, students undertaking an extended, paid final placement.
3. Imagine that you are a second-year student nurse on placement. Your practice supervisor is asked to redeploy to support the intensive care unit. What factors would you have to consider when making your decision to follow your supervisor? Health Education England's (2020a) *Student Support Guidance During COVID-19 Outbreak* may help provide you with some prompts to guide your thinking (see the Web resources section at the end of this chapter for the link). Access and use to reflect on the options.
4. You may also want to think about your own skill set and whether your knowledge and skills could be used in another clinical area.
5. As a further activity, continue to access and read your university support and advice pages, as these offer direct information concerning your placement environments on an ongoing basis. This includes any change as the learning environments begin to return to previous patterns of practice.

There is little empirical evidence at the time of writing, regarding the numbers of students who decided to follow their supervisor or the impact this had on those students, but some studies do describe the tensions involved in being a paid member of staff and a student nurse. As paid members of staff there were sometimes reduced access to learning opportunities, but for some that resulted in increased self-confidence (Goldbold et al., 2021).

In May 2020, Health Education England (2020b) undertook a survey as part of its Reducing Pre-registration Attrition and Improving Retention (RePAIR) project to capture the experience of pre-registration nurses, midwives and allied health professionals during one wave of the COVID-19 pandemic. A total of more than 14,000 students responded to the survey. The majority of those had chosen to 'opt in' to clinical service-facing environments, and 85 per cent appeared to be well supported in the clinical environment (see the Web resources section at the end of this chapter for a link to the key findings of the study).

At a time of a global nursing shortage, for many students, the completion of their studies was delayed by the pandemic as timelines became uncertain (Agu et al., 2021) and the lack of opportunity to achieve proficiency (Douglas, Kennedy and Torrance et al., 2021) took its toll.

Learning opportunities normally made possible through exposure to clinical environments became limited as health services rapidly changed to accommodate more individuals requiring treatment for the virus.

The ICN (2021) suggests that 46 per cent of countries experienced delays or cancellations to nursing students' clinical placements; 57 per cent of countries reported delays in student graduation, including 7 per cent that reported major delays of 12 months or more. This means that the impact in terms of nurse education will be felt for some years to come.

As planned surgeries and medical investigations ceased, this meant that placement learning opportunities diminished and an abundance of students were competing for the few opportunities that remained (Agu et al., 2021). Opportunities for learning enhanced infection control procedures, however, were plentiful (Townsend, 2020) and, in some cases, students became very conscientious regarding hand hygiene, the use of gloves and the application of preventive measures (Ulenaers et al., 2021). Opportunities to be involved in vaccine administration were also abundant.

For the students who 'opted in', the transition to the world of work took place overnight with little opportunity for lengthy adaptation to the new role (Monforte-Royo and Fuster, 2020).

Students entered chaotic conditions in health care settings that were struggling to cope with the sheer volume of high patient mortality and where treatment protocols were updated frequently (Monforte-Royo and Fuster, 2020). According to Monforte-Royo and Fuster (2020: 1), due to the enormous demand for health care services and personnel, students were deployed across the full range of settings (hospital units, intensive care units (ICU), A&E, field hospitals, repurposed hotels and care homes). Although the students were supervised by registered nurses, the pressures on the health system meant that they had to work as full team members.

Activity 14.2 provides an opportunity to think about these issues in relation to your own situation and whatever decision you took at the time. It is also a time to reflect on your learning experiences in the past two years and consider how it has impacted on your current role (see Chapter 4 on Reflection). Some of you may already be working as a newly qualified nurse.

Activity 14.2

1. You may have decided to undertake an extended paid final placement or made a different decision. What factors did you take into consideration when you made your decision?
2. What support did your university and/or practice learning setting provide if you decided to opt in or opt out?
3. If you are experiencing any challenges in your ongoing learning experiences, either academically or clinically, it is very important that you have someone to talk to about this. Your academic supervisors or personal tutors will be an invaluable point of contact for you, as will your university's student support services.

As we write, the situation is still unfolding, and the updated recovery standards (NMC, 2022) are in place. The full impact of deciding to opt in and spend the final placement as a paid member of staff, working as a (Band 4 graded employee) health care support worker while finishing a pre-registration nursing programme will not be fully realised for some time.

More studies are required over the coming years to investigate the early career pathways of those who became registered nurses during the pandemic. It will be interesting to see if those who became registrants during the pandemic feel ready to take on the supervisory role themselves, and how their own experiences as students will impact on their role as future supervisors of others.

The Context of University Learning: Engaging with Technology

As the impact of the pandemic swept across the world, Higher Education institutions adapted their programmes so that students could continue with their studies. For most universities, as noted earlier, this involved a rapid transfer to online or e-learning options (Haslam, 2021). Some universities enabled nursing students to continue with some limited clinical skills and immersive learning (ICN, 2021).

In the UK, nurse educators transferred their face-to-face delivery to online approaches using sometimes unfamiliar education technology and working from home (Haslam, 2021; Leigh et al., 2020).

The NMC's (2021) iterations of the emergency standards actively supported the use of distance learning approaches.

According to the ICN report, as noted earlier, for students in some parts of the world, these heightened inequalities of digital access, but there were some gains made, too, as 'the modalities have several positive outcomes, including increased flexibility, student-centred learning and easier access to learning' (2021: 3). The modalities noted here refer to the online learning approaches to delivery of learning activities. It is still important to recognise, however, that not everyone has access to the Internet and/or digital technology. Similarly, the environment in which students are studying may not always be conducive to learning.

For some student nurses, everything changed, as they then worked as paid health care personnel, tried to complete their educational studies and, given the impact of the pandemic on the whole education system in the UK, also home-schooled their children, but mostly managed to make it work (see the Web resources section at the end of this chapter for the links to several nurses' stories).

It is perhaps unsurprising that many students relied heavily on digital group messaging technologies (such as WhatsApp), involving friends, family members and peers to alleviate frustrations and anxieties, rather than university-based formal support mechanisms (Douglas, Kennedy and Torrance et al., 2021). It has been found that students' anxieties were further heightened as communication regarding the pandemic, associated restrictions and advice from the universities and indeed the government 'were perceived to lack clarity and consistency' (Douglas, Kennedy and Torrance et al., 2021: 1), leaving some students feeling isolated and distressed (Douglas, Kennedy and Torrance et al., 2021).

There are positive and negative aspects of messaging and social media. Take a moment to think about the positive aspects of messaging and also consider how to use it responsibly in Activity 14.3.

Activity 14.3

1. How do you (or might you) use digital groups such as WhatsApp as a way to obtain and provide peer support?
2. How is professionalism maintained when using closed groups or digital groups that are not set up by the university?
3. What key accountability and confidentiality issues will you need to consider?

The NMC issued its *Guidance on using Social Media Responsibly* (n.d.) and how this relates to *The Code*. Reading the guidance together with *The Code* provides a helpful framework that can help nurses to avoid the pitfalls of messaging and social media. (See also Chapter 5 and 6 for additional support regarding social media and the student nurse.)

For those student nurses in the second or final-year of their studies who decided not to 'opt in' to an extended paid final clinical placement, the NMC's emergency standards facilitated other innovative routes through their pre-registration programmes. First-year students could not opt in, but (in some cases), entire cohorts were unable to go on placements for their clinical practice learning. These students may have to make up their practice-based learning later in the programme in order to meet the required learning hours for both practice and university. The decision-making process for those who did not volunteer to remain in clinical areas was multi-faceted; reasons included living with people from an at-risk group, that they themselves were in such a group or, simply, they felt unprepared for the challenges posed by the pandemic (Monforte-Royo and Fuster, 2020). While the study by Monforte-Royo and Fuster (2020) was conducted in Spain, the sentiments expressed by the students are likely to be replicated elsewhere. McSherry et al. (2021) undertook an evaluation in the UK of the experiences of students who had opted in to paid clinical placements and found both positive and negative consequences for their decision. The experience of opting in equipped the respondents with increased confidence because they felt they were valuable members of the workforce. Equally, some participants experienced role confusion as their student role was eroded. None the less, the students wanted to help and support their registered nurse colleagues.

Haslam (2021) provides a detailed description of moving to online learning by nurse educators in the UK. He argues that the changes were necessary prior to the pandemic, but the situation accelerated the inevitable transition to the development of resources such as videos, lecture capture, podcasts and so on.

Online learning facilitates accessibility and widening participation in nurse education, but Haslam (2021) calls for a collective commitment to evaluating these strategies (particularly for struggling or failing students) as the impact of the large-scale shift to this mode of learning may have an impact on attrition as home-based learning could exacerbate 'ineffective learning strategies, poor motivation, and reduced communication skills' (Haslam, 2021: 2). Also, while asynchronous online learning may suit some students, as they juggle the demands of being a student nurse, worker and parent or carer, for example, for others the effect on student engagement and satisfaction may be detrimental (Haslam, 2021).

Some nurse educators are questioning whether the situation is sustainable in the long-term, particularly if the pandemic continues (Dewart et al., 2020; Haslam, 2021). However, a blended or hybrid approach to nurse education is likely to exist at least for the foreseeable future.

Challenges for Educating the Future Global Nursing Workforce

The long-term effect of the pandemic on nurses' education globally is unknown at this time. It seems that there has been however a recognition for nurse education for the future to include some acknowledgement of the role of the nurse in large-scale emergencies, be they pandemic, terrorist, or natural disaster (Cusak, Arbon and Ranse, 2010). Cusak and colleagues (2010) were eerily prophetic when they suggested that student nurses could be called on to fill an urgent and sudden workforce gap.

More recently, Gómez-Ibáñez and colleagues call for future nurse education programmes in Spain to include elements relating to 'managing complex situations, placing significant emphasis on decision-making under pressure to increase preparedness for pandemic response' (2020: 6). Another team from Spain has also called for students to 'have adequate education in infection prevention and control and the opportunity to develop the skills and attitudes required to provide care to infected patients during a pandemic' (Goni-Fuste et al., 2021: 53).

The NMC's (2010) *Standards for Pre-registration Nursing Education*, which preceded its current standards of proficiency – *Future Nurse: Standards of proficiency for registered nurses* (2018a) – acknowledged the role of the nurse in disasters, major incidents and public health emergencies. This requirement continues within the new educational standards but perhaps now, more than ever, the overarching statement about the role of the nurse in the 21st century, which then encompasses all the proficiency standards about outcomes, is important:

> Registered nurses provide leadership in the delivery of care for people of all ages and from different backgrounds, cultures and beliefs. They provide nursing care for people who have complex mental, physical, cognitive and behavioural care needs, those living with dementia, the elderly, and for people at the end of their life. They must be able to care for people in their own home, in the community or hospital or in any health care settings where their needs are supported and managed. They work in the context of continual change, challenging environments, different models of care delivery, shifting demographics, innovation, and rapidly evolving technologies. Increasing integration of health and social care services will require registered nurses to negotiate boundaries and play a proactive role in interdisciplinary teams. The confidence and ability to think critically, apply knowledge and skills, and provide expert, evidence-based, direct nursing care therefore lies at the centre of all registered nursing practice. (NMC, 2018a: 3)

It will be important for future student nurses, midwives and other health care workers that their programmes of learning engage with the global context of health and social care in order to be able to actively respond to emergency health care needs that impact on societies and share in collaborative initiatives to ensure risk and safety is managed effectively and with positive outcomes.

Let us consider the full meaning of the NMC statement on the role of the nurse of the twenty-first century through undertaking the following activities in Activity 14.4.

Activity 14.4

1. Consider the meaning of 'proficiency' (see Chapter 1) in terms of the key elements noted for the future nurse: working with others in teams (both nurses and those from other professions) to manage and prioritise actions and care, and provide expert, evidence-based, direct nursing care.
2. Write down what you think these proficiencies are. (See Chapter 3 on EBP and Chapter 7-10 on the four fields of practice)
3. There is clearly an acknowledgement here that nurses cannot work in silos but, rather, complex teamworking relationships are required. There will undoubtedly be times when nursing expertise will come to the fore and there will be times when others will take the lead to prioritise and manage a situation. For example, consider what is the nurse's role in providing information to the general public on the benefits of wearing a mask or being vaccinated?
4. What is the evidence base that will help you to engage with people in a community placement, for example?

The wearing of masks and being vaccinated have been highly sensitive issues that could potentially have had an impact on engaging with people generally and other members of staff (see the Web resources section at the end of this chapter for a link to the RCN's information regarding mandatory vaccination). Both student and registered nurses need to be able to offer patients and others an explanation of the current guidance as an essential part of upholding the NMC's (2018e) *The Code: Professional standards of practice and behaviour for nurses, midwives and nursing associates*, but that information needs to be delivered in a non-judgemental way: nurses should not make a judgement on what is right or wrong for another person.

An interesting discussion is provided by de Campos-Rudinsky and Undurraga (2021), who provide a very interesting position as they discuss the shifting nature of evidence that emerged during the pandemic. Furthermore, they suggest that having access to empirical data does not necessarily mean that good decisions will be taken. In terms of public health policy, sound ethical reasoning is more important alongside evaluating normative judgement.

The ICN (2019) published an updated framework outlining competencies for disaster nursing. The framework acknowledges that epidemics, pandemics and violence are major global health challenges that can have a negative impact on health. In such circumstances, nurses are the largest group of health professionals 'serving as first responders, triage officers and care providers, coordinators of care and services, providers of information or education, and counsellors' (2019: 3). As such, the ICN (2019) framework suggests that nurse educators and all nurses working in hospitals, clinics and public health centres require Level 1 competency, which in the framework is defined as follows:

At Level 1, the basic or generalist nurse is not expected to be an expert in response to any single kind of emergency or work in isolation of the response team. It is possible that outside of the working day, a nurse as a member of the community might be on the site of an emerging disaster or event; in which case the nurse should use basic first aid and professional skills until additional responders arrive and a team structure is organised.

While every nurse develops greater proficiency in those competencies used in every-day practice; the acute care nurse may make little use of community-focused competencies and the public health nurse may make little use of cardiac resuscitation competencies. (2019: 6)

The context in which you work therefore impacts on the way in which you might be asked to respond to large-scale emergencies. Interestingly, the framework also highlights the nurse as an employee in a professional context and as a member of the community.

Let us consider how these ICN competency statements support the student nurse through considering the activities in Activity 14.5.

Activity 14.5

1. Consider the following competency statement for a student nurse as given in the ICN's framework:

    Competency I.4.2, the learning objectives to move a nursing student toward competency would include knowledge of the germ theory of disease; methods of transmission of infectious organisms; means of disrupting transmission of organisms; influence of cultural practices on spread of micro-organisms; and skills laboratory experience with hand cleansing, use of gloves and protective gowns or aprons, and/or the use of masks and breathing apparatus. (2019: 6)

2. Reflect on your own theory and practice in relation to these issues and how your programme of learning has already changed to accommodate some or all of these. Make a note of the key issues and your own learning needs.
3. How different is your current experience of this ICN competency statement?
4. See the Further reading section and other resources given at the end of this chapter and use them to enhance your understanding of why these topics are important in relation to nurses' competencies given the COVID-19 global pandemic and the rise in other diseases, such as TB (Tuberculosis), which have been increasing in countries such as the UK.

The ICN's framework underlines the importance of nurse education in preparing the nurses of the future to plan, respond to and manage such inevitable disasters. So, it seems that disaster planning preparedness of student nurses to adapt and contribute to large-scale health incidents will need to be a feature of future nurse education.

The Changing Patterns of Care and Impact on Ethical Decisions in Practice

Carolan et al. (2020) suggested that the global COVID-19 pandemic will 'indelibly transform the content of curriculums.' They also call for curriculums to include epidemiology and the need to understand the evolving nature of viral pandemics, public health and health promotion. They go on to suggest that 'advanced understandings of intensive care nursing and supportive care for patients who experience abrupt transitions to end-of-life care, and a greater appreciation of ethical complexities' are required (Carolan et al., 2020: 2).

They poignantly also point out the need for educational preparation for negotiating difficult end-of-life conversations with frightened patients and their distant families through layers of personal protective equipment (PPE) as nurses break bad news over the telephone; challenges which they say would put pressure on even the most experienced nurses (Carolan et al., 2020). Nurse educators who work in clinical practice as well as those in universities will need to ensure that skilled clinical supervision and pastoral support is in place for all future nurses.

Jeffrey (2020) describes the key ethical challenges for health care workers during the pandemic as being:

- isolation and social distancing;
- duty of care to patients;
- access to treatment when resources are limited.

Jeffrey (2020) presents a moral response to these issues and suggests that ethical frameworks will continue to evolve but the mainstay of these should be trust and solidarity, to aid decision-making.

Ethical decision-making can include time sensitive issues: for example, a potential delay to commencing cardiopulmonary resuscitation (CPR) while appropriate personal protective equipment (PPE) is put on. Starting CPR without adequate PPE could possibly result in aerosol-generating procedures (AGP, which are procedures that stimulate coughing and so promote the generation of tiny droplets, requiring additional infection prevention and control precautions when an increased risk of infection has been identified).

The pandemic also prevented hospital visits from family members taking place; this has particular consequences for end-of-life care as often nurses were the only individuals present towards the end-of-life. Nurses relayed messages often received over the telephone between family members and their hospitalised loved ones. Weaver et al. (2020) describe human touch through a touchscreen when telemedicine approaches were used by hospice nurses with rural paediatric patients and their families at the end-of-life. The following excerpt from their study provides a detailed picture of the impact of distance during palliative communication:

> multi-face screen function allowed for coparents or grandparents or other relatives, local paediatricians, and interdisciplinary palliative care team members to join. With this inclusion came a caution of creating a mass presence while missing the intimate, personal touch each family deserves. This sense of personal touch was not only depicted as physical handholding or hugging but also expanded to the deeper personal touch of attentiveness and healing presence for each individual in the room. Although the screen fostered a community gathering, this risked missing moments of attending to each participant's personal needs. Nurses recommended finding ways to check in with each person who had been present at the tele-health visit after the visit, as one would in person. Although this is a time commitment, this sense of personalised care was notably essential when using a less personal communication format. (Weaver et al., 2020: 1029)

Providing nursing care at the end-of-life can be emotionally difficult, but the situation can be magnified when relatives rely on nurses to convey important and sometimes intimate messages of love. In addition, not being able to engage in face-to-face communication due to the physical barriers of a face mask and PPE equipment further increases the trauma for nurses.

In Activity 14.6, you can consider your experiences during the current pandemic and reflect on your thoughts about this challenging aspect of looking after patients and their families. Consider, also, how you would have normally managed communicating with patients and relatives, and especially how making decisions would occur.

Activity 14.6

1. Think about how you would follow up on difficult conversations with family members, as suggested by Weaver et al. (2020). There may be policies in place to help direct what you would do. Discuss with your practice supervisors to ensure you are following best practice.
2. You may also want to talk to your practice supervisors about how they manage such difficult situations and whether they have any advice regarding self-care. If a clinical placement has already set up reflection periods for students experiencing such situations, this may be an essential part of those shared learning sessions. There should,

of course, be short periods of time and space made available whenever possible for all health care team members during non-pandemic situations as well.

3. Access and read the key research report from the Marie Curie (2021) organisation and partners in relation to end-of-life care during COVID-19 to enhance your learning (see the Web resources section at the end of this chapter for the link).

Conclusion

This chapter has outlined the impact of the global pandemic caused by the COVID-19 virus on the student experience of learning to become a nurse, in particular in the UK. Technology enhanced and online learning is likely to remain in some form, and further studies will be required to investigate the effectiveness of these in learning to become a nurse. Agile responsive decision-making is a feature of nursing, and we are still discovering ways to ensure that we prepare the future nursing workforce in the best way possible.

In this sense the chapter also reflects the situation in which nursing globally has found itself, as a response to a situation that has not been seen previously and in particular has impacted the needs of all nurses in relation to each other and to those that they care for. As a result of a major commitment by nursing's professional body in the UK, collaborating with the other professional bodies, the government and the Health and Social care departments, student nurses have been able to maintain their journey to becoming a qualified nurse. Incredible teams of practitioners and academics collaboratively supported them to achieve their proficiencies and a graduate award which are the expectations of the future nurse.

References

Agu, C. F., Stewart, J., McFarlane-Stewart, N. and Rae, T. (2021). COVID-19 pandemic effects on nursing education: Looking through the lens of a developing country. *International Nursing Review*, 68: 153–158.

Appleby, J. (2021). NHS sickness absence during the COVID-19 pandemic. *British Medical Journal*, 372: n471.

Campos-Rudinsky, T. C. de and Undurraga, E. (2021). Public health decisions in the COVID-19 pandemic require more than 'follow the science'. *Journal of Medical Ethics*, 47: 296–299.

Carolan, C., Davies, C. L., Crookes, P., McGhee, S. and Roxburgh, M. (2020). COVID-19: Disruptive impacts and transformative opportunities in undergraduate nurse education. Guest Editorial. *Nurse Education in Practice*, 46: 102907.

Cusak, L., Arbon, P. and Ranse, J. (2010). What is the role of nursing students and schools of nursing during disaster?: A discussion paper. *Collegian*, 17: 193–197.

Deep, A., Knight, P., Kernie, S. G., D'Silva, P., Sobin, B. et al. (2020). A hybrid model of pediatric and adult critical care during the coronavirus disease 2019 surge: The experience of two tertiary hospitals in London and New York. *Paediatric Critical Care Medicine*, 22(2): e125–134.

Dewart, G., Corcoran, L., Thirsk, L. and Petrovic, K. (2020). Nursing education in a pandemic: Academic challenges in response to COVID-19. *Nurse Education Today*, 92: 104471.

Douglas, F., Kennedy, C., Torrance, N., Grant, A., Adams, N., Butler-Warke, A., Kidd, A. and Cunningham, S. (2021). *An Investigation of Health and Social Care Students' and Recent Graduates' Clinical Placement and Professional Practice Experiences and Coping Strategies During the Wave 1 COVID-19 Pandemic Period*. Edinburgh: Chief Scientist Office. Rapid research in COVID-19 Programme, Robert Gordon University, Aberdeen.

Goldbold, R., Whiting, L., Adams, C., Naidu, Y. and Pattison, N. (2021). The experiences of student nurses in a pandemic: A qualitative study. *Nurse Education in Practice*, 56: 103186.

Gómez-Ibáñez, R., Watson, C., Levya-Moral, J.M., Aguayo-González, M. and Granel, N. (2020). Final-year nursing students called to work: Experiences of a rushed labour insertion during the COVID-19 pandemic. *Nurse Education in Practice*, 49: 102920.

Goni-Fuste, B., Wennberg, L., Martin-Delgado, L., Alfonso-Arias, M., Martin-Ferreres, L. and Monforte-Royo, C. (2021). Experiences and needs of nursing students during pandemic outbreaks: A systematic overview of the literature. *Journal of Professional Nursing*, 37: 53–64.

Haslam, M. B. (2021). What might COVID-19 have taught us about the delivery of nurse education, in a post-COVID-19 world? *Nurse Education Today*, 97: 104707.

Iheduru-Anderson, K. and Foley, J-A. (2021). Transitioning to full online teaching during COVID-19 crisis: The associate degree nurse faculty experience. *Global Qualitative Nursing Research*, 8: 1–14. Available at: https://journals.sagepub.com/doi/full/10.1177/23333936211057545 (accessed 24 May 2022).

International Council of Nurses (ICN) (2019). *Core Competencies in Disaster Nursing: Version 2.0*. Geneva: ICN.

International Council of Nurses (ICN) (2021). *Nursing Education and the Emerging Nursing Workforce in COVID-19 Pandemic, Policy Brief*. Geneva: ICN.

Jeffrey, D. I. (2020). Relational ethical approaches to the COVID-19 pandemic. *Journal of Medical Ethics*, 46: 495–498.

Leigh, J., Vasilica, C., Dron, R., Gawthorpe, D., Burns, E., Kennedy, S., Kennedy, R., Warburton, T. and Croughan, C. (2020). Redefining undergraduate nurse teaching during the coronavirus pandemic: Use of digital technologies. *British Journal of Nursing*, 29(10): 566–569.

McSherry, R., Eost-Telling, C., Stevens, D., Bailey, J., Crompton, R., Taylor, L., Kinston, P. and Simpson, A. (2021). Student nurses undertaking acute hospital placements during COVD-19: Rationale for opting in?: A qualitative enquiry. *Healthcare*, 9: 1001.

Monforte-Royo, C. and Fuster, P. (2020). Coronials: Nurses who graduated during the COVID-19 pandemic: Will they be better nurses? *Nurse Education Today*, Editorial, 94: 104536.

Nursing and Midwifery Council (NMC) (n.d.) *Guidance on using Social Media Responsibly.* London: NMC.

Nursing and Midwifery Council (NMC) (2010). *Standards for Pre-registration Nursing Education.* London: NMC.

Nursing and Midwifery Council (NMC) (2018a). *Future Nurse: Standards of proficiency for registered nurses.* London: NMC.

Nursing and Midwifery Council (NMC) (2018e). *The Code: Professional standards of practice and behaviour for nurses, midwives and nursing associates.* London: NMC.

Nursing and Midwifery Council (NMC) (2020). *NMC Response to the COVID-19 Emergency.* London: NMC.

Nursing and Midwifery Council (NMC) (2022). *Current Recovery Programme Standards.* Updated 24 January 2022. London: NMC.

Townsend, M. J. (2020). Learning to nurse during the pandemic: A student's reflections. *British Journal of Nursing*, 29(16): 972.

Ulenaers, D., Grosemans, J., Schrooten, W. and Bergs, J. (2021). Clinical placement experience of nursing students during the COVID-19 pandemic: A cross-sectional study. *Nurse Education Today*, 99: 104746.

Watts, G. (2020). COVID-19 and the digital divide in the UK. *The Lancet*, 2(8): 395–396. Available at: https://www.thelancet.com/journals/landig/article/PIIS2589-7500(20)30169-2/fulltext (accessed 23 August 2022).

Weaver, M. S., Neuman, M. L., Navaneethan, H., Robinson, J. E. and Hinds, P. S. (2020). Human touch via touchscreen: Rural nurses' experiential perspectives on telehealth use in paediatric hospice care. *Journal of Pain and Symptom Management*, 60(5): 1027–1033.

Further Reading

Cushen-Brewster, N., Barker, A., Driscoll-Evans, P., Wigens, L. and Langton, H. (2021). The experiences of adult nursing students completing a placement during the COVID-19 pandemic. *British Journal of Nursing*, 30(21): 1250–1255.

Garcia-Martin, M., Roman, P., Rodriguez-Arrosta, M., Mar Diaz-Cortes, M. del, Soriano-Martin, P. J. et al. (2020). Novice nurse's transitioning to emergency nurse during COVID-19 pandemic: A qualitative study. *Journal of Nursing Management*, 29: 258–267.

Loke, A. Y., Li, S. and Guo, C. (2021). Mapping a postgraduate curriculum in disaster nursing with the International Council of Nursing's Core Competencies in Disaster Nursing V2.0: The extent of the program in addressing the core competencies. *Nurse Education Today*, 106: 105163.

Nursing and Midwifery Council (NMC) (2008). *Standards for Competence for Registered Nurses*. London: NMC. Available at: https://www.nmc.org.uk/globalassets/sitedocuments/ standards/nmc-standards-for-competence-for-registered-nurses.pdf (accessed 23 August 2022).

Web Resources

HEE (2020a). *Student Support Guidance during COVID-19 Outbreak, Version 1.0*: www.hee. nhs.uk/sites/default/files/documents/Student%20support%20guide%20master%20. pdf (accessed 3 June 2022).

HEE (2020b). Reducing Pre-registration Attrition and Improving Retention (RePAIR) project's report, *The 'Impact of COVID-19 on Students' Survey Key Findings*: www.hee. nhs.uk/our-work/reducing-pre-registration-attrition-improving-retention (accessed 23 June 2022).

International Council of Nursing (ICN) *Policy Brief: Nursing Education and the Emerging Nursing Workforce in COVID-19 Pandemic* (April 2021): www.icn.ch/sites/default/files/ inline-files/ICN%20Policy%20Brief_Nursing%20Education.pdf (accessed 23 June 2022).

King's College London (2020) – new research to examine student nurses' educational experiences during COVID-19: www.kcl.ac.uk/news/new-research-to-examine-student-nurses-educational-experiences-during-covid-19 (accessed 23 June 2022).

Marie Curie (2021). *Better End of Life 2021: Dying, death and bereavement during COVID-19*, research report: www.mariecurie.org.uk/globalassets/media/documents/policy/ policy-publications/2021/better-end-of-life-research-report.pdf (accessed 23 June 2022).

NHS (2020). *COVID-19: Deploying our people safely*: www.wsh.nhs.uk/covid-staff-zone/ Working-differently/docs/Deploying-staff-safely/C0143-COVID-19-Deploying-our-people-safely-4-April.pdf (accessed 23 June 2022).

Nursing and Midwifery Council (NMC) (2020), *NMC Response to the COVID-19 Emergency*: www.nmc.org.uk/globalassets/sitedocuments/councilpapersand documents/council-2020/item-6-nmc-response-to-the-covid-19-emergency.pdf (accessed 23 June 2022).

Paediatric Critical Care Society (PCCS) – PICS and ICS Joint Position Statement (12 March 2020): https://pccsociety.uk/news/pics-and-ics-joint-position-statement-12-mar-2020 (accessed 23 June 2022).

RCN guides and advice regarding redeployment due to COVID-19 and for students on COVID-related issues:

www.rcn.org.uk/get-help/rcn-advice/redeployment-and-COVID-19 (accessed 23 June 2022).

www.rcn.org.uk/get-help/rcn-advice/students-covid-19 (accessed 23 June 2022).

RCN guide regarding COVID-19, mandatory vaccination and vaccination as a condition of employment: www.rcn.org.uk/get-help/rcn-advice/covid-19-and-mandatory-vaccination (accessed 23 June 2022).

Robert Gordon University – supporting the rapid transition to professional practice in response to COVID-19: www.rgu.ac.uk/news/news-2020/3102-supporting-those-rapidly-transitioning-into-professional-health-and-social-practice-in-response-to-covid-19 (accessed 23 June 2022).

University of Plymouth – returning to practice to provide critical care for COVID-19 patients: www.plymouth.ac.uk/about-us/civic-impact/supporting-national-effort-against-coronavirus/returning-to-practice-to-provide-critical-care-for-covid-19-patients (accessed 23 June 2022).

World Health Organization (WHO) (2016). *Three-year Regional Prototype Pre-service Competency-based Nursing Curriculum: Prototype curriculum for the African region:* https://apps.who.int/iris/bitstream/handle/10665/331657/9789290232629-eng.pdf?sequence=1&isAllowed=y (accessed 23 June).

INDEX